Praise for *Mo* TØ186930

'A book that will inspire today's new par[ ]
Conaboy promises a new route through th[ ]

'A compelling book that upends popular notions about becoming a parent . . .
Mother Brain reminds us why scientific research is a feminist issue'

New Statesman

'I wish I'd had this book when I first became a mother. If I'd known what was coming, I might not have been so blindsided by how different I felt in my own head.
Conaboy has done a great service to parents and brains everywhere . . . I am so grateful for her work, insight, courage and generosity'

Emma Jane Unsworth, author of *After the Storm*

'Conaboy presents a vital new narrative of what it means to parent, and to care.
Meticulously researched and deeply personal, *Mother Brain* explores how parenting and caregiving shapes us, changes us and makes us human. Compelling and compassionate, this is the book we need as we look towards a future where parenting, in all its diversity, is valued and celebrated'

Elinor Cleghorn, author of *Unwell Women*

'An awesomely detailed and refreshingly positive review of brain science as a rich source of explanations for the often surprising, commonly bewildering, routinely criticised experiences of parenthood . . . Powerful, honest and reassuring'

Professor Gina Rippon, author of *The Gendered Brain*

'Fearlessly researched and deeply empathetic . . . Every page pruned away sexist, guilt-inducing assumptions about the 'maternal instinct'. If every new parent, boss and lawmaker read this book, we would make a century of progress overnight'

Lauren Smith Brody, author of *The Fifth Trimester*

'If I had read *Mother Brain* in the early days of my recovery from postpartum psychosis, it would have been more than medicine – reassuring, legitimising and qualifying all those negative feelings that I thought were "just me"'

Laura Dockrill, author of *What Have I Done?*

'A generous, engaging, deeply researched book that will change the way you think about your own parents, your children and yourself'

Rebecca Traister, author of *Good and Mad*

'Vital reading for anyone who wants to understand more about how and why the maternal brain changes during such an important life event'

Melissa Hogenboom, author of *The Motherhood Complex*

'*Mother Brain* uses science to confirm a truth known to adoptive and other non-gestational parents: becoming a parent rewires our brains to love and care for children, just like biological parents. This physiological change anchors us to our children and makes space for society to see us as real parents. Thank you for including our mother brain in your tome about parenthood'

Nefertiti Austin, author of *Motherhood So White*

'Takes direct aim at the damaging and false narratives of morality and biology that have shaped our thinking about women and mothers for centuries. Fascinating and relatable . . . A must-read'   Brigid Schulte, author of *Overwhelmed*

'Shines a bright light on the truth of parenthood, and the way it changes us . . . Insightful, generous and wise'

Jennifer Finney Boylan, author of *She's Not There*

'Conaboy fearlessly pours herself into the silence surrounding the open secret of mothering and caregiving – how we are profoundly remade by it, in both beautiful and destabilising ways'   Angela Garbes, author of *Like a Mother*

'Part memoir, part scientific sleuthing, *Mother Brain* is storytelling at its very best'   Amy Ellis Nutt, author of *The Teenage Brain*

'Becoming a parent often comes with an influx of overwhelming feelings, and beliefs that result in guilt and shame. Conaboy dissects the research of what is truly going on inside our brains through storytelling to help us remove the unrealistic parenting expectations and get true support'

Eve Rodsky, author of *Fair Play*

MOTHER
BRAIN

MOTHER BRAIN

SEPARATING MYTH FROM BIOLOGY –
THE SCIENCE OF THE PARENTAL BRAIN

CHELSEA CONABOY

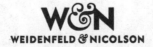
WEIDENFELD & NICOLSON

First published in the United States in 2022 by Henry Holt and Company
First published in Great Britain in 2022 by Weidenfeld & Nicolson
This paperback edition first published in Great Britain in 2024 by
Weidenfeld & Nicolson,
an imprint of The Orion Publishing Group Ltd
Carmelite House, 50 Victoria Embankment
London EC4Y 0DZ

An Hachette UK Company

1 3 5 7 9 10 8 6 4 2

A CIP catalogue record for this book is
available from the British Library.

ISBN (Mass Market Paperback) 978 1 4746 1838 0
ISBN (eBook) 978 1 4746 1839 7
ISBN (Audio) 978 1 4746 1840 3

Typeset by Input Data Services Ltd, Bridgwater, Somerset

Printed in Great Britain by Clays Ltd, Elcograf S.p.A.

MIX
Paper | Supporting
responsible forestry
FSC
www.fsc.org   FSC® C104740

www.weidenfeldandnicolson.co.uk
www.orionbooks.co.uk

For my boys.

CONTENTS

CONTENTS

PREFACE

What does it mean to become a mother?

Certainly, every person's experience is different. It is shaped by one's circumstances, and those circumstances can vary in infinite ways, even from the very start, depending on whether a pregnancy is planned or not, agonized over or agonizing to discover, undertaken with or without a partner, begun with a donor, with assistance, or with ease. But parenthood in general, and motherhood in particular, is viewed often as something hyperpersonal. A mother is sacrosanct, love embodied. Motherhood is too precious to look at directly, to dissect. Instead, we see it sideways. We celebrate the transformative power of a child—"Having a baby changes everything," according to Johnson & Johnson—without really naming what is changed.

For many women, the question feels dangerous. To answer it directly would require us to acknowledge just *how* we are changed by motherhood, altered from the person we were before and distinct from those who do not have children. Distinct from men. Different, in this context, has most often meant lesser. Forgetful. Frazzled. Consumed. Hindered by our own biology, perpetually at the edge of moral delinquency, and certainly less interesting. Better not to consider it.

In the forty or so weeks of pregnancy—many more if you account for the months spent attempting conception or struggling with pregnancy losses—birthing parents are bombarded with information about what pregnancy means for our body, our breasts, our hips, our waist-line, our cardiac function, our pelvic floor, our sex drive. We are over-whelmed with guidance about what our behavior will mean for our children, how the choices we make will affect their developing bodies and their lifelong physical and mental health. How little we learn about ourselves. Even less about our partners. Among all the information we take in during the run-up to motherhood, what do we learn about how parenthood changes us, our inner lives? What does it mean to *become* a mother?

For nonbinary parents, fathers, or same-sex partners, the question—what does it mean to become a parent?—might seem unacknowledged, their stories treated like footnotes to a "truer" narrative about the tran-sition to parenthood, the distinctly maternal one. Science has given us a whole new way of answering these questions, of asking them, even.

The first time I tried, I was four months postpartum and sitting in a tiny windowless room at the newspaper where I had recently returned from maternity leave to my job as an editor. I had just pumped a mea-sly two or so ounces of breast milk that, with two more trips from my desk in the newsroom to this closet—which had a table and a chair and a scrawled "do not enter" message on the door but no lock—would become just one of the two bottles I needed in order to feed my infant at day care the following day. I had reporters to meet with and deadlines to manage, and the clock was ever ticking toward the precise minute by which I needed to leave the office to fetch my baby from day care. But as desperate as I was for more time in my day and fewer things on my to-do list, I was desperate for information, too.

I wanted to understand what I was experiencing as an anxious new mother. I was sure there was far more happening in my brain and my body than what I had learned over the months when I was reading books and taking classes that I thought would prepare me for this time. So I turned off the *wah-whir-wah-whir* of my breast pump, dropped the milk into a cooler, opened my laptop, and called Peter Schmidt.

Schmidt has researched the influence of hormones and reproduc-tive state on a person's mood and mental health since about 1986—when misogynistic doctors thought postpartum mood disorders were simply further evidence of women's impairment by their reproductive system, feminists worried (not without cause) that male researchers were pathologizing their normal biological processes, and Schmidt's peers in science viewed these conditions as "soft quality of life issues" rather than a real public health concern. When I talked to Schmidt in July 2015, those barriers to studying the parental brain had begun to fall, and he was now chief of behavioral endocrinology at the National Institute of Mental Health.

Schmidt was the first person I heard describe new motherhood as a distinct developmental stage with long-lasting effects, in which each of the body's systems thought to regulate social behavior, emotion, and immune responses—"all of those things get drastically changed." Schmidt affirmed what I was feeling, that the way we talk about postpartum experiences is really limited. Making postpartum depression a mainstream concern had taken so much effort. Next, he said, the challenge was broadening the understanding of just how much change a person goes through when they become a parent and what's at stake in the process.

This was revelatory to me then, though to be honest, I barely knew what he meant. This book is the result of my effort to figure it out, through interviews with dozens of researchers and nearly as many parents, with a deep dive into the research on the human parental brain and the foundational animal literature, and by taking a critical look at the stories we live with about parenthood and how they came to be.

I had thought I would write an essay about my own realization of motherhood as a developmental stage and how expectant mothers deserve a more complete understanding of how the postpartum period could go for them. And I did that, but then I got hooked. The more I learned, the bigger this science felt, capable of changing not only our individual experiences but also how we view and talk about parenthood overall and so much of what it touches—sex and gender, work, equity in science, social policy and politics, the time spent engrossed in our children and the time spent apart from them.

This is a book about the parental brain, but you should know that I am neither a "parenting expert" (whatever that means) nor a neuroscientist. The expertise I bring to these pages is twofold. First, I am a journalist with nearly two decades of experience translating complicated topics for readers, with a particular focus on health care. And I am an expert at parenting my two particular children with their particular needs alongside my particular husband in our particular time and place. I've tried to make sense of the science in the context of my own life as a parent, with the hope that what I've learned will be meaningful to others, too.

In the years since I interviewed Schmidt from that lactation closet, the number of neuroimaging studies focused on the parental brain has grown significantly, as has scrutiny of the technologies and the methods of analysis used in those studies, particularly regarding functional magnetic resonance imaging, or fMRI. Mindful of these criticisms, I've aimed to highlight findings that hold up across disciplines or have been replicated, and to be transparent about the places where the research is thin or conflicted.

Science is not static. The parental brain has been neglected as a subject worth studying for a long time. The story it tells today is well worth exploring. But in truth, this research is just getting started. The findings here will change—already are changing—and will raise new questions. I've tried to point in the direction those questions might lead.

For now, this research is still overwhelmingly focused on cisgender, heterosexual women who are gestational mothers. This is changing, too, but slowly. In writing about specific studies, I've deferred to the authors' description of study participants. Otherwise, I've used inclusive language to describe parents, because it is most accurate. Transgender men and nonbinary parents who don't identify as mothers give birth, and their brains change across pregnancy and the postpartum period, too. And importantly, it's not only gestational parents who experience profound neurobiological changes, but rather anyone who is deeply invested—with their time and their energy—in caring for children.

The "mother brain" is not synonymous with the female brain nor with the birthing brain. Rather, it is the brain that is "earned by care," as feminist philosopher Sara Ruddick might have described it. It is the one engaged in the life-supporting practice of mothering, which "is older than feminism," as Alexis Pauline Gumbs wrote in *Revolutionary Mothering: Love on the Front Lines*. "It is older and more futuristic than the category 'woman.'" The *capacity* for this kind of connection is a fundamental characteristic of our species—and others—possessed by all. The development of that connection is the thing that defines parenthood in practice. This book is an exploration of the neurobiological mechanisms and the lived experience that makes it so.

To new or expectant parents reading: if you are struggling in any way, please get help. The brain goes through a massive change in pregnancy and new parenthood. Struggle is common, and it is normal to need support. Seek it out from your doctor, online, or in your local area.

Finally, this book will not offer advice about how to care for your child or about what kind of parent to be. It may not answer any of the questions recurring in your Google search history about sleep or day care or how exactly to get your preschooler to put on his snow boots without anyone in the room losing their cool. I hope this science will help you, as it did me, to understand what kind of parent you already are and the one you are becoming. We are not hardwired for this work, but must grow into it. How does that happen, and why, and what does it mean for our lives today and in the long term?

We owe it to ourselves to consider those questions with all the information available to us. We owe it to one another.

MOTHER
BRAIN

CHAPTER 1

At the Flip of a Switch

Year after year, a nest appeared in early spring, tucked inside a wreath on the front door of my childhood home. The mother robin didn't seem to mind that I would peek at her from just inside the glass, inches away. At least, I didn't think so. After all, she kept coming back. And I was glad. She was a marvel to watch, tireless as she set twig to twig, layering in mud and then fine grass to make a safe space for those beautiful, fragile blue eggs. Her devotion to her scraggly, gape-mouthed chicks seemed complete. She was alert and vigilant, patient and selfless. She knew just what to do to care for them, to protect them, as mothers are supposed to.

That's what I thought. Because that's how the story goes, the one told across time and through generations, carried forward in fable and in myth until it becomes a part of how we measure the world around us, how we see ourselves. We are the dedicated mother bird, the story tells us, guided by a maternal instinct perfected through the ages into something solid and certain, like a smooth red marble hidden beneath a feathered breast. We nest. We nurture. We defend. Naturally.

Then something happens. We have a baby of our own. And we realize, that sweet story line that seemed full of truth and beauty—it's bullshit. Broken. Either that, or we are.

* * *

FOR SO MANY OF US, maternal instinct doesn't show up, at least not in the ways we expected it to. Caring for a newborn does not feel innate. There is no switch that flips when we become pregnant or when our baby arrives. Too often, we don't question the narrative, the one that says we should know just what to do and how to feel. The one that discounts how parenting requires a whole set of practical skills that we may or may not already possess. The one that omits the facts and circumstances of our individual lives before pregnancy and afterward, that says we will transition seamlessly (but for a bit of sleep deprivation) from a person committed first and foremost to sustaining our own survival to one who is now also entirely responsible for a tiny, nonverbal creature that depends on us for their every need. Instead, we question ourselves.

That's what Emily Vincent did.

Vincent had been certain, as the end of her first pregnancy approached, that she wouldn't want a full twelve weeks of maternity leave. She loved her job as a pediatric nurse. By eight weeks, she figured, she would miss her coworkers and her patients. She would be lonely with all that time at home. Then baby Will arrived, and she couldn't imagine being apart from him. Eight weeks came and went, and she didn't want to go back to work full-time, not yet and maybe not even after her twelve weeks were up. She worried about day care. Would he be safe there? Would his caregivers pace his feedings correctly? Would they leave him to cry for too long? Would he be OK outside the cocoon of protection and care that she and her husband had woven for him, with love, yes, but also with urgency and with worry? Those are common concerns for a new parent. But for Vincent, they felt like a symptom of something bigger. Her work had been her identity. That identity was in crisis.

It wasn't just about Vincent's job, either. There was also Dawn, the baby from the movie *Trainspotting*, whose image—one particular image—kept popping into her head, though she hadn't seen the movie in at least a decade. If you've seen the film, you know the one I'm talking about, though Vincent had urged me not to watch it. She didn't want it to live in my head as it had in hers. (Watch *Bao* instead, she told me—"with tissues"—referring, as if it were an antidote, to Pixar's Oscar-winning animated short film that imagines a boy as a plump dumpling with an overprotective but loving mother.)

Dawn and Will have nothing in common except that they are both babies and, by nature, vulnerable to their circumstances. Fictional Baby Dawn died neglected in Edinburgh, the adults in her life lost in the abyss of heroin addiction. Will is lovingly cared for at home in Cincinnati by parents who have the means to commit themselves to raising him. Still, the image of Dawn lying motionless in her crib was there in Vincent's mind when her son napped during the day or as she lay in bed in the wee hours of the morning after feeding him, telling herself over and over, "He's fine. He's in his crib. He's fine"—a mantra of truth against her worst fear. She couldn't explain it.

"I felt really silly for being so upset about that movie scene," she told me when Will was nearly six months old. "I felt really silly about suddenly not wanting to go back to work full-time." She felt afraid of how she was feeling, she said, of what it meant about her ability to be a good mother and about her sense of herself.

Alice Owolabi Mitchell questioned herself, too.

She had prepared for many possible outcomes of her daughter's arrival. She was acutely aware of the fact that, as a Black woman living in the United States, she was at considerably higher risk than a White expectant mother for suffering complications, including fatal ones, through pregnancy and the postpartum period. Her own mother had died of cardiac arrest two weeks after giving birth to a son when Owolabi Mitchell was a teenager. That baby boy had grown into a fourteen-year-old whom she and her husband were raising. Her mother's story and her own—they were a lot to carry. While pregnant, Owolabi Mitchell had started seeing a therapist and enlisted the help of a group of doulas. She made plans to go to a diverse mothers' group in nearby Boston, as well as one close to her home in Quincy.

Then, Everly was born early, about a month before her due date. Owolabi Mitchell didn't have a chance to make final preparations for leave from her job as a fifth-grade teacher or to say goodbye to her students. She felt she hadn't fully been able to shift her frame of mind to focus on her baby's arrival. Days after Everly was born, shelter-in-place protocols began to roll out across the United States in response to the coronavirus pandemic. Owolabi Mitchell's breast milk was slow to come in, and she and Everly struggled to get the latch just right. She worried about whether Everly was eating enough, about whether her own stress was hampering her milk supply, about the myriad threats the pandemic posed to her family. In-person support groups were canceled. With doctors' offices mostly closed, six weeks—then seven and eight—passed, and Owolabi Mitchell wasn't able to see her ob-gyn for her standard postpartum visit.

In those first weeks, one worry seemed to surmount them all: Why didn't she feel connected to her baby? She had anticipated a flood of warm emotions when Everly was born. She expected she would fall in love at first sight with such force that it would sustain her through those disorienting first days and make her forget about the pain of her own recovery, even carry her through the turmoil of a pandemic. "I was expecting that automatic switch, and that didn't happen," she told me. She wondered, "Am I already a bad mom because I don't have this?"

My experience of brand-new motherhood was different in the details, but so much about Owolabi Mitchell's and Vincent's stories, and so many that I've heard from other new parents, is familiar to me. Our expectations of ourselves did not match reality. In the days and weeks after my oldest son, Hartley, was born, I felt joy and awe. But I did not feel any sort of natural calm, no sense of certainty or clarity in my thoughts or actions. Instead, I felt a kind of roiling, a constant, unfamiliar motion. Each of us had stepped through the portal of childbirth and were startled to realize that the topography of the map we had been given to guide us in unfamiliar territory barely resembled what we found. Where we expected land, there was water, and we were unmoored.

* * *

IN MY FIRST WEEKS AND months as a mother, worry became a kind of ceaseless static in my mind, never not there. With the worry came guilt. And with the guilt, loneliness. I didn't feel like the parent my son deserved or the naturally nurturing mother I had been told repeatedly I would be. The orbit of my life had shrunk to encompass little more than the chair in which I nursed my son and the room where his bassinet stood next to our bed. Feeling overwhelmed even in that felt like failure.

None of this—the all-consuming nature of it, the devastation that accompanied the joy—was how I had imagined it would be. Close friends who had young children reassured me that the early months were hard, that things would get better when the baby started sleeping more at night, but they never talked about this thing I felt that I couldn't quite name, a kind of untying. Neither did I.

Even as the months passed and my worry began to fade some, the sense remained that I had stepped into a disorienting new reality in which everything sat a few degrees off-center. In some ways, it was thrilling. I recognized a new power in myself. I would stand in the mirror, holding my son, in awe of our two bodies, of the thing I had done. Other times, when I waited in line at the grocery store behind a mother with a toddler in her cart or when I spotted someone else walking to work with the same ugly breast pump bag that I had, I would wonder, did they feel it too? Had they become familiar with the same soundtrack of what-ifs, crescendoing in absurdity? (What if that sniffle is the start of pneumonia? What if I fall down the stairs while carrying him? What if my child chokes, someday, on one of those dreaded laundry pods?) Did they find themselves crying uncontrollably as they read about the capsizing of a boat full of refugees in the Mediterranean—or the latest school shooting or hate crime—the news not only tragic but now something visceral, an agony for somebody else's babies? Did they know the strange tug between the urge to run from the shower to comfort their crying child in the next room and the desire to climb out the bathroom window, so desperate for a moment to themselves, with their old selves?

I feared that their answer was no. That I was an outlier, that the maternal instinct that was supposed to provide equilibrium in the tumult of new parenthood was broken. Or, worse, that something deep within me had been altered. Set loose.

Pregnancy and parenting books seemed only to gloss over the questions I now had about myself as a mother. I found an inkling of something different first in a tattered hand-me-down copy of *Infants and Mothers: Differences in Development* by famed pediatrician T. Berry Brazelton, originally published in 1969. Brazelton wrote that many new mothers face emotional and psychological challenges, that those struggles are normal and "may even be an important part of her ability to become a different kind of person." Soon after, I read other people's writing about the maternal brain and, because I am a questioner by nature and a health journalist by training, I dug into the research myself.

I would think of Brazelton's words often as I pored over studies documenting the change in the volume of gray matter in a mother's brain or what one paper describes as the "wholesale remodeling of synapses and neural activity." Half a century ago, Brazelton sensed what researchers today are establishing using human brain scans and animal models: parenthood creates "a different kind of person."

Birthing a baby doesn't simply turn on a long-dormant circuit marked for maternal instinct and specific to the brains of females. Researchers studying the neurobiology of parents have begun documenting the many ways having a child reorganizes the brain, altering the neural feedback loops that dictate how we react to the world around us, how we read and respond to other people, and how we regulate our own emotions. Becoming a parent changes our brain, functionally and structurally, in ways that shape our physical and mental health over the remainder of our life span. Scientists have found such significant change in gestational mothers, by far the most studied group, that they now recognize new motherhood as a major developmental stage of life. And they've begun mapping how, in *all* parents who engage in caring for their children, no matter their path to parenthood, the brain is changed by the intensity of that experience and the hormonal shifts that accompany it. We are, in a very real sense, remade by parenthood.

Most pregnancy books and health care providers pay lip service at least to the fact that hormone levels rise steeply during pregnancy and childbirth and plunge soon after. New parents are discharged from the hospital with pamphlets gently warning about the "baby blues," a period of moodiness and mild depression that most birthing parents experience in the first weeks after childbirth. But rarely do we learn what that jolt of hormones sets in motion.

This hormonal surge around childbirth acts like a rush order on the remodeling of the brain, sensitizing it for the creation of new neural pathways aimed first at motivating parents—despite self-doubt or lack of experience—to meet baby's basic needs in those tenuous first days, and then setting them up for a longer period of learning how to care for their child. Babies change like the weather and then grow, before we know it, into walking, talking beings with complex physical and emotional needs. Parents need to be able to change with them. The brain adjusts in ways that account for that, becoming more moldable, more adaptable than it typically is, maybe even more so than at any other point in adulthood.

The physiological changes are dramatic. Using brain imaging technology and other tools, scientists can clearly detect and measure changes in the physical structure of new mothers' brains. They've found that regions key to the work of parenting, including those that shape our motivation, attention, and social responses, change significantly in volume. These structural changes are complex. Some regions seem to shift in size, growing or shrinking as the brain responds to the rapidly changing nature of new parenthood, especially through pregnancy and the first few months with a newborn, in a process thought to represent a fine-tuning of the brain for the demands of parenting.

Researchers have identified a general pattern of activity across birthing parents' brains that builds over time, a caregiving circuitry that is activated as they listen to recordings of their baby's cry, for example, or respond to images or videos of their child smiling or in distress. The imprint of that circuitry is present even when a mother is doing nothing in particular, lying in an fMRI scanner and letting her mind wander. Caring for a baby changes what researchers call the functional architecture of the brain, the framework across which brain activity moves. And remarkably, those changes last, not only weeks or months after a baby is born but perhaps even decades later, over a person's whole life span, long past what we think of as the child-rearing years.

Taken together, the science suggests that remodeling of the parental brain involves much more than rearranging furniture to make room for one more role in a busy life. Becoming a parent moves weight-bearing walls. It tweaks the floor plan. It changes the way light enters the space.

As I learned more, my worries seemed to quiet some. Having a baby changes the brain. Not only for the one in five birthing parents who develop a perinatal mood or anxiety disorder, but for *all* of them. For *all parents*. I had felt adrift in new motherhood, and this anchored me. The turmoil I felt might be normal, an intrinsic part of the reorientation of the brain for parenthood. This prompted a slew of new questions: What else was I missing? How exactly did the brain change, and what could those changes mean for my life? And then, why hadn't I known about this earlier?

The story I found in the science was decidedly not one of a woman girded by the magic of motherly love, who responds to her baby's every need reflexively, accepts the self-sacrifice required of her without question, and taps into a well of mother-knows-best wisdom. That narrative, it had become clear to me, was about as representative of new motherhood as the someday-your-prince-will-come Disney stories are of dating and marriage.

Instead, the science tells us that to become a parent is to be deluged. We are overwhelmed with stimuli, from our changed bodies and our changed routines. From the hormonal fluxes of pregnancy and childbirth and breastfeeding. From our babies, of course, with their newborn smell, their tiny fingers, their coos, and their never-ending needs. It is brutal, in a sense, how completely engulfed we are by it and from multiple fronts, like a rock at the ocean's edge, battered by waves and tides and sun and wind. Some researchers refer to this as the environmental complexity of new parenthood. All the new input our brain must take in, suddenly and all at once, may feel disorienting and distressing. But it has a point.

This flood of stimuli compels us to care for infants in their most vulnerable state, because a parent's love is neither automatic nor absolute. In a sense, the brain works to keep our babies alive until the heart catches up. It transforms us into protective, even obsessive caregivers when so many of us lack any skill whatsoever in actual child-rearing. If that were all, the parental brain would be worthy of awe. That's just the start.

Scientists have begun tracking how the neural reorganization caused by parenthood affects a person's behavior, their way of being in the world, their life at large. Ask any researcher what exactly they know to date, and they'll likely tell you, "far too little." This work is just beginning. But the findings so far and the questions they point to are deeply meaningful in themselves. For me, studying them has been like seeing my own reflection in a storefront window along a bustling sidewalk—a chance to recognize myself.

Researchers studying women have found that new motherhood seems to alter how they read and respond to social and emotional cues, not only from their babies but perhaps also from their partners and other adults. It may change their ability to regulate their own emotions, helping them to stay calm—in a relative sense—in the face of a screaming infant (or a stubborn preschooler or a moody teenager), and to plan a response. While many people experience real but generally temporary memory loss during pregnancy and the postpartum period, motherhood in certain contexts also has been found to enhance executive functioning, affecting a person's ability to strategize and her capacity to shift attention between tasks. Though the results are somewhat complicated to date, a small number of studies suggest motherhood may even protect cognition later in life.

The questions at the forefront of this field are urgent and, in a frustrating sense, basic. Parenthood has been neglected by science, seen more as a subject of morality and the soft laws of nature than as one worthy of rigorous investigation. For a long time, beyond pregnancy and the act of breastfeeding, human maternal behavior was thought to be determined wholly by social and individual factors, with little physiological basis. But parenthood is all those things, psychosocial and neurobiological, a change in lifestyle and a change in self.

Researchers leading the field today—notably, many of them women—recognize that and are pursuing answers that could have far-reaching effects. Why do the brain changes directed at making parents into motivated caregivers also make them vulnerable in ways that can undermine that very goal? What does a person's reproductive history, even one in which they have no children, mean for their long-term health? How does the brain-altering disease of addiction interact with the brain-altering period of new parenthood? Do pregnancy-related brain changes alter the effectiveness of antidepressant medications in the postpartum period? How does trauma, in all its forms, including the extremely common experiences of pregnancy loss and childbirth trauma, affect a person's postpartum development and mental health over time?

"Mommy brain" jokes aside, what really happens to a person's cognitive function after they have children? What about their creativity and their emotional state? How does having a child affect a person's life, beyond their aptitude to parent?

It has become clear to me that the parental brain is an essential topic not only for people taking prenatal classes or navigating the first weeks at home with a newborn. It's one that grandparents and policy makers, health care providers and advocates, any working parent and any manager of working parents should understand, too, along with any person who is considering whether to become a parent and looking for information, beyond mythology, to help them decide. This science can play a role in shifting gender norms at home and at work, in building public policies that actually support parents of young children, in securing reproductive rights, and in reimagining the relationship between parenting and society. At the very least, it alters the stories we tell ourselves about our individual experiences of parenthood and about the world around us, stories that so desperately need rewriting. Stories about the inner life of that mother robin, or my own brokenness.

This science has exposed something essential that is so obviously missing from the old story of maternal instinct: time. Becoming a mother, a parent, is a process. Unless we've previously done the intensive work of wholly caring for another vulnerable person, our fundamental capacity for parenting is not preexisting. It grows. That growth can be painful and powerful. And long-lasting. All sorts of factors determine just how it will occur. How would our expectations change—the ones we hold ourselves to, the ones we judge others by—if we could see that fundamental truth?

* * *

IN FACT, WE'VE KNOWN THIS for a long time. Many people who experience this transition have recognized it for what it is. Feminist scholars have been saying for generations that much of what we are told about motherhood, and especially the notion that maternal instinct is something hardwired, universal, and essential to female identity, is false. In the early 1960s, a gentle-spirited researcher at Rutgers University and his colleagues built on work he had done studying domestic kittens and added evidence to that claim.

Jay S. Rosenblatt was somewhat unusual in that, through much of his career, he studied the psychobiology of maternal behavior in mammals, in all its complexity, while also seeing patients as a psychoanalyst. He was a painter, too, having served during World War II painting camouflage, perhaps a hint at his ability to see what was hidden.

For decades, many of his peers and most of his predecessors had looked at the patterns of behavior carried out by mothers across species—their propensity even as first-time mothers to build nests and to feed and protect their young—and found them to be so uniform, so particular to females, that they had to be an inborn characteristic of the sex. Maternal behavior was "indisputably innate," Frank A. Beach Jr., a founder of the field of behavioral endocrinology, wrote in 1937. That view was widely held. "Without exception investigators studying maternal behavior in the rat have classified the activity as native," he wrote. Native, as in the opposite of learned or acquired. Built in.

For a while, newborns were viewed in a similarly static way, as creatures who grow and develop motor skills, but who don't develop in any social way until they have passed the newborn stage. The authors of one 1950 study tracked the development of puppies and wrote that the dogs' ability to learn in the first weeks of life "must be extremely limited." The human condition was much the same, they found. At the start of a new life, it seemed, mother and baby acted almost wholly by instinct.

Instinct has always been a somewhat loosely defined thing, generally thought of as those behaviors that members of a species perform, nearly all in the same way, without ever having been taught them, such as a bird's regular migration path or a bee's very particular role in constructing a hive. Psychologists writing the theory of instinct in the late nineteenth and early twentieth centuries often disagreed on the definition of an instinct or just how it worked. By the early 1950s, Austrian ethologist Konrad Lorenz and others popularized the idea that species-typical patterns of behavior occur through inherited, machinelike mechanisms in the central nervous system. Lorenz famously described the process of imprinting, by which newly hatched birds of certain species attach to the first moving creature they see, typically their parent but possibly a member of a different species or an inanimate object in motion. Lorenz's observations of birds that imprinted on him formed the foundation for his theories on instinct across the life span, but especially regarding links between mothers and babies.

Lorenz believed instinctive behavior was the result of inherited impulses that build up in designated areas of the brain until an animal encounters a particular stimulus that triggers the release of a set action. In her book *The Nature and Nurture of Love: From Imprinting to Attachment in Cold War America*, science historian Marga Vicedo explains that Lorenz often used a lock-and-key metaphor to describe an innate behavior and the corresponding stimuli that would release it. "The form of the key-bit," he wrote, "is predetermined." To Lorenz, the instinctive behavior of mothers and babies was a complex system of such locks, a heavy key ring of releasers forged long ago.

There are many aspects of Lorenz's work and writing that have proven essential to the study of behavior across species. He was one of three ethologists awarded the Nobel Prize in 1973 for his work on imprinting and the broader subject of how genetics shape behavior. Some of his peers said the award was inappropriate, given that Lorenz had joined the Nazi party in 1938—a decision he later said he regretted—using his theories about behavior to support the idea of a racial state and to advocate against the spread of "socially inferior human material." Still, he is cited throughout the modern literature on the parental brain for his foundational work on how social bonds are built in biology and especially for his theory on how a baby's cuteness prompts a powerful response in an adult's brain.

Lorenz suggested that the factors that make a baby cute—big head, chubby cheeks, clumsy movements, and a body like a "half-inflated football"—release the instinctive movement, most strongly in women, of taking that baby up in one's arms, as evidenced by his own daughter's loving reaction to a cute doll. Recent and more rigorous research has borne out the idea that cuteness has a powerful, measurable effect on the human brain, though the modern framing is quite a bit different and, thankfully, less reliant on the socialized idea that dolls automatically are to girls what babies are to women.

The rigidity with which Lorenz defined instinct, however, as something separate from a person's environmental context or experience, built into an individual much like an organ, has been profoundly detrimental to mothers. Lorenz's work captured the public imagination. There he was, bare-chested in a pond and chattering to his own baby goslings, above a 1955 *Life* headline, "An Adopted Mother Goose." And he gained a following among child development specialists who saw his theories as validation for their own nascent ideas about bonding and attachment between human babies and their mothers. Vicedo documents just how much bolder Lorenz became as his career progressed, despite—perhaps even because of—the building criticism he faced from fellow scientists studying animal behavior. Where he once said it was likely that the same kind of mechanistic imprinting he observed in geese also occurred in human children, he later held that out as a fact and one that, if unheeded, spelled doom for humankind. Mothers were spending too little time with their infants, he said, disrupting "genetically anchored social behavior." As a result, he told the *New York Times* in 1977, "the capability of creating personal ties is atrophying," and violence and crime in human societies are on the rise. In Lorenz's view, mothers must act in line with their inherited instinct or risk endangering the species.

Scientists today have dismissed the entirely unilateral influence of genetics on behavior. Our understanding of the brain—as a complex web of reactions shaped also by our lived experiences and our physical and social environments—no longer accommodates the simplistic idea of energy building in a specific neural center waiting for a specific, predetermined trigger. Yet so much of Lorenz's view on the fixedness of maternal instinct has stuck.

Expectant parents so often anticipate that, in those first few moments with their newborn, they will feel an overwhelming rush of warmth, that setting eyes on their own child's face will trigger in them the kind of automatic, all-consuming love they've long been told they have in waiting. So many of us are confused by what may come instead. Shock or sadness. Ambivalence. Love, plus fear. Joy, plus dread. If something goes wrong during pregnancy or at the start of our child's life, if we experience complications, or if other stressors—say, from a strained relationship, financial stress, or a global pandemic—alter our postpartum experience in ways we couldn't have anticipated, we may worry that we've already failed. Lorenz's voice echoes through every wrenching internal debate about how to balance childcare and career. It's there, too, when we try unsuccessfully to comfort a wailing newborn in the disorienting hours of the early morning and we wonder what is wrong with us, or with our baby, or with our bond. How can it be that lock and key don't match?

* * *

JAY ROSENBLATT SAW THINGS DIFFERENTLY. Rosenblatt was influenced by animal psychologist T. C. Schneirla, who rejected Lorenz's ideas about innateness and instinct. Schneirla believed an individual's development, even at the earliest stages of life, is driven not only by what some saw as gene-determined physical maturation but also by that individual's over-all experience, in the broadest sense. Development, he said, occurred in a progression, with one phase of life influencing the next, so that the effects of all sorts of stimuli, including genetics and environmental factors, "inseparably coalesced." Today, this is taken as fundamental—the complexity of one's environment influences gene expression so that a particular set of genes (a genotype) can result in varying characteristics and behaviors (a phenotype), depending on the context.

For such a theory to hold, it would have to be true that even days-old mammals could, in fact, respond in a meaningful way to their environment. Along with a colleague, Rosenblatt and Schneirla studied the behavior of kittens, documenting their normal, efficient suckling and weaning patterns. Then they set up a study to isolate some kittens from their litter for designated windows of time, removing them to a pen with a kind of artificial mother, a brooder with a fuzzy platform from which they could suckle formula. Those isolated in the first week of their lives adjusted easily to feeding from the brooder but then struggled, when returned to the litter, to physically orient themselves alongside their mother cat and find their way to her nipple. Kittens isolated when slightly older could more readily locate their mother but then nuzzled her all over, including on her face, searching for the source of milk. Those isolated after spending about five weeks with their litter had trouble adjusting in a different way when they returned.

In their absence, the mother cat had become more mobile and their littermates had started taking more initiative to feed. The returning kittens had a hard time keeping up. They hadn't been there to adjust as the litter's habits had changed. In isolation, the kittens had missed opportunities to learn how to nurse in a group and from a living, purring mother cat, whose fur pattern and smells and subtle prompts would have guided them. They hadn't been able to develop typically, in a progression and in response to their environment, alongside their siblings.

Rosenblatt's work in kittens informed how he saw animal mothers, too: not as a stake in the ground around which a growing baby circles, but as an organism who is herself developing and changing in tandem with her baby. In 1958, Rosenblatt joined the Institute of Animal Behavior at Rutgers University, founded by Daniel Lehrman. A few years earlier, just as Lorenz was gaining a popular following in the United States, Lehrman had published an incisive analysis calling many of the conclusions Lorenz drew about human behavior "patently shallow." Rosenblatt and Lehrman devised a series of studies using laboratory rats that would chart a very different theory about the nature of behavior in mothers than the one Lorenz had posited.

Before a lab rat is ever pregnant, it is generally averse to pups. Once a rat has a litter, her demeanor changes quickly. She engages in behaviors that *are* typical across the species. She builds a nest. She licks her pups and crouches over them to allow them to nurse. If she finds one outside the nest, she retrieves it. She can do all those things immediately after her pups are born. But Rosenblatt and Lehrman found that, if they removed the pups from a nest soon after birth, those behaviors in the mother quickly disappeared. Even when the mothers were later briefly given foster pups to care for, they mostly couldn't do it. Hormones and the physiological changes of pregnancy and birth prompt the onset of maternal behavior, but in order to maintain those behaviors, "the presence of the young is required," Rosenblatt and Lehrman wrote in a 1963 chapter that became a landmark publication for the field. In other words, childbirth jump-started things. But fully developing as mothers required interaction with pups. It took time.

Rosenblatt and Lehrman went on to document, in various ways, how the behavior of mothers and pups was not fixed but flexible. The development of each responded to the needs and behavior of the other. Removing pups from the nest at particular points in the postpartum period or swapping a rat mother's own pups for foster pups of a different age would alter her behavior. Conversely, when older pups were placed into the care of a brand-new rat mother, the foster mother gave the pups more attention than they typically would have received, and their development effectively slowed. A mother rat, they found, was not a rigid lock against which a key turned. She was growing and changing, too.

In 1967, Rosenblatt published findings that further rocked popular ideas about motherhood. Quite by accident, he and his colleagues at the Institute of Animal Behavior found that virgin female rats would begin caring for pups if they had enough exposure to a litter. After ten days or more with the babies, almost all the virgins they studied began building nests and even crouching as if to nurse, though they weren't actually producing milk. So did male rats, which normally would not care for offspring outside the laboratory. Given time with pups, the males began to lick and retrieve and crouch to nurse in nearly equal measure as the female virgins.

Certainly, the hormones that mother rats experience when having a litter seemed to fast-track the development of maternal behavior. But those same behaviors could develop in the absence of those hormones and irrespective of an individual's sex. "Maternal behavior," Rosenblatt concluded, "is therefore a basic characteristic of the rat." Not of the female rat alone. Of all rats. Rosenblatt found that the compulsion to care for young, to tend and protect them, was a basic characteristic of the species as a whole.

Humans parents and lab rat parents are not the same. Their brains share a common mammalian architecture and the same building blocks, but they also are different in many ways. The human cerebral cortex is wrinkled in complexity and the rat's is smooth, for example. Rodents rely heavily on their sense of smell and have an outsized olfactory bulb, which in humans is relatively tiny. Maternal behavior in the laboratory rat occurs in a very predictable pattern, in which licking is a prominent facet, and comes to a sharp end at about four weeks postpartum. Rats may cycle through many pregnancies and litters in a given year. In humans, maternal behavior extends over years or, often, decades and can involve simultaneously caring for multiple offspring at different ages, who may have dramatically different needs. Human parenting is notable for its variability, from family to family, between one generation and the next, influenced by innumerable social, political, and economic factors. Simply to draw direct correlations between Rosenblatt's findings in lab rats and human behavior would be to repeat Lorenz's folly.

Yet the basic tenets that Rosenblatt and colleagues first proposed in the early 1960s and built on in the years that followed have held true through decades of research and across mammalian species, so much so that Rosenblatt is now considered by many to be the "father of mothering" research, both for his groundbreaking work and for his skill in mentoring others. Nearly every major paper on the human parental brain in the past thirty years includes one of Rosenblatt's students, or his student's student, as an author. Those papers have borne out the idea that all mammal mothers go through very similar physiological changes in pregnancy, labor and delivery, and lactation, and that the hormones driving those changes also prime the brain in ways that make mothers hyperattentive to their babies, who arrive with their own genetic makeup and sense of agency.

Then the baby takes over, becoming a powerful stimulus that drives a dramatic reorganization of a mother's brain for the long term, to help her to balance the needs of her child alongside her own, even as those needs continually change. Babies and birthing parents develop together at a neural level, not only in response to their genes and their environment but in response to one another, with each new stage building on the last, in a process that doesn't end at six weeks postpartum or when a baby weans or walks or starts kindergarten. It is ongoing. This kind of growth, intense to start and reciprocal, may be unlike any mothers have experienced before, or at least not since they were on the other side of it. And it's not just mothers.

Following in Rosenblatt's footsteps, researchers today have clarified that "maternal behavior" is, in fact, a basic human characteristic, not uniquely maternal after all. Studies of fathers, including nonbiological fathers in same-sex couples, have found that the brains of men who are regularly engaged in caring for their children change in ways that are strikingly similar to gestational mothers'. Those changes are clearest in brain regions related to how fathers process their own emotions and read and respond to others' cues. Researchers suspect that similar brain changes occur for other nonbiological or nongestational parents and likely anyone who does the work of intense caregiving.

Certainly, things happen differently for parents who don't carry their children, at least at first. No pregnancy. No lactation. But they also may experience a significant shift in hormones upon becoming a parent, and researchers believe that shift, plus practice caring for a baby—exposure— drives the creation of a universal caregiving circuitry that has profound implications for how we perceive the bounds of family. Parents, according to the brain, are defined almost entirely by the attention and care they provide.

Rosenblatt's early work feels radical to me even today. I suppose that's because so much of the research that has given me a sense of awe and relief in this moment, in my own motherhood, can be traced to his work more than six decades ago. His research so elegantly obliterates the notion of a mechanistic maternal instinct and the gender norms built upon that lie. It suggests that the onset of parenthood is intense by design and requires fundamental, ongoing change. That process can be disrupted by trauma or stress or other obstacles, but perhaps unlike a rigid instinct, it also can be repaired and redirected. I wondered, did Rosenblatt, who died in 2014, see it that way? Did he consider his work to be radical? To be feminist?

To a point, according to Alison Fleming, who earned a doctorate under Rosenblatt's mentorship in 1972 and went on to run her own lab at the University of Toronto at Mississauga for a quarter century. Rosenblatt's work on male rats was published at a time when people involved in the women's liberation movement, including some men who wanted a more engaged experience of fatherhood, were calling for an overhaul of cultural norms and public policy to create more gender equity in child-rearing. Some seized on Rosenblatt's research as valida- tion, to say, "See? Fathers can be parents, too," Fleming told me. But if Rosenblatt's intent was at all political, its aim was at his peers.

Rosenblatt and Lehrman believed that the Lorenzian view of instinct was "completely wrong." Maternal behavior is "not like a fixed action pattern," Fleming said. "It's not like a mechanistic thing that happens automatically. It has its own development. And that was an important political point for Jay." It became an important point for Fleming, too.

Fleming has a massive body of published work that continues to grow in her retirement as she publishes ongoing studies with her own mentees (I also have heard Fleming called the "mother of mothering" research, which I suppose would instead make Rosenblatt a grandfather of the field). She has studied the nuances of maternal behavior in lactating laboratory rats and in first-time human mothers, tracked the role of cortisol and other hormones, and documented correlations between behavior and changes in neural circuitry. When she talks about what motivates her work, she talks about her daughters.

Fleming's own mother worked at the United Nations and was a strong role model of an intellectual and independent woman, not necessarily a nurturer. Fleming lived apart from her through much of her childhood. When Fleming was pregnant with her first daughter in 1975, she said she had no expectation of love at first sight. She hadn't had a model for that, she said. And it didn't come. But with time spent as a mother, she became deeply connected to her daughter, with whom, along with her sisters, she is "completely obsessed," Fleming said. "I really believe in experience," she told me.

Experience matters. That is the counterpoint to Lorenz. Of course, the biology of new parenthood matters, too, including the hormonal fluctuations of pregnancy and childbirth and the species-typical response patterns that follow. In 2015, Fleming and two other senior researchers wrote a comparison of studies on the maternal brain across human and nonhuman mammals. Human behavior is profoundly shaped by language and culture in ways that may make humans unique among mammals. That does not mean that the biological basis of mothering is less important in humans, they wrote. It means that the full context of a person's life—the physical environment in which they live, their relationships with other people, the cultural pressures and expectations they carry, among many other factors—has a stronger influence on those biological processes than it might in a rat. The psychological experience of being a parent and the neurobiological transformation it entails are, to borrow Schneirla's phrase, inseparably coalesced. If we devalue one and ignore the other, how can we ever really understand ourselves as parents, as people?

If we're lucky, when we are cast off from the old story line about maternal instinct, there's someone there who can help us find our way. Alice Owolabi Mitchell confided to a close friend that she was struggling to connect with little Everly, and her friend told her what she needed to hear: it's OK. Sing to her, the friend suggested. Look into her eyes. Rub her hand while you breastfeed. With a little time, Owolabi Mitchell said, she started to feel like Everly trusted her. And that gave her joy where before there was only worry. "We're learning each other," she said.

* * *

As it turns out, writing about the maternal brain while in the trenches of early motherhood is hard. My sons were two and four when I started writing this book. Many days, I have sat at my desk writing and rewriting the same sentence or two, too bleary-eyed from a night of wakings to focus on the mechanisms of maternal motivation, too conscious of the time ticking by before I have to wake my toddler from a nap and rush to pick up his brother at preschool, or, once the coronavirus pandemic hit, too distracted by impending doom and the sound of the boys roaring like dinosaurs just outside the door of my tiny home office. Sometimes I lose my temper with them in the morning, only to cry at my desk later over a study about how a mother's emotional control shapes her children's brain circuitry for regulating their own emotions.

On the best days, I get a chance to talk to someone like Jodi Pawluski, who researches the neurobiology of maternal mental health at the University of Rennes 1 in France. She primarily studies rodents, but she also produces the *Mommy Brain Revisited* podcast. It made perfect sense to me when, in 2020, she began offering counseling services to human mothers. Our many phone and email conversations, about whatever aspect of the research I was reporting on that day, often felt a bit like therapy. We would talk about the societal expectations placed on birthing parents and what the neurobiology reflects about the actual experience of motherhood. "It's OK to have bad days," she'd tell me. Or, "you learn as you go." In just about any other context, these phrases would be more or less meaningless to me, feel-good catchphrases. Coming from her, they felt different. They felt true.

Pawluski and coauthors Craig Kinsley and Kelly Lambert published a literature review in a January 2016 edition of the journal *Hormones and Behavior* in which they wrote about mothers in a way I had never seen before. The maternal brain, they wrote, is "a marvel of directed change" shaping a mother's life well beyond child-rearing. The brain is made flexible and "more complex" by the "endocrine tsunami that accompanies pregnancy," by the "enriching experiences" of motherhood itself, and by the long path of evolution. Pregnancy, the authors wrote, marks a "developmental epoch as significant as sexual differentiation and puberty."

Whoa, I remember thinking the first time I read that line. *As significant as puberty?*

Parents and educators understand much more about teenagers today than they did when I was one, growing up in a conservative suburban family in which the pressure to be a good girl was high and I felt as though I was perpetually folding and unfolding, like an origami fortuneteller, wondering who I would become and fearful I would never arrive at that person. We have a whole cultural canon of teenage characters celebrated for slouching their way through their own coming-of-age or for masking internal turmoil with rebellion or quiet. And today, the science of the teenage brain has reached the mainstream, serving teens themselves and the adults who care for them. It has shaped public health campaigns related to mental health and substance use. It has guided the national movement to delay school start times so that teens can get the sleep their changing brains require. In some places, it is changing how principals and school counselors think about discipline and support students in distress. The science has become a kind of coping mechanism for parents and teens alike to get through the tumult of adolescence, which we now understand reaches later into life than previously thought. In other words, we see that becoming an adult takes time.

We have long treated the hormonal upheaval around childbirth as something to wait out, until things level off in short order and return to normal. We expect birthing parents to simply carry on, to be who they always were—and more, to be fulfilled—all while their bodies may feel broken and their brains are being kneaded into shape. We don't tell teenagers to wait out puberty, as if it is simply a passing rainstorm.

We often do just the opposite, in fact. If we are doing right by them, we acknowledge and celebrate the young adults they are becoming. We give teens guidance and offer them compassion when things are hard. We create milestones in schools and on playing fields and in houses of worship just so we can stand up and say to them, "Look at you! Look how you are growing and changing. We are so proud."

For new parents, there is no return to normal, but the profound changes they experience in themselves often go unacknowledged. When Pawluski made those sweeping, generous statements about motherhood and the need to cut ourselves some slack, she wasn't being trite. She was conveying what she knew, based on the research. New parenthood is a period of monumental change for the brain, "a major event," as she puts it. On social media and in popular culture, we're getting better at talking about the range of emotions it brings. We're moving beyond bliss. That's good. "But," Pawluski said, "sometimes if people can put a finger on the fact that, oh my brain actually *physically* changes, that can help give— not an excuse—but give more weight to your feelings."

New parenthood is a developmental stage that takes time. Yet the lock-and-key idea that a woman is a mother waiting for a baby sits at the core of our cultural convictions about parenthood, still. As we'll see in the next chapter, dogma holds that belief in place, even while science has shown it to be old-fashioned. Outdated. Debunked. Seven decades of research suggest a new way of looking at things, one that truly acknowledges the turbulence of new parenthood and celebrates it as a time full of potential. Gather round and say it with me: "Look at you! Look how you are growing and changing. We are so proud."

In July 2018, an article I wrote about the science of the maternal brain and my own transition to motherhood was published in the Sunday magazine of the *Boston Globe*. Many readers wrote to me to say the piece helped them understand what they went through during the postpartum period and beyond. Among them was Emily Vincent, the pediatric nurse and new mother. Her sister-in-law had sent her a reprint of the article, published in the magazine *The Week*, with a question: Have you seen this? Vincent told me later that reading it helped her to realize the worry she felt over her return to work was not an unreasonable overreaction. Neither was the never-far image of baby Dawn. They were part of a physiological response, with a purpose. "I am not stupid or crazy for having these emotions," she said. "It *is* important to work through them and to put them in their place, but I didn't have to feel ashamed of myself for having them."

Will was enrolled in day care. Vincent went back to work, with slightly reduced hours, to a job where she felt a whole new level of compassion for the parents she works with, especially those overcome with worry; she was able to do this in part because of a newfound intensity of focus she felt in managing her life at home. It wasn't always easy, but understanding how her brain was adapting to help her to continue caring for herself while also caring for her precious baby boy made her feel proud. She could more fully recognize how she was changing. She could see who she was becoming.

CHAPTER 2

The Making of a Mother's Instinct

Around the same time that Mimi Niles became a new mother, a woman who lived upstairs from her in her New York City apartment building had twins. Occasionally, the two women would run into one another in the hallway or on the sidewalk, and Niles would ask the neighbor how she was faring. "Fabulous," Niles remembered her saying. "I'm so happy."

Niles was dumbfounded. She was not feeling fabulous at all. She slept little and cried a lot. She struggled to figure out what her daughter needed. She'd given birth at home, with support from a midwife. She was breastfeeding and co-sleeping and wearing her baby in a sling as often as possible. She had grown up in a Hindu household that embraced pain and struggle as an essential part of life, and her mother regularly told Niles stories of being a midwife in India, before she and her husband had emigrated to New York. Niles was on a path to become a midwife herself. The fact that new parenthood felt so hard left her feeling surprised and angry in equal measure. She had expected it to be different.

Her neighbor's cheeriness must be a facade, Niles thought. How could it be true? "There's no way," she told herself then, "because this is a miserable experience." It wasn't only miserable, of course. But, then and later, Niles felt there was so little room for that part of the experience— the struggle—within the social construct of motherhood. By the time

Niles's children were teenagers, she had cared for birthing parents at Woodhull Medical Center in Brooklyn for more than a decade. She earned a doctorate in nursing and began researching birthing parents' autonomy and how midwifery care practices can best serve marginalized communities. Niles told me she sees birth and new parenthood as transformational—difficult and powerful, a chance to consider the full capacity of your body and your relationships. That's what she tells anyone she knows who is pregnant, patients and friends alike. But she also knows that transformation is so often limited by cultural expectations, by the focus on a mother's capacity to get her child to sleep, to keep them content and quiet, to look good doing it, and to feel good, too, to feel "fabulous." To have a "good baby," and to do it all independently, within one's own individual family.

"Is there a wizard behind the machine?" Niles said. "Because it doesn't feel right. And I—I think about that all the time."

In a sense, there *is* a wizard behind the machine, a man behind the curtain. Many of them, actually.

Take Charles Darwin, for one, neither the first nor the last man behind the curtain in this case, but a leader of the pack. Darwin was strongly influenced by the mothers in his life—by the absence of his own, who died when he was eight years old, and by the constant presence throughout his adult life of Emma, his wife and the mother of their ten children, whom he considered a grounding force and who gave him a critical push to publish his seminal work, *On the Origin of Species*, in 1859. It's hard to fathom, then, why Darwin paid so little mind to mothers when it came to their place within his scientific theory and the social creatures he studied.

The theory of evolution upended how the world saw human nature and gender. Darwin explored how sexual selection shapes the future of a species, but he mostly ignored the role that parents play once their choice of mate bears fruit. Instead, within his revolutionary work, he codified very old ideas about the inferiority of women, rooted in their essential role as childbearers and their unquestioned self-sacrifice. "What a strong feeling of inward satisfaction must impel a bird, so full of activity, to brood day after day over her eggs," he wrote in *The Descent of Man*. Forget the hunger she feels or the angst that may come once she has more mouths to feed and new predators to fend off. Ignore that sense of wasting where wing meets body, from her own unending still-ness.

In the long history of the idealization of motherhood, the notion that the selflessness and tenderness that babies require of their caregivers is ingrained in the *biology* of women, and only women, is a relatively mod-ern one. It has been crafted by men upholding an image of what a mother should be, diverting our attention from what she actually is, and calling it science. We may have a broader, more generous understanding of what it takes to be a parent today and of who is capable of doing it, but the legacy of maternal instinct as scientific fact is all around us. It has stuck despite the best efforts of feminists trying to debunk it from the moment it entered public discourse. And it continues to shape political and per-sonal ideology about what a mother does and how she feels—what she *should* do and how she *should* feel. Those ideas dictate how everyone else involved in child-rearing is expected to act as well, including parents who are not gestational mothers, and they shape the motivations of people drafting policies that affect young families.

We often accept maternal instinct as outdated in the details but hard to set aside entirely. We may see evidence of it in the intense love mothers have for their children, or in the nesting impulses they feel as a baby's due date approaches. For generation after generation, mothers have cared for babies. Something compels them to do that. If not an instinct inherent to women, then what is it? Maternal instinct gives some com-fort. It offers romance and peace, the promise of falling in love at first sight and the certainty of natural order in the face of the unknown. Even the idea that this inborn drive can undermine a woman, leaving her with "mommy brain," feels uncomfortably true.

Maternal instinct was meant to work this way, to use women's own complicated emotions about themselves and their children and their place in society to compel them to fit a certain mold. It is a classic case of disinformation. An idea that has the illusion of plausibility gets repeated over and over, despite evidence to the contrary, until believing it becomes reflexive. To understand just how much we need to rewrite the story about what it means to become a mother, how very fundamen-tal and necessary this research on the parental brain is, it's important to know how we got stuck with the old telling of it, the old stories that are so profoundly wrong—based not in science, but in belief.

* * *

IT MAY SEEM THAT MOTHERS have been cherished for as long as humans have made babies—the mother is queen of the home, the emotional heart of the family, the maker of chocolate chip cookies. It hasn't always been so. Throughout most of recorded history, a mother's social status has been raised and lowered depending on which tool, the bludgeon or the prize, the people in charge choose to influence women's labor. In some societies mothers have been shut away in the home, unwelcome in public spaces or in politics, while in others they've been held up as representative of the best of human nature. In *The Myths of Motherhood: How Culture Reinvents the Good Mother*, psychologist Shari Thurer documented how the womb has been, by turns, celebrated as a source of fertility and rejuvenation, or reduced to a mere vessel for the father's child and considered the root of hysteria. Breastfeeding has been represented as a source of womanly power, or as a task that, among those who can afford the option, is best relegated to a wet nurse chosen and paid for by a child's father so the mother can return to full fertility or to her social schedule. Maternal love itself has been deemed suffocating and damaging, or pure and holy.

Modern Christian notions of motherhood were shaped by two women. There was Eve, the first woman, made from Adam's rib, who ate the forbidden fruit and in doing so caused the suffering of every human to come. And there was the Virgin Mary, the unwitting actor in a great miracle who became the most virtue-laden symbol of motherhood there is, her inner life and actions entirely consumed by the glory of her maternal love. I was raised Catholic, and I often wonder about how things—the faith itself, the power dynamic within my own family, the history of the world—might be different had Mary been granted space in the Bible to offer her own take.

For many women, the Virgin Mary has been a source of comfort, a mentor in motherhood. But Mary's story, combined with Eve's— unattainable goodness, plus perpetual servitude—created a moral model for motherhood that has proven stifling and unforgiving. It deemed women property of their husbands and denied them basic rights. It allowed them to be castigated or called witches if they couldn't produce children, or subjected to a full lifetime of pregnancy and nursing if they could. It linked women's destinies, in this life and the afterlife, to their reproductive capacity and the degree to which they met an impossible ideal.

Yet across time and cultures, the status of a mother within religious society was not entirely self-limiting. From ancient Israel to the early colonies of America, women saw their struggles in pregnancy and child-rearing as fate, ordained by God. But there was little sense yet of maternal identity being so singular, so narrow. The home was the seat of economic production, as well as a place of politics, education, and religious activity. As keepers of that home, women's lives reached beyond maternal duties.

Among the White women of colonial America, mothers had too many children and faced too many threats of death from disease or food shortages to focus intently on caring for any one child. "Mothering meant generalized responsibility for an assembly of youngsters rather than concentrated devotion to a few," Pulitzer Prize–winning historian Laurel Thatcher Ulrich wrote in her book *Good Wives: Image and Reality in the Lives of Women in Northern New England, 1650–1750.* It was "extensive rather than intensive." Plus there was other important work to be done, including making bread and cheese and beer, tending gardens, stoking fires used for cooking and for warmth, overseeing servants, and caring for neighbors when a crisis hit or a baby arrived. Mothers counseled their husbands in matters of politics and participated in stereotypically masculine work as "deputy husbands" or as surrogates in business dealings, all of which, Ulrich wrote, gave them power that often has been overlooked by historians.

Of course, the history of motherhood is not linear. While those "deputy husbands" were stoking the fire, other women living on the land that would become the United States saw morality imposed on their experience of motherhood in very different ways.

Among the Indigenous people of North America, the role of mothers was diverse to such a degree that it defies simple explanation here, but it often was characterized by power and appreciation, the maternal body thought to be synonymous with creation (a reverence once shared by early human societies around the globe). Many Indigenous people didn't see gender as rigid or categorical, to start with—and many still don't—so it followed that gender roles were generally more fluid and valued equally. Some looked to the mothers among them to choose the men who would become their chiefs, Indigenous scholar Kim Anderson wrote in her essay "Giving Life to the People." When White Christian settlers wanted to eliminate or assimilate Indigenous people, they targeted the family. Children were taken from their families and sent to boarding schools where girls were taught domestic skills and boys were trained in farming and trade—the process, including forced removal from families, carried out largely by White women. Many of those children never returned. Women were stripped of their roles as spiritual leaders. Traditional ceremonies honoring the maternal went underground. "'God the father' took over from 'mother the creator,'" Anderson wrote.

Black women enslaved in the colonies and in early America saw no reprieve from the brutality of slavery when they became mothers. Instead that violence was compounded, as they frequently birthed the children of their enslavers and rapists, and as they saw their children sold off or forced to labor alongside them under fear of the whip. They were treated, traded, and talked about as "breeders." This was especially true during and after the 1820s, as cotton production in the South spread westward, in part to feed the growing New England textile industry. Congress had already banned US participation in the international slave trade, so enslaved women were the only means of growing the enslaved labor force, and a woman whose fertility was proven—by motherhood—was valued far more at auction. Yet within their quarters, mothers also were the makers of a domestic life, often created equally alongside men, Angela Davis wrote in *Women, Race and Class*. In opposition to "an environment designed to convert them into a herd of subhuman labor units," Davis wrote, they built extended families, maintained traditions, and plotted rebellion.

From the late eighteenth through the nineteenth centuries, two major events shifted the White motherhood ideal in North America and Europe in ways that would have far-reaching effects for all mothers. Darwin brought one of those events into being. But first came the Industrial Revolution. It changed the nature of the home and, in doing so, dramatically altered a woman's role there. The industrial economy moved people from farm to factory. It separated work from home, public life from private. The home was no longer a place of economic production but of consumption. Home became sacred, "a place 'where the heart is' as well as, in its ideal manifestation, the locus of intimacy, peace, spontaneity, and unwavering devotion to people and principles beyond the self," Thurer wrote. The importance of such a place grew as capitalism focused work and politics on individual competition and created a ladder for the "self-made" man. The family was seen as the backstop against such self-interest, "the one place where interdependence, noncalculative reciprocity, and gift giving prevailed, the arena in which people learned to temper public ambition or competition with private regard for others," wrote historian Stephanie Coontz, in *The Way We Never Were: American Families and the Nostalgia Trap*. Women were the keepers of that place of reprieve from all that might be wrong with the world outside. Their moral imperative was inflated, as their role in society shrank.

The Enlightenment and the gendered science it produced had already laid the groundwork for such a separation of spheres. Children were newly recognized as children rather than simply small versions of adults, and they were full of potential goodness rather than original sin. They required love and nurturing, to which women were thought to be naturally suited. Men and women were different. Women were the source of morality and stability, linked to predictable cycles of fertility, and motherhood was core to their being. Deviation from that role was considered a subversion of nature. So the men went to work to earn money to buy goods they once had traded for or produced alongside their wives. And the women stayed home.

Except, of course, many didn't. Attracted by reliable wages and a chance to support their families, lots of young, single women went to work in cities as factories grew in number. Married women went to work, too, though often their participation in the labor force has been downplayed or overlooked by historians. A close reading of census data in England found that between about one-third and one-half of all working women in late-nineteenth-century London were married or widowed, depending on the district, and similar figures were found in outlying towns and cities.

Separately, economist Claudia Goldin looked at labor trends in seven southern US cities that were growing quickly after slavery was officially abolished, and found that more than a third of married Black women were in the labor force in 1880, about five times the rate among married White women. Black mothers with young children were more likely to be working, too, even when measured against White mothers of similar means. Goldin attributed that difference to various factors, including that for Black women earning wages wasn't shameful but necessary, a hedge against all sorts of uncertainties that White women didn't face, including housing discrimination and the fact that the men in their families faced even more severe workplace discrimination than they did themselves.

The Victorian notion that a woman should be the "angel in the house" was not the reality for many women. Not in Victorian London and not elsewhere. Middle-class families in the United States through much of the nineteenth century were able to dedicate more time to child-rearing specifically because of their ability to hire help, typically young immigrants, Coontz wrote. For every family "that protected its wife and child within the family circle, then, there was an Irish or a German girl scrubbing floors in that middle-class home, a Welsh boy mining coal to keep the home-baked goodies warm, a black girl doing the family laundry, a black mother and child picking cotton to be made into clothes for the family, and a Jewish or an Italian daughter in a sweatshop making 'ladies' dresses or artificial flowers for the family to purchase."

Yet this unrealistic ideal had profound and long-lasting consequences for working mothers. It empowered their bosses—and so many other judging eyes—to see them as lesser. Amy Westervelt put it this way, in her book Forget "Having It All": How America Messed Up Motherhood—and How to Fix It: "Employers tended to be white, middle- or upper-class men who took the view that all women were married and being supported by a husband, and thus could be paid less because their income was merely supplemental, or that women who were working when they had children at home were inferior women, an assumption bolstered by racism and xenophobia if they happened to also be women of color or immigrants (and most were)."

Many men simply didn't want women at work. They didn't want to see the patriarchal norms of their homes turned upside down. Plus, women's cheap labor meant competition. Some factories ran on long hours worked by women in dangerous conditions for pitiful pay. Around the turn of the twentieth century, labor rights advocates pushed a slate of laws aimed at improving conditions for those women workers, some of them explicitly citing the need to protect current or future mothers. But, Westervelt noted, those "protective" laws also had the effect of making women less appealing to employers, more costly and more complicated. Women were edged out of the job market even as unions worked to establish the "family wage"—enough to support a wife and children at home—as the working-class standard for the White men in their membership.

Yoking women to the home has long been in the state's interest, for supplying the numbers necessary for nation building, for controlling the demographics of race, class, and faith, and for quelling political opposition. In 1839, the powerful Reverend Francis Close of England condemned women for rallying in support of political reform and workers' rights in his parish church. He told them they debased themselves when they became political agitators: "The fountain of all your influence in society, is your home—your own fire-side—it is amongst your children, it is in the bosom of your family, and in that little circle of friends with whom you are more immediately connected, there your legitimate influence must be exercised; there you are born to shine."

In the decades after America threw off the British, its founders were actively searching for a role for women in the new nation. One woman had the audacity to write, in an essay published in 1801 under the name "The Female Advocate," that women should be granted full citizenship, with representation in church and government. Instead, White "republican mothers" were urged to educate their children on civic virtue and thereby shape the future of the nation. For some women, this new charge felt like an improvement on their political status, even while it built the walls of domesticity around them ever higher. The effects of that paradox, wrote historian Linda Kerber, would last well into the twentieth century. And on into the twenty-first.

Maternal instinct grew up as a belief in God-given differences between men and women, in their temperaments and in their purpose, to serve their family and to serve their nation. Soon, the same message about a woman's rightful place was reframed for a changing world, not as a matter of religion but as a truth borne out by science.

* * *

THE THEORY OF EVOLUTION CHALLENGED traditional ideas about gender in dramatic ways, the biggest and most obvious being that it discredited Adam and Eve as the mold from which we are all made. Certain religious leaders responded to the threat by promoting a "muscular Christianity," with an emphasis on Genesis. Others embraced the notion that evolution was a kind of complement to the Bible, further evidence of human dominance and progress toward perfection. That was an idea the White elite could get behind, wrote historian Kimberly Hamlin, in *From Eve to Evolution: Darwin, Science, and Women's Rights in Gilded Age America*. It was seen as proof that their place at the top was justified not only by their faith but by natural law.

Darwin wasn't really trying to dispel the biblical notion that men rightfully dominate women. Quite the opposite. He simply shifted the focus from faith to biology. Darwin believed it was precisely a mother's powerful maternal instinct that made women intellectually inferior to men. Women are specialized to care for other humans and men to compete with them, he wrote. By that basic fact, men achieve "higher eminence" in virtually all things, from the use of their senses to reason and imagination. Social Darwinists seized on that idea as justification of continued male dominance, as more women demanded their own identities under the law. Among them was Herbert Spencer, an English philosopher who coined the phrase "survival of the fittest" and wrote that childbearing costs women "vital power," stunting them emotionally and intellectually.

Despite this, women's rights advocates saw opportunity in evolution, precisely because it moved the gender debate away from biblical ancestors and the status of a person's soul, to biology with a focus on reproduction. That posed its own challenges. Male and female reproductive biology *is* different. But women fighting for a more equal standing in society previously had to put their word up against God's. Evolution changed the terms. Now, they had to prove that different does not equal lesser. Science, Hamlin wrote, "offered the promise of objectivity."

Among those early Darwinian feminists was Antoinette Brown Blackwell, who was no stranger to bucking the gender norms of her day. She had distinguished herself as a frequent speaker on the issues of slavery and women's rights before being ordained in 1853 in the Congregational Church, the first woman to serve as pastor in a mainstream Christian denomination in the United States. She left the church less than a year later, in part because of a crisis in faith, and later joined the more liberal Unitarian Church. When she married at the ripe old age of thirty and began having children—she would have seven, two of whom died as infants—she spent more time writing than speech making. Women's rights became her primary focus—especially the idea that a woman could be a mother and engage in a productive public life.

In 1875, Blackwell published *The Sexes throughout Nature* and marked another first. It was the first feminist critique of evolution published by a woman. It wasn't the theory of evolution she took issue with, so much as its interpretation. Blackwell criticized the great thinkers of her day for being unable to see beyond their own sense of male superiority. Darwin, she wrote, had simply found "a fresh pathway to the old conclusion" about women's inferiority. With evolution as a new lens, Blackwell looked across species and instead saw a system that "favors the female": "Nature's sturdiest buds and her best-fed butterflies belong to this sex; her female spiders are large enough to eat up a score of her little males; some of her mother-fishes might parody the nursery-song, 'I have a little husband no bigger than my thumb.'" Of course the men of evolution saw it differently, she wrote. According to her experience, "Men see clearly and think sharply when their sympathies are keenly enlisted, but not otherwise."

Science would be the judge, Blackwell believed, particularly science conducted by women. She and her peers imagined a future in which women would represent themselves in the field of science, tapping into their lived experience to identify the most urgent questions and advancing their own scientific skill in order to answer them. That future didn't arrive. At least, not in their lifetimes.

Science was rapidly walled off to women. The study of biology and science as a whole became professionalized, dictated by rigorous protocols and blessed by institutions to which women were typically denied entry. To feminists in the late nineteenth century, evolution had meant "freedom from stories about virgin mothers and evil temptresses," Hamlin wrote. It offered the idea that human development happened through "an orderly, knowable process," one that could be revealed through careful study. To the men within the scientific establishment at the turn of the century, however, science was too often a means of affirming the status quo.

This was particularly evident among men who were writing the theory of instinct in the late nineteenth and early twentieth centuries. Darwin had suggested that natural selection acts on instincts much as it does on the physical characteristics of a species, with a preference for those that ensure survival. "Lower" animals had long been thought to be driven primarily by instinct and, by tearing down the wall between them and humans, Darwin propelled the study of how instincts shape human behavior.

As early psychologists explored the nature of human instincts, the number of things that could qualify as an instinct seemed to grow. Included in the list William James published in his *Principles of Psychology* in 1890 were instincts toward cleanliness, belligerence, jealousy, and sex; toward hunting and building and climbing; and away from strange men and strange animals. Then there was the instinct for parental love, "stronger in woman than in man" and one that alters her instantly from the person she was into the Virgin Mary–like figure her species requires of her. "Contemning every danger, triumphing over every difficulty, outlasting all fatigue," James wrote, "woman's love is here invincibly superior to anything that man can show." William McDougall took things one step further in 1908, writing that the instinct to protect and cherish her children—along with the "tender emotion" required of the task—becomes "the constant and all-absorbing occupation of the mother, to which she devotes all her energies." It is an instinct stronger than any other, he wrote, "even fear itself."

But maternal instinct apparently was never as strong as a woman's education. In the same book, McDougall wrote that, as a person's intelligence grows, parental instinct declines, unless countered by "social sanctions" enforced by moral institutions to discourage, for example, birth control, divorce, and the erosion of gender roles. This was a big concern for McDougall, who would go on to become an outspoken promoter of eugenics and to write a deeply racist book on the topic. A subtext of his writing on maternal instinct is the maintenance of White supremacy. He wrote, "those families and races and nations in which it weakens become rapidly supplanted by those in which it is strong."

As Darwin had his Blackwells, McDougall had his dissenters, too: women who called maternal instinct what it was, not a scientific theory but a social device, a means of controlling how they thought and acted. Leta Hollingworth, a trailblazing psychologist (who also embraced certain eugenic ideas), wrote to her peers in the *American Journal of Sociology* in 1916 that women were compelled to believe that their highest use was as a mother through the same means that soldiers were compelled to go to war. Social norms idealized a "womanly woman" who dwelled enthusiastically in her maternal duties. Art revered her, with galleries "hung full of Madonnas." The laws of her day prohibited deviation from that norm by limiting women's control of property and money, which ensured financial dependence on a husband, and by forbidding the distribution of information about birth control. Then there were the many ways that the hard parts of motherhood were hidden, made taboo. The rate of maternal mortality, then at least sixty times higher than it would be at the end of the century, was rarely made public, Hollingworth wrote. The monotony of a mother's work was barely mentioned. But the joys—those were celebrated at every opportunity.

Many women of Hollingworth's day had embraced a reverence for motherhood—or at least the White ideal of motherhood—as a means of elevating women's social status. Hollingworth put it bluntly: "There is no verifiable evidence to show that a maternal instinct exists in women of such all-consuming strength and fervor as to impel them voluntarily to seek the pain, danger and exacting labor involved in maintaining a high birth rate." She suggested that political leaders should give up on "cheap devices" and instead provide women with fair compensation for their contributions to "national aggrandizement." Such a change would result in significant social gains, she wrote, "assuming always that the increased happiness and usefulness of women would, in general, be regarded as social gain."

* * *

IT'S DISMAYING, REALLY, TO THINK about how relevant Hollingworth's comments are all these years later, how obvious the myth of maternal instinct was to some people then, and how long it has held on, becoming perhaps even further ingrained in our beliefs about family and about ourselves. Anthropologist Sarah Blaffer Hrdy (rhymes with birdie) described the hopes of Darwinian feminists as "the road not taken." Instead, our early understanding of the biology of motherhood "was built on patriarchal assumptions introduced by earlier generations of moralists," she wrote in *Mother Nature: A History of Mothers, Infants, and Natural Selection.* "What was essentially wishful thinking on their part was substituted for objective observation." That wishful thinking has had lasting consequences.

Scientists today recognize that human parental behavior is far too variable to be dictated by a rigid maternal instinct. The idea of instinct as a whole is problematic in many cases. What may look entirely innate is instead the subtle influence on genes by one's inherited environment, learning, life experience, and lessons passed, for better or worse, across generations. The natural order of things is far less orderly. Popular culture has mostly relinquished that old science of femininity that Blackwell railed against. We know that motherhood is neither duty nor destiny, that a woman is not left unfulfilled or incomplete without children. But even as I write those words, I doubt them. Do we, collectively, believe that?

Whether or not we call maternal instinct by its name today, its influence is everywhere. The idea survived an era in the 1920s and 1930s during which a generation of psychologists favored the idea that babies could be trained, believing, as Thurer put it, that "children are made, not born" and that women could hardly be trusted with the task. It resurged following World War II, when mothers in the United States saw wartime job opportunities and federally funded childcare disappear and were told, once again, that it was their role to be a steadying force, to reaffirm humanity after the horrors of battle. Around the middle of the century, a growing chorus of psychoanalysts, psychiatrists, and child development experts declared that mother love is as important to a child's emotional development as vitamins are to his physical development.

British psychoanalyst John Bowlby built on Lorenz's work on imprinting in birds to write a new theory of mother-child attachment that remade how we think about infancy for the better, while almost entirely ignoring the broader context of family life and the needs and development of mothers themselves. Now it was not just a mother's behavior but her maternal love that was the powerful key to unlock a child's proper development. The historian Marga Vicedo wrote, "In earlier times, a mother could enable or constrain her children's capacities. Mothers could temper, control, and educate their children. But now, according to Bowlby, children have a uniform, universal need for a specific type of mother love, while a mother's feelings determine her children's minds."

Bowlby's work was popularized by William and Martha Sears in the 1990s as "attachment parenting," seen by some as intuitive and natural, and by others as overly prescriptive and extreme in its demands of mothers over others. But long before that, a belief in maternal instinct and the deterministic value of mother love had fueled "pro-family" conservative politicians for decades. That belief proved effective at blocking so many of the initiatives of second-wave feminists who sought a dramatic reimagining of gender roles at home and at work—not simply a status-quo world in which women could "have it all." Bowlby told the *New York Times* in 1965 that the only people interested in challenging his theory that a child suffers if deprived of maternal love were communists and professional women, and the latter "have, in fact, neglected their families."

We are still fighting an uphill battle for even modest paid family leave policies in the United States, and universal childcare remains far out of reach. The Comprehensive Child Development Act of 1971 was the country's last serious attempt to establish a national day care system. President Nixon vetoed it, saying it was a "family-weakening" bill and the government must "cement the family in its rightful position as the keystone of our civilization." Implicit in that statement was a belief about a woman's natural place. Families have struggled in all the years since with the high cost of childcare and long wait lists for quality programs, a problem that intensified when the coronavirus pandemic caused huge numbers of day care centers to close or shrink. The United States has never invested in childcare infrastructure in any reasonable, serious way, because the powers that be have always seen childcare as a woman's job, one determined by her biology.

It can be hard to see the way forward. In March 2021, a group of US Senate Democrats introduced a resolution calling for a "Marshall Plan for Moms," to include improved access to childcare options, paid leave, and mental health support, acknowledging the toll the pandemic took on the working lives and financial stability of women, especially women of color. Just one day earlier in Idaho, lawmakers had refused a $6 million federal grant to support early childhood education, with one lawmaker saying—in remarks he later said he regretted—that he wouldn't support anything that makes it "more convenient for mothers to come out of the home and let others raise their child." This is the exact same sentiment Pat Buchanan, right-wing commentator and political adviser, expressed to Nixon when he persuaded the president to kill the 1971 bill. And it's the same one that continues to be parroted by those opposed to national investment in policies that support young families. (As of early 2022, President Biden's Build Back Better plan and its nearly $400 billion investment in affordable childcare and universal preschool had stalled indefinitely in the Senate.)

Belief in maternal instinct also drives opposition to birth control and abortion, for why should women limit the number of children they have if it is in their very nature to find joy in motherhood, if caring for children is their essential biological destiny? It divides the routes to parenthood into categories of "natural" and other. It has grown the modern parenting-advice industry, which often capitalizes on the self-doubt of parents who find themselves experiencing something other than Hallmark-card-quality contentment. It maintains culture wars around the "right" way of child-rearing and can make parents feel defective if they want to breastfeed but struggle to do so, for example, or if childbirth doesn't go according to plan.

Maternal instinct has long fueled discrimination against those families that do not consist of one woman and one man of at least moderate means. It sustains outdated ideas about masculinity that teach fathers that they are secondary—assistants, babysitters—and that encourage mothers to see them that way, too. It undermines the rights and recognition of same-sex couples and transgender and nonbinary parents, who see their ability or desire to care for their children questioned or criminalized. It creates a hierarchy of caregiving in which the importance of the birthing parent is immutable, no matter the circumstances, and that often diminishes the value of adoptive parents and other loving adults in a child's life.

The "good mother" ideal never has been fully extended to women of color. Or to women in poverty. Or to anyone less likely to hew to the "angel in the house" model because they have to work or because they choose to. Or because it is important to them that their children be raised by a circle of family and friends that stretches beyond themselves. Or, as Mikki Kendall wrote in her book *Hood Feminism: Notes from the Women That a Movement Forgot*, because the reality of parenting in a marginalized community requires that parents not only hold the center of their home but also face the real threats of deportation, hunger, eviction, violence in the neighborhood, police brutality, underfunded schools, and systemic racism in all its forms.

The angel narrative obscured so many stories about other ways of caring for children—ways of being a nurturer *and* a fighter, of protecting your family *and* building your community. This has been especially true in the United States, where the motherhood ideal has been central to our social infrastructure. "Family holds a place of honor in the American Dream—a 'good family' has some of the status of a successful career, but with the added weight of morality and virtue," Mia Birdsong, a scholar on family and community, wrote in *How We Show Up: Reclaiming Family, Friendship, and Community*. "By American Dream standards, a 'good family' is an insular, nuclear family comprising a legally married man and woman raising biological children. This family is self-sufficient— and as such, functions as an independent unit. It's toxic individualism, but in family-unit form."

By propping up an ideal grounded in White, well-off motherhood, maternal instinct continues to shape women's economic and political value, collectively and individually. For proof, just look at the extreme attention paid to the number of Amy Coney Barrett's children—

seven—during her 2020 confirmation to the highest court in the United States. Senate Republicans "fetishized" Barrett's motherhood because doing so blunted attacks from Democrats about what her nomination could mean for the future of things mothers are supposed to care about, like accessible health care, Lyz Lenz wrote in *Glamour* at the time. It was strategic to celebrate having a mother on their side— especially this one. Lenz wrote, "America has long lauded this certain kind of mother—white, successful, walks into church holding hands with her husband, has dinner on the table at 6 p.m., with a circle of children around her."

Just a few years ago, the executive editor of the newspaper I worked for asked me and two other senior editors, all women, whether women are more collaborative in the workplace because we are more naturally nurturing. It was a statement rather than a question, really. I'd wonder later, with cause, whether by "collaborative" he meant "willing to con-tribute ideas without getting credit for them." In ways that are subtle and not so subtle, the myth of maternal instinct has defined the place of women in the workplace. It has the potential to designate every woman a possible mother and every mother of lesser value to her employer once her children have stolen her focus, her time, or even her intellect (cue the "mommy brain" meme, with echoes of Herbert Spencer).

The gender pay gap is real, but a large chunk of it is actually attribut-able to reproduction. Mothers make less money than men and childless women, not just in the years right after they have children but over time—another dynamic exacerbated by the pandemic. That's true even in countries with generous paid parental leave and other policies to support new families. And this is not a problem that women can fix simply by working harder. Researchers have found that mothers who are viewed as highly competent and hypercommitted to their jobs may be judged for those exact qualities, viewed as cold and selfish, and paid less because of that. Men meanwhile, especially those who are already high-wage earners, gain professional reward for their fatherhood.

* * *

THE HOSPITALS WHERE MOST PEOPLE deliver their babies are gener-ally staffed by committed, passionate caregivers, but they are also part of long-standing medical systems whose histories are woven through with racism and sexism. Those in medicine like to think of their field as objective and based only on science and evidence. "Nowhere is that less true than in reproductive and sexual health and perinatal care," Mimi Niles told me. "That's just not true."

The idea that women arrive at motherhood prepared for the job has contributed to the perception that childbirth is a medical procedure focused entirely on delivering a healthy baby. The fact that a birthing parent also experiences a fundamental biological and psychological change often is ignored, or recognized but not acted on—sometimes with tragic consequences. The US maternal mortality rate is more than double the rate in most other high-income countries, at about seventeen maternal deaths per hundred thousand live births as of 2018. The risk to Black women of dying during pregnancy or within forty-two days of delivery is two and a half times what it is for White women, and the disparity may be greater when deaths up to a year postpartum are taken into account.

The cause seems to be a collision of some of the worst effects of systemic racism, as journalist Nina Martin and her colleagues made clear in their important ProPublica/NPR series *Lost Mothers*. Before pregnancy, Black birthing parents already are at higher risk for health conditions that can make pregnancy more dangerous, including heart disease and diabetes. They face higher rates of complications during and after pregnancy, including for preeclampsia, heart failure, and postpartum depression. They are less likely to have health insurance and more likely to deliver their babies at hospitals that grew out of segregation and today are underfunded and have lower quality of care. They face bias among doctors who don't acknowledge their pain or complications even when they advocate for themselves. And higher socioeconomic status or education level does not seem to protect them from these risks.

There is a double threat in these numbers—the risk itself plus a denial of joy. Niles told me that birthing parents in marginalized communities, especially those who face higher risks of conditions such as gestational diabetes and preeclampsia, often see their pregnancies pathologized, with caregivers and public health experts focused so intensely on what could go wrong with the baby that pregnancy feels laden with blame, and the parents are never given a chance to under-stand their own transformation. "It should be held out in front of you, to say, 'This is the potential of what this could be for you,'" she said.

Normalizing the biological and psychological—as well as the social and cultural—processes of new parenthood is central to midwifery. In midwifery care, the same provider may see a birthing parent from before pregnancy on into the early days of parenting, with more of that care occurring in community clinics or at home, instead of in a hos-pital. Evidence from around the world has found midwife-led care to be effective and affordable, resulting in fewer interventions in healthy pregnancies and birthing parents reporting a greater sense of control and satisfaction with their childbirth experience. The United States has been slow to reinstitute midwifery as the standard of care it was before the rise of the professionalized field of obstetrics, which was long dominated by White men (now, by women, most of them White).

The shortage of maternity care providers in general and of mid-wives in particular is a significant factor in the high maternal mor-tality rate in the United States, according to a 2020 Commonwealth Fund report. In recent years, the country had just four midwives per thousand live births, while the rate was thirty in France, fifty-three in Norway, and sixty-eight in Australia. In those countries, midwives care for families during pregnancy and childbirth, but they also do the essential work of visiting families after a baby has arrived, recog-nizing the postpartum period as a time of need. German birth parents can receive daily visits from a midwife—covered by national health insurance—for the first ten days postpartum and up to sixteen visits in the weeks that follow.

Add to all this the patchwork system of US health insurance and the fact that, in some states, people may be kicked off their Medicaid plan about sixty days after having a baby, leaving them without access to help when they need it. (The Build Back Better Act would have required Medicaid coverage to extend to one year postpartum.) Even for those with good health insurance, the standard of care is one visit with an ob-gyn—one!—by about six weeks postpartum. The American College of Obstetricians and Gynecologists has advocated for a more holistic and ongoing approach to postpartum care, noting that the typical single, six-week visit "punctuates a period devoid of formal or informal maternal support."

New parents in the United States are mostly on their own after they leave the hospital. Many hospitals are working to integrate midwives into their care teams, but still, childbirth is typically "castrated" from the experience of parenting, Niles said. Support groups and at-home services are often seen as a privilege, rather than a necessity. In Maine, where I live, a program that sent public health nurses to the homes of new parents was decimated under Republican governor Paul LePage. It was a particular blow to the state's rural communities and came just as the number of babies and mothers affected by the opiate crisis skyrocketed.

In labor, the body often knows what to do. Niles tells birthing parents that they could labor while standing on their heads or fully anesthetized, and their bodies may still do what's necessary to deliver a baby. "But parenting is so different," she said. "It's so, so different."

How, exactly? The ghost of maternal instinct is in how we answer that question, too, in the stories we tell one another and in what we withhold. Poet Hollie McNish captures the incredulity of brand-new parenthood in the opening pages of her memoir in poetry and prose, which is full of raw bits: "Nobody told me you can't use toilet paper / Nobody told me that you bleed / Nobody told me you might need a secret place / where you can scream." Ali Wong's second Netflix special, *Hard Knock Wife*, performed after her first daughter was born and with a second on her way, is fueled hilariously by the outrage of the unprepared, over the physical trauma of birth and over the stupid things people say to working mothers, over breastfeeding. "I thought it was supposed to be this beautiful bonding ceremony where I would feel like I was sitting on a lily pad in a meadow and bunnies would gather at my feet while the fat-Hawaiian-man version of 'Somewhere over the Rainbow' would play," she said. "No! It's not like that at all. Breastfeeding is this savage ritual that just reminds you that your body is a cafeteria now. It don't belong to you no more!"

Social media is full of posts from mothers sharing stories about pregnancy loss and infertility, or about the reality of their postpartum body, their sense of themselves, the anxiety and monotony of parenting. Often, there is a disconnect between the frankness of the words and the glossed-up photograph above it, as if it's OK to get real if you still look good, in natural light, while doing it. Increasingly, though, there's rawness in the images, too: stretch marks and C-section scars, tears and spit-up, the reality of pumping, an awkward feeding, a hand cupping the feet of a baby who arrived as a stillbirth. More and more, that work is being done by nonbinary and transgender birthing parents. Such posts frequently are made with a direct acknowledgment of the risk that each person is taking by revealing a story line that does not match an idealized view of motherhood.

In February 2020, the company Frida, which makes products for new parents and babies, announced that its ad depicting a newly postpartum mother trying to use the bathroom was prohibited from airing during the Oscars because it was deemed "too graphic." The video garnered nearly four million views in its first two weeks on YouTube. Friends and I passed around the link and marveled at how it made us weep. The ad itself is simple. A woman switches on a lamp, reaches over to comfort her newborn crying in the bassinet next to her bed, then hobbles to the bathroom, in pain. She struggles to use the toilet and replace the postpartum pad held up by her hospital-issued mesh underwear. There is no narrative arc. It is a snapshot, one that hits us because it *is* us. We know the smell of the witch hazel pads and the squish of the peri bottle full of warm water, the agony and the relief, the sharpness of the physical pain against the haze of sleeplessness and emotional upheaval.

Frida's chief executive told the *New York Times* that the Academy had suggested Frida consider a "kinder, more gentle portrayal of postpartum." Such a portrayal would have been false, one more obfuscation. The ad worked because we thought no one had seen us there in the bathroom, alone and adrift, in that moment when we began to realize how far from shore we were. And yet there we are on the screen. There we all are. Lost together.

How can so much of parenthood be unspoken? So much of it deemed unspeakable, still? I imagine this whole situation like a massive billboard depicting some Virgin Mary–like image of a mother rested and at peace, her baby plump and contented. All of this—the Frida ad,

the rise of the confessional social media post, Ali Wong onstage screaming about the need for maternity leave so that mothers can "hide and
heal their demolished-ass bodies"—like bits of garish graffiti scrawled
around the edges. Yet the picture still looms large. We've become really
good at protesting the parts of this story that feel wrong to us. But we
haven't replaced it. Not yet.

* * *

THE SCIENCE OF THE PARENTAL brain has the potential to pull back the
curtain, exposing old biases and outdated norms, revealing how they
are woven throughout our individual and societal definitions of mother
or parent or family, and offering something new. But it can do that only
if we are diligent in preventing this new science from being riven by old
thinking. Only if we look at it clear-eyed.

In 2019, a group of researchers published a very specific finding on
differences between male and female mice in the distribution of certain estrogen-related oxytocin receptors in a part of the medial preoptic
area, a brain region important to mammalian caregiving. The research
was publicized with a press release under the headline, "Scientists Find
Clue to 'Maternal Instinct'"—words that never appeared in the paper
itself. In a 2017 editorial, a pediatrician from the Netherlands reviewed
some of the literature on the maternal brain and, remarkably, came to
this conclusion: "The notion of a maternal brain explains why so many
brilliant and ambitious women, capable for a top career, lose interest in
pursuing such careers after childbirth. Their new maternal impulses are
at odds with their original ambitions, and for many mothers stress and
frustration will be the result." One could argue that an oppressive patriarchal system that lacks necessary supports for new parents explains
why brilliant women drop out of the workforce, often with their ambition intact and newly laden with bitterness.

Already, the neuroscience has been cast in some cases as validation of an old-fashioned maternal nature, much as Darwin and others
remade moral motherhood into something scientific. In other cases, it
has been rejected for its potential to do just that, for the perceived threat
it poses to women's progress.

When Hrdy, the anthropologist and primatologist, started graduate school at Harvard University in 1970, biologists still held tight to the notion that the whole purpose of mothers "was to pump out and nurture babies." The belief was especially strong in the field of primatology, according to Hrdy, "where the creatures being studied were so similar to ourselves" and the people more prone to impose beliefs upon them. Hrdy would soon become part of a first generation of women in her field, many of them also mothers to young children, who found themselves repeatedly running into questions that couldn't be answered by the evolutionary theory they'd been taught.

Jeanne Altmann, along with her husband, Stuart, studied baboons in Kenya and recognized them as "dual-career mothers." Baboon mothers spend three-quarters of their day doing what Altmann described as "making a living," walking with their group to feeding areas and digging for bulbs and grass corms to eat, all while avoiding predators and tending to their infants' needs. Altmann wanted to know, how did they manage their time? How was their social status changed by motherhood? How did reproductive history affect their lives over the long term? Meanwhile, anthropologist Barbara Smuts wondered about the purpose of the long-running friendships that develop between male and female baboons, and sometimes between adult males and infants who are not their offspring. (Altmann called these males "godfathers.") Smuts asked, "What were these large, ruthless fighters doing in the 'female domain,' looking slightly out of place as they cuddled and carried tiny infants?"

Hrdy herself began asking provocative questions about langurs, a type of leaf-eating monkey, and the males among them who would sometimes kill infants with apparent "collusion" from the mothers, who would later mate with those same males. What role could such incidents of infanticide possibly play in advancing the survival of a species? And, looking across the animal world, what about those species in which mothers are the ones doing the killing or, more commonly, abandoning offspring under pressure from food shortages or predation or so they can be free to mate again?

A female, in Darwin's thinking, is generally sexually passive, choosing among the mates who compete for her attention and beyond that having little influence on the fate of the species. But nearly a century after Blackwell's call to action, the work of these women and many others made the idea that maternal biology renders a female "coy," wholly self-sacrificing, or inherently inferior seem downright silly.

Slowly, a new picture emerged of primate mothers who plot, in a sense, for evolutionary success and rely on others to help them achieve it. Mothers, Hrdy wrote, were "just as much strategic planners and decision-makers, opportunists and deal-makers, manipulators and allies as they were nurturers." Female sexual and maternal behavior varied across and within species, shaped by competing demands. Maternal care—let alone maternal love—was not automatic. Within that framework, babies had to become agents of their own survival, compelling parents to care for them.

If Rosenblatt's work cracked open the door, allowing researchers to look with fresh eyes at the biological transformation that comes with new parenthood and the ways that babies and parents act on one another, the work of evolutionary biologists in Hrdy's era pushed it open. "More women in evolutionary studies changed science," Hrdy told me. "It wasn't that we were doing science differently. It was that we were—we had different starting assumptions."

But the work of these primatologists, especially Hrdy, also has drawn the ire of some feminist thinkers. Ten years after Hrdy published *Mother Nature*, her 1999 tome on the biology and behavior of mothers and babies, she followed it up with a book about the roles extended family members and other caregivers have played in child-rearing throughout evolutionary history. French writer and philosopher Élisabeth Badinter called the determinism she saw in Hrdy's work "loathsome." In 2010, Badinter published *The Conflict: How Modern Motherhood Undermines the Status of Women*, in which she objected to the rise of attachment parenting and its promotion of a "return to a traditional model" at the expense of a woman's identity. She made many good points about the jumps in logic required to sustain maternal instinct as a tool for social control. She also faulted the evolutionary biologists who study primates and see in them clues about human mothers.

Although Badinter declined to be interviewed for this book, she told me by email that she thinks there may be room for neurobiology in the study of motherhood, but only as a factor secondary to societal influences. In her book, she wrote that the link between human and primate is weak. Environmental context, social pressure, and a mother's individual psychological experience all carry more influence than "the feeble voice of 'mother nature,'" she wrote. "As soon as we bring nature into the discussion," she told the magazine *Le Nouvel Observateur* in 2010, "there is no way out."

I see Badinter's point. The natural history of motherhood has proven too often to be a cage. Maternal instinct, to twist Lorenz's metaphor, has been the impenetrable lock on the door. But becoming a mother *is* a major biological event rooted in evolutionary history. New parents *do* experience a dramatic neurobiological change, and that change is particularly intense for gestational parents. Failing to acknowledge that is a trap in itself, if only because it leaves space for the specter of those old ideas to fill.

The transition to parenthood builds on the inherent flexibility of the brain, molded by both hormones and experience, influenced by the inherited coding of our species and by the peculiarities of our own brand-new babies. It is a process—one of short-term upheaval and long-lasting, continual change. Overwhelming and purposeful. In the early months, as the next chapter makes clear, it can be shaped as much by worry as by love. When you are in it, the voice of nature may sound like many things, but it is certainly not feeble.

What happens if we look at this new science of parenthood with full knowledge of how the old science was manipulated? What if we examine it with urgency and with an awareness of the cultural baggage we bring to the task?

Then, what story will we tell?

CHAPTER 3

Attention, Please

Soon after my husband, Yoon, became licensed to fly a drone, he took his aerial camera out for a test run over Scarborough Marsh. All summer long here, tourists paddle flocks of brightly colored kayaks through the narrow channels of the saltwater marsh that stretches over more than three thousand acres. We occasionally walk across it as a family, along a path built over an old railroad bed that cuts a straight line through the landscape's soft curves. We drive around it even more frequently, its reliable cycle from new-growth green in spring to the whites and grays of winter a steadfast mark of time. It is a familiar part of the place where we live. Yet the footage Yoon captured that day made it seem new.

From above, I could see how the great mats of grasses are not uniform and whole but variegated. Blades make up clusters that meet in great swirls and layers, circling pools of water and tracing the curves of rivulets. Smudges of color highlight hummocks of grass or gullies where the water has dried and the sun has crisped the salt that remains. The water becomes the sky, the reflection of puffy white clouds visible through long narrow panes between the grasses. From this vantage point, up is down. Space and time seem indistinct. Big is made up of so much little.

This is what I thought of when I stood outside an MRI room at Yale School of Medicine in February 2020 while a technician captured images of the brain of a young woman, a mother, lying inside the machine. A powerful magnet pulled the woman's hydrogen protons into alignment and released them, creating radio signals that the machine translated into black and white images of her brain that moved in sequential cross sections across the technician's screen. The stop-motion curves of white and gray matter in her cerebrum reminded me of the passing topography of the marshland, the seemingly more amorphous inner structures of the brain like the vast mats of grass, incredibly complex and interconnected if you look at them right. This is not a perfect metaphor. But it is useful.

A marshland is always in flux. Water perpetually moves salt and sediment, sluicing soil from the banks in one place or depositing it somewhere else. When a storm comes, the change is big. Fresh water floods in from upstream. Or a storm surge brings ocean waves farther inland, where they might literally fold pieces of the marsh upon itself, or sweep away chunks from the cliff edge. The influx of water from either side can change the salinity of whole sections, causing some plants to die off once the storm has cleared and allowing others to thrive. A big storm is a kind of jolt to the ecosystem, marking the start of a new epoch as nutrients are redistributed and water forms new paths. Salt marshes are championed by climate scientists—and, increasingly, by the people who live nearby—for their ability to absorb floodwaters. Inherent in the landscape's adaptability is its potential for destruction and for growth.

The brain is like this, too. In every person, it is always changing, adapting to the circumstances of life, propelling a person's behavior and responding to the outcomes. The brain was long thought of as a "nonrenewable organ," where things were more or less fixed once a person reached adulthood and cells could only be lost, in contrast with skin or blood, where cells are constantly replaced. Scientists today know that things happen differently in the brain, but it has its own remarkable, lifelong ability to change and to adjust, even to create something that wasn't there before or to make up for what was lost.

Our conscious and subconscious life is made up of signals transmitted across the physical structures of the brain, from neuron to neuron, between some eighty-six billion neurons that are always chatting. Those neurons change in form and function, in the number of connections each makes with other neurons, in the strength or nature of those connections, and in the pathways along which they send their messages. A neuron is made up of branching dendrites on one end, which receive signals from other neurons and pass them down the stemlike axon to endings called axon terminals, another bunch of branchy bits that produce just the right chemicals to convey those messages to the next neurons, across the space between them, called the synapse.

Every part of that process is subject to change. Axons are coated in a fatty substance, called myelin, that speeds up transmission and can be lost or regenerated. Dendrites can shrink and be pruned away, or they can grow stronger and more complicated. New synapses are formed. Others are eliminated. And constant shifts in the neurochemicals that carry signals across the synapse—or inhibit their transmission—change the strength and function of those synapses instantaneously, and over time. In some parts of the adult brain, whole new neurons are created, something scientists thought was impossible until relatively recently (though many questions remain about the extent and purpose of neurogenesis in humans).

Then there's the fact that the overall organization of the brain makes room for change. Neural activity is organized around critical centers in the brain to maximize efficiency in communication. But it also is diffuse in the sense that repeated movements or perceptions can involve a different set of neurons each time a person makes them. Neuroscientist Lisa Feldman Barrett compares the complexity of the brain to air travel, with certain airports serving as hubs and others primarily directing local traffic, to maximize resources and options, with numerous ways, for example, to get from Boston to Cairo.

The makeup of the brain, from the overall architecture to the size and function of each neuron, is shaped by a person's experience. The brain is plastic. It is anatomically flexible. It can be changed through learning, when a person moves to a new place or takes up a new hobby, for example. But the brain's rewiring also occurs on a more subconscious level, propelled by the stimuli a person is exposed to and by shifts in hormones. By the very progression of one's life. The wiring of the brain is not unlike the grass roots in a salt marsh and the ecological systems that support them, woven into a complex, ever-changing system that is, by nature, adaptable.

Researchers have described pregnancy and delivery as a kind of storm for the brain. The hormonal surge, particularly in the weeks and days before labor, is incredible. Progesterone levels can increase up to fifteen times what they are during the peak in a person's regular menstrual cycle and drop precipitously at the start of labor. The rise in certain estrogens is even more dramatic, with a whopping three-hundred-fold increase in estradiol as the end of pregnancy approaches. The development of a whole new organ, the placenta, introduces hormones that are entirely novel to the human body, never before experienced. And oxytocin surges near labor, accompanied by an increase in prolactin, and generally remains high postpartum. Nearly all mammals follow a similar pattern of hormone fluctuations, though they differ in the timing of hormonal peaks and valleys.

Prenatal education typically addresses these rising waters in terms of what they mean for maintaining pregnancy and supporting the mechanisms of labor. We may learn that estrogen helps grow the uterus and amps up overall blood supply to support a changing body and to nourish a new one. We might think of progesterone as a hormone that causes the lining of the uterus to thicken and elsewhere softens things, promoting breast tissue growth and, along with relaxin, loosening ligaments to help the body expand and ultimately be able to deliver a large baby through a small birth canal. We understand prolactin as a milk-making hormone. And, likely, we have read about oxytocin's role in uterine contractions, milk letdown, and a feeling of closeness once a baby arrives.

This is certainly a lot more than my own mother learned about the mechanisms of her body when she began having children in the early 1970s. But these mostly below-the-neck, pregnancy-specific changes are only part of the picture. The massive hormone fluctuations that come with having a child, likely more extreme than at any other point in a person's life, also go to work in the brain, acting as neurotransmitters or regulating the production of other neurochemicals that alter the way neurons are wired together, setting off a cascade of effects that unfurl over time and that last. They are a kind of weather front, which passes and leaves behind a still-changing landscape. In a strictly metaphorical sense, they soften the brain so that it can be molded into something different. In a literal sense, they make it more plastic and more responsive to the world around it, which now includes a baby.

* * *

IN LABORATORY RODENTS, THERE IS a clear story developing about how the hormonal surge of pregnancy and childbirth acts on the brain. Estrogen and progesterone work in concert with each other and with oxytocin and prolactin—no single hormone can do it on its own—to turn up a rat mother's sensitivity to cues from her young, creating what Alison Fleming and her colleagues, Joseph Lonstein and Frédéric Lévy, call "a maximal state of responsiveness." That responsiveness begins to build even before her pups are born, as her previous impulse for avoiding baby rats is replaced by attraction toward them. In preschool terms, we could say that hormones turn on the brain's "listening ears," tuning a rat mother to the particular cues her baby gives off and prompting her to respond to their direction by adjusting her behavior.

Then, the babies bring the noise. According to animal models in mammals, mothers can have all the necessary hormones that pregnancy and labor provide, but without sensory input from babies, they won't develop maternal behaviors as typical gestational mothers would. A first-time mother mouse must be able to smell her pups. If her olfactory bulb is removed, she may not build a nest and is less likely to nurse them. Newly maternal sheep are similar—without smelling their lambs, they perform poorly in caring for them. Mice and sheep with previous experience parenting—and smelling—young, however, will do just fine with subsequent babies after they've been rendered smell-blind. (Experience matters.) Tactile cues seem to matter equally, if not more, for laboratory rats. Mother rats need to be close to their pups. They need to lick them, to mouth and nuzzle them in order to develop motivation to care for them and to nurse them.

This convergence of hormone-induced sensitivity and baby-induced sensory overwhelm prompts a reorienting of the brain toward caregiving. The circuitry involved in parenting is complex and multidirectional. But animal studies in the 1970s—and many more since—pointed to the medial preoptic area, or the MPOA, as an important center of activity. We could think about the MPOA as a receiver. This tiny part of the hypothalamus contains receptors for all the hormones important for reproduction, and those receptors generally increase in number in late pregnancy and in the early postpartum period. The MPOA also receives all kinds of sensory data—meaning lots of input from the babies. It's thought that the MPOA acts as a critical hub in the parenting circuitry, taking in a massive amount of baby-related information and sending out messages organized into actions and inhibitions. The neurobiology of parenting, across species, is a careful mix of do's and don'ts. *Do pick up that distressed pup and carry it to your nest. Don't eat it.* As you'll see, it's a tricky balance.

A few years ago, researchers discovered a key piece of information about *how* the MPOA translates all that noise into signals for the rest of the brain. A group of researchers at Harvard University, led by neuroscientist Catherine Dulac, found that a subgroup of neurons in that area of the brain was essential to parenting behavior in mice—males and females, mind you. These neurons produce galanin, a neuropeptide. Neuropeptides are similar to neurotransmitters in that they carry messages from neuron to neuron, but peptides are especially potent and their signals far-reaching. The researchers found that mice whose galanin neurons are deactivated, through genetic modification and injection of a toxin, show dramatically reduced parenting behaviors. Unlike rats, virgin female mice spontaneously care for pups when presented with them. But virgins who have lost more than half of their galanin neurons don't. Instead, they become aggressive. Mother mice fail to retrieve their pups. Male mice that previously showed parental behaviors lose them. The discovery offered a promising window into the parental brain, "a precious entry point," as the researchers described it.

For one thing, it added nuance to the MPOA story. At least in the early postpartum period, damage to that area of the brain generally or to the galanin neurons specifically makes mice much less likely to do the things that their pups need them to do. Conversely, injecting the MPOA with estrogen or biologically activating those neurons speeds the onset of caregiving behaviors, in both male and female rodents. The fact that the galanin neurons are present and meaningful in the MPOA in both male and female mice added evidence to the idea that all members of a species have the capacity for a core parental brain circuitry that may be activated differently under different physiological circumstances.

Importantly, the findings gave Dulac's group an opportunity to follow the galanin. That's just what the researchers did, an effort that earned Dulac a 2021 Breakthrough Prize in Life Sciences, a $3 million award started by internet entrepreneur Yuri Milner and his wife, Julia Milner, and funded by some of the biggest names in science and technology.

The researchers found that the galanin neurons of the MPOA send signals, in males and females, to about twenty areas of the brain, many of them already known to be important for caregiving. All the galanin neurons in the MPOA are active when a mouse is engaged in parenting behaviors, but the researchers found that subsets of neurons form pools that influence specific components of parenting. The researchers tried activating individual galanin pools and found that those neurons that project signals to the periaqueductal gray, a midbrain region, increase pup grooming, for example. Activation of a pool that projects to the ventral tegmental area increases a mouse's drive to climb a barrier to be near pups. Projections to the medial amygdala don't affect interactions with pups at all but do influence interactions with other adult mice, seemingly rendering anything that's not pup-related uninteresting to the mouse.

The work of Dulac's lab uncovering this "modular architecture" of the MPOA is a powerful example of how much researchers can learn by manipulating rodent behavior and physiology in precise ways and, quite literally, putting the animals' brains under the microscope. They can inject the rodent brain with herpes or rabies virus as a tool for tracing neural circuits. They can remove female rats' ovaries, where estrogen and progesterone are produced, to test what happens when they go without those hormones. They can use receptor-blocking drugs to prevent neurotransmitters from working as they typically would. They can lesion areas of the brain or remove the olfactory bulb or anesthetize a rat's mouth or nipples and watch to see which components of maternal behavior are impaired as a result. They can stress a pregnant rodent, or separate a mother from her pups, and test the long-term effects. They "sacrifice" mother mice at particular points in pregnancy or the postpartum period and freeze slices of brain tissue for analysis.

Creating that cause-and-effect picture in humans is far more difficult. For one thing, human parenting is quite a bit more complicated and less predictable than that of a rat, especially one in a controlled laboratory setting. Human maternal behavior is harder to measure. Rat mothers and human mothers do share many basic functions. They feed their babies and tend to them. They must give them enough interaction to enable them to grow and develop. They notice their baby's needs and respond. But human parental behavior is influenced by culture and language, by lifestyle and sociopolitical context, by individual and family history, and by genetics that are far more diverse than in rats bred for science. (Wild rodents also are far more complex and variable than those in the lab.) Plus there are other people to consider—spouses and partners, grandparents, other adults and children in the household who may or may not be biologically related, even neighbors and teachers and friends—all of whom can influence a person's entry into parenting and their child's entry into the world.

Then there's the fact that researchers can't, for good reason, perform the same kind of manipulations on human parents and newborns that they can on laboratory animals. (There are people who would say such manipulations shouldn't be performed on any animals, a worthwhile discussion for a different book.) In humans, researchers rely on different techniques. They observe and measure the behaviors of parents and their interactions with their children, at home or in the lab, during normal interactions or during assigned tasks. They collect parents' self-reported information about how they feel and what they do. They assess levels of hormones in the bloodstream across pregnancy and the postpartum period. They review clinical diagnoses and symptom severity. And increasingly, in the past two decades, they use technology to assess what's happening in the parental brain, especially during tasks that are related to or meant to mimic parenting behaviors. When they are lucky, with time and funding, they can collect images of the brains of parents several times over a span of months or years to see how they change in structure or activity or connectivity. Even then, they are constantly hedging their results against the reality of human parenting and the changing circumstances of a person's life.

During my kindergartner's remote pandemic schooling, he often was assigned a lesson that involved watching a short video story and then sorting a series of picture cards that appeared on his iPad screen into the sequence in which they occurred in the film. The story of the parental brain in rodents is a little like that video, and the story of the human maternal brain is more like those cards. Each group of researchers is working, through some combination of measurements and with what they've learned from laboratory animals always in the background, to capture a snapshot of the human story, to identify where it fits in the sequence and why it matters. Eventually, they may have enough cards to tell a story. They're adding more all the time, filling in the details, and, more often than not, affirming just how much of the parental brain has been conserved across species, through evolutionary history. They are beginning to see the plotline of human parenthood, and to understand the scale and scope of the drama.

* * *

THE MOTHER IN THE fMRI was fast. As the woman lay inside the scanner, Madison Bunderson, a postgraduate research associate with the Yale Child Study Center, led her through a series of tasks. First up, the mother would see the words "win" or "lose" pop up before her. If the command said "win," Bunderson told her, she should press a key with her index finger when she saw a white box appear on the screen. For "lose," press the middle finger. Do it fast enough and, according to the directive, the mother would win a bit of money or avoid losing money from her pot of earnings. This is a common neuroscience test, called a monetary incentive delay task, designed to evaluate how the brain processes reward.

The computer from which Bunderson controlled the task was time-stamped to the brain scans, so researchers could precisely track brain activity alongside a person's responses. And the test was titrated to the test taker, meaning the speed with which she had to respond in order to win was adjusted to how quickly she had performed in earlier practice tests, when she'd sat at a desk before a computer. The point was for her to win some and lose some, so that the researchers could evaluate not just how her brain responded to the reward itself—the money, in this case—but also how her brain responded to the anticipation of it and the drive to obtain it. Then, the money was swapped out for a baby. And not just any baby, but this mother's cherubic baby girl.

The mother had brought her daughter with her during an earlier visit to the lab, so researchers could observe and evaluate how they played together, looking for measurements of the mother's sensitivity to her child's behavior. They also took pictures of the baby, lots of them, in all emotional states. This time in the scanner task, "win" was correlated with happy or calm faces and "lose" with neutral or sad faces. The white box appeared and, if the mother was fast enough, she would earn an image of her happy daughter, or avoid seeing the girl with an open-mouthed screech or a pouty lip. After almost every test, a chubby-cheeked smiling baby girl appeared. "She's really good at this," Bunderson said.

Lead researcher Helena Rutherford and her colleagues planned to analyze the data to see how the mother's neural circuitry responded, looking broadly at the brain and also specifically at the nucleus accumbens, which is thought to be active during reward anticipation and when a person is striving toward a goal, and at parts of the brain's frontal lobes recruited in processing receipt of rewards and the pleasure they generate. In tests using money, researchers have found that the brain responds differently in its drive to obtain that money than it does when receiving the reward itself. The researchers wanted to see whether the same was true in the parenting context. This mother was part of a group of mothers and fathers, about half of whom were smokers, who would be included in the study.

Prior studies have established that addiction generally tamps down the brain's reward response to money. Rutherford's group wondered whether the same effect was present when parents with addiction, in this case to nicotine, process baby-related rewards, with the goal of using that information to tailor parenting-support programs. But there is something implicit in this research that's relevant to all parents, smokers or not—a question, really.

What is it that compels us to care for children?

Perhaps the answer seems obvious: it's love. There is joy in loving and being loved by a child. That is the reward. Except, as Rutherford's framework shows, it may not be quite that simple. Certainly, there is pleasure in a baby—the joy of seeing your own sweet-cheeked daughter appear on the screen before you, or in the flesh. But there is something else, the urge to make that child happy or to keep her from ever being sad. A compulsion to keep her well and safe and growing and thriving. A drive to look at her, to listen to her, and then to act on her behalf. There are neurobiological mechanisms at work to shape that drive because the reality is that, from an evolutionary perspective, love alone is not enough. Love is neither universally reliable nor automatic. We know this by looking at extremes and at averages.

It is a difficult truth that, across history and societies, infanticide has been a part of human parenthood. Its prevalence rises and falls in relation to poverty, a person's ability to control their own reproduction, and societal norms. For generation after generation, for example, many thousands of babies in European cities were left in foundling homes known to have abysmal survival rates. In Florence, where the historical record is especially clear, the rate of baptized children who were abandoned never fell below 12 percent in the sixteenth and seventeenth centuries, Sarah Blaffer Hrdy writes in *Mother Nature*. In the 1840s, 43 percent of baptized children in that city were abandoned. Rates of infanticide in Europe generally fell with the rise of contraception in the nineteenth century. As writer Sandra Newman put it, humans "stopped killing our babies only when we started having fewer of them."

Of course, birth control—still nowhere near universally accessible—was never an elixir capable of assuring every mother is a devoted one or guaranteeing that every child is safe and well cared for. In the United States today, hundreds of thousands of children suffer from neglect or abuse every year. Caring for vulnerable children has always been a balancing act of so many factors, including parents' and families' ability to grapple with stress, poverty, oppression, mental illness, addiction, or other aspects of life that do not align with a baby's best interests, measured against the degree of social support a person has to mitigate those factors. Parents are not automatically committed to caring for every baby born. "Nurturing has to be teased out, reinforced, maintained," Hrdy wrote. "Nurturing itself needs to be nurtured."

Then there is the very ordinary but too-little-acknowledged truth that, for many birthing parents, a rush of love does not attend a baby's delivery, or it comes with equally powerful waves of fear or dread. Studies examining first-time mothers' frame of mind at birth often describe feelings of guilt over the sudden weight of responsibility that comes where they expected pure affection. One study found that, of 112 first-time mothers interviewed a week after birth, 40 percent said that what they felt the first time they held their baby was "indifference." I wonder about that word and if what respondents were referring to wasn't so much a lack of interest in their child as a kind of cool shock where they had anticipated warmth. The feeling of affection came for those mothers, as it does for most birthing parents, with just a bit of time. Still, when it does come, affection can be disorienting in its own way. The demands of a baby are immense and relentless, and the desire to fill them may be as big as the anguishing prospect of failure.

It is, in fact, entirely normal to feel a mix of all these things. In a 2005 paper arguing that new motherhood can lead to spiritual awakening, psychologists Aurélie Athan and Lisa Miller wrote that conflicting emotions are "natural and purposeful." Ambivalence is, in fact, "the defining feature of this transitional process." Psychotherapist Rozsika Parker wrote a whole book on the balance of hate and love in motherhood, one for which the scale tips differently from person to person. "A mother needs to know herself, to own up to the diverse, contradictory, often overwhelming feelings evoked by motherhood," she told the *Guardian* in 2006. "It's only by accepting that at times you are a bad mother, that you can ever be a good mother." And in 1949, psychoanalyst Donald Winnicott somewhat famously listed eighteen reasons why a mother hates her child—"even a boy"—from birth. The truth in it stings, even as Winnicott's tone makes me laugh. "The baby is not magically produced," he wrote. "The baby is a danger to her body in pregnancy and at birth. . . . He is ruthless, treats her as scum, an unpaid servant, a slave. . . . After an awful morning with him she goes out, and he smiles at a stranger, who says: 'Isn't he sweet!'" And, "If she fails him at the start she knows he will pay her out for ever."

There are costs to being a parent, financially of course, but also to a person's general well-being and bodily resources. When caring for a newborn, especially in those weeks before he smiles or can focus his eyes, before those inklings of social reciprocity, the costs are especially high. New parents pay with their sleep, their time, their attention, their emotional equilibrium. They pay with their energy, with what they expend in feeding and bouncing and shushing, in coping through days that seem to last weeks and through lonely early morning hours during which time disappears entirely. Then there is the required internal investment, a reorienting of resources needed to balance their own physiological processes in order to be the arbiter of the very factors that shape those processes for their babies: food, rest, safety. This is no small thing.

The parental brain makes love for our children possible, and that love can be big and generous and lifelong. But it unfolds with time, and a baby cannot wait to be cared for. So at the very start, the parental brain does not rely entirely on love, or at least not the version of it we may know. Its first mission is to capture—and to keep—a parent's attention. "We always think about the pleasure of parenting," Rutherford told me, "and we don't always think about the drive or the motivation of parenting."

The "we" Rutherford is referring to is parents and society. Researchers, on the other hand, think a lot about that motivation. Rutherford leads the Yale Child Study Center's Before and After Baby Lab, in which researchers study the transition to parenthood. Its name acknowledges right up front that there is a "before baby" and an "after baby," and they are not the same. When researchers talk about parents in the "after," they often start with all the ways that babies set that drive in motion.

* * *

BABIES BRING THE NOISE, FOR humans, too. They are inherently powerful stimuli for all adults, with variation from person to person of course. And while it's commonly thought that women respond more strongly to babies—you know, because of their maternal instinct—research has not entirely borne that out.

This is where Konrad Lorenz's work has been most clearly carried forward into modern parenting research. Lorenz wrote about the *Kindchenschema*, the makeup of a baby's face that compels an adult to act on that child's behalf. It is the power of cuteness, where "cute" in this case is a technical term, though one that might apply about equally to your Memoji, your kitten, or your chubby-cheeked nephew. Cuteness is a measurable set of characteristics shared to some degree by babies across mammalian species, including a big head and proportionally large eyes, plus a small chin and round cheeks. Frequently co-opted by illustrators and marketing experts, these characteristics trigger particularly strong reactions in the adult brain and give babies the best chance of securing the care they need to survive.

Researchers often have found that men and woman respond similarly to cute baby faces. In one study, adults without children were asked to rate a group of babies by cuteness. The women in the group gave the babies higher marks, when consciously rating the faces. Yet the men and women worked equally hard in a key-pressing task to continue viewing cute infant faces, versus adult faces of "average attractiveness." Separately, cute baby faces, but not adult faces, have been found to trigger a very fast surge of activity in a part of the brain, the medial orbitofrontal cortex, important in detecting and responding to positive, or rewarding, stimuli. In at least one small study—with just twelve participants in all—those results held true in men and women, parents and nonparents.

Today, scientists understand that the power of *Kindchenschema* encompasses much more than how a baby looks. It includes all those other sensory channels through which babies announce themselves and lay claim to their caregivers. Parents are generally really good at identifying their *own* newborns based on how they smell or the sound of their cry, or at picking their babies out of a lineup of newborn photographs after only a couple hours together. On some such measures, mothers' responses are strongest. In others, mothers and fathers perform equally.

More recently, researchers have begun looking more deeply into just how a parent's brain responds in the postpartum period to the parent's own baby's face, her coos, or what some call the "biological siren" of her cry, with the understanding that a baby's development depends on the ability of the adults in her life to interpret those cues and deliver the food or the comfort or the developmental stimulus—including play and baby talk—that she needs.

In study after study, parents have looked at images of their own babies or other babies, or listened to recordings of their own precious child's cry or that of a stranger's baby, or they've been asked to engage in some more-active task involving those cues, as in Rutherford's study. They do so while lying inside an fMRI machine, or while attached to electrodes that measure activity in the brain's outer layers, or while seated with their head inside a massive cone-head-like machine that measures the magnetic fields generated by brain activity. Sometimes researchers study how a group of parents changes over time. Sometimes they compare them to people who are not parents. The large majority of time, they have studied only cisgender, heterosexual women who carried their babies, though that is beginning to change.

In truth, the baby cues used in these studies are paltry substitutes for the real thing. A recording of a baby's cry can't possibly capture in full how parents react when their baby is crying with his whole body and they not only hear him but also feel his chest vibrating against their own. Or, what about the specific kind of joy that comes when you see, for the first time, what might be a tiny, purposeful smile form on your baby's face, when you squeal and coo and are rewarded with an undeniable, open-mouthed grin? How about when a breastfeeding parent is out for a walk with a baby sleeping on their chest and that baby begins to stir? You know what's coming, those first gurgles as a tiny fist finds a mouth and, soon, a cry. The baby is hungry. Can a laboratory machine really capture the whole-body drive to find a park bench or to make it back home in time to nurse? Can it document the flush of relief in getting there, in filling that need? No. But what those tests can do is record the fingerprint of those real-life responses, the shape of the groove they've worn in the brain's circuitry.

These studies repeatedly found heightened activity and connectivity across two interrelated networks involved in processing infant cues and attaching meaning to them—the networks most implicated in a birthing parent's "maximal state of responsiveness": the dopamine-driven reward network and the salience network.

The reward system actually has outgrown its name. It is sometimes referred to in this context as the maternal motivation system—a better fit, though it is involved in motivated behavior generally, and not only in mothers. Key hubs include the ventral tegmental area, in the midbrain, which sends signals via the neurotransmitter dopamine to the nucleus accumbens, mentioned before. Both are also connected to the amygdala, medial prefrontal cortex, and hippocampus, among other regions essential in caregiving responses.

In animal models of motherhood, the MPOA—the receiver—is an important starting point for this network. In humans, the MPOA often gets left out. It was long thought that, because the human cortex is about one thousand times bigger than a rat's, it must have more influence over human maternal behavior than the tiny MPOA, whose small size makes it hard to measure. Researchers told me they can't really tell whether the limited and variable activity they capture in that area during brain scans is an indication that the MPOA is less involved in driving human motivation, or that there's plenty happening there that's just out of sight. There are some indications that it's the latter. Because its projections lead to the complex prefrontal cortex, the MPOA seems to be an important generator of motivated caregiving in humans, too.

This motivational system runs on dopamine, regulated by oxytocin. Dopamine often is cast as the "feel-good" hormone linked to the pleasure people get from sex, a runner's high, or the smell of cupcakes baking in the oven. That's mostly a misnomer, and one that won't quit. Scientists used to think dopamine responded only to rewarding stimuli, but animal research over several decades has found that it often responds to negative stimuli, too. Dopamine is, instead, a gambler. It reads the table—one's environment—and helps the brain make constant predictions about how things are going to go. Based on its wins or losses, when things go better or worse than expected, it drives signals to circuitry that direct action, emotion, and learning.

One fascinating set of studies from Alison Fleming's lab found that the hormonal priming of pregnancy lowers the baseline dopamine level in mother rats. Then the spike of dopamine the mothers receive from interacting with pups is more extreme and more meaningful. The pups become a "discrete signal," Fleming told me. The payoff is bigger, speeding the onset of the maternal behavior the pups require.

Oxytocin influences dopamine production. This neuropeptide, which is released in the brain of birthing parents during labor and in *all* parents as they interact affectionately with their babies, stimulates production of dopamine in the ventral tegmental area. In animal models and in humans, oxytocin has been shown over and over to be important in parenting. Rat mothers with more oxytocin projections to the ventral tegmental area show greater levels of maternal care, and it's thought that oxytocin's work in the reward system is key to switching the smell of pups from offensive to appealing. In one study with a very, very small sample size—just twelve mothers tested a few weeks after birth— researchers found that when they listened to their babies cry, mothers who delivered their babies vaginally had greater neural activity in brain regions related to reward and motivation, including the amygdala, than mothers who delivered by C-section. The study authors hypothesized that this difference had to do with the "vaginocervical stimulation" and surge of oxytocin that are particular to vaginal delivery.

Researchers are still puzzling out just how the dopamine pathway works, but the key here for parents is responsiveness. Good gamblers adjust quickly when the circumstances on the table change. Dopamine contributes to the flexibility of human behavior and may even drive much of the plasticity that occurs as a parent navigates this time of constant prediction errors.

The salience network plays a very related role in regulating responsiveness, though in a parenting context it's often framed in terms of vigilance and threat detection, serving the fundamental goal of keeping a vulnerable baby safe. The salience network includes the amygdala and key cortical structures, including the anterior cingulate cortex and the anterior insular cortex, which respond to infant cues in healthy postpartum women. It is thought to play an essential role in separating the wheat from the chaff when it comes to the deluge of input the brain receives, particularly in a complex social environment. It directs attention and working memory toward events or stimuli that are most essential to regulating the basic functions of the body—or *bodies*, in the case of caregiver and child—and facilitating fast responses from the motor system. You can see why it's important in the care of babies, those fire hoses of need that require attention and fast action.

The amygdala may be the most studied part of the brain in the context of human maternal behavior. You might know the amygdala as the center for flight-or-fight reactions. It was long seen as the brain's fear detector. Now it is more often called a "salience detector." A meaning maker. It serves as a mediator between—and an instigator of—systems that detect infant cues, interpret a baby's emotional state, and direct appropriate responses to them. And it does seem to give preferential status to signs of distress. In parents, the amygdala and interconnected areas involved in emotion processing are activated more by baby cries than by baby laughter. Notably, the reverse is true for people without children, with stronger activation to laughter.

One 2019 study looked at the "resting state" connectivity between the amygdala and other brain regions. In this case, researchers didn't give the participants—forty-seven first-time mothers, with babies between a few weeks and almost ten months old—a task to perform. Instead, they examined the blood-oxygen level across the brain while they were simply resting in the scanner. Scientists think this approach can reveal the brain's intrinsic or baseline connectivity—not just how neurons fire together in response to a specific stimulus, but how they are prepared to fire together even before there is a task in mind. It shows the functional architecture of the brain—not just how the subway moves, but how the tunnels are constructed.

The researchers found the more experience a mother had—the further along she was into the postpartum months—the more connected her right and left amygdala were to key brain regions while she was in that resting state. And mothers with more connectivity between the amygdala and the nucleus accumbens were better able to engage in what researchers call "maternal structuring," which involves reading a baby's interests and guiding them without overwhelming the baby. Essentially, paying attention and responding thoughtfully.

The findings add evidence to the importance, as parenting progresses, of reward and salience and their influence on one another, according to Alex Dufford, lead researcher on that paper. "So, you look at baby, it causes this flood of dopamine. You're really interested—you know, this baby looks very cute," Dufford said. "And then you sort of begin your maternal behaviors somewhat not knowing what to do maybe, and then you get this—it's this feedback loop. Baby may respond positively when I do this. They may respond negatively when I do this." Motivation and salience, he said, drive learning.

Researchers give these networks names and put them into categories, but the networks don't actually operate in discrete ways. They overlap with each other and with circuitry involved in interpreting others' emotional states and regulating our own, in decision-making and directing attention. Recent studies in humans have found that connectivity within the salience network depends on dopamine function and its role in assigning value to stimuli. Other brain regions influence and interact with these networks, too, helping to tag baby cues as important even before a person is consciously aware of them. Among them are that fast-acting orbitofrontal cortex, which sometimes is included as part of the salience network; a midbrain area called the periaqueductal gray that's been found to be similarly fast at detecting infant sounds; and the cerebellum, whose exact role in parenting is still relatively unknown.

Babies need us to respond quickly. We need to comfort them and to meet their basic needs, even when we don't have a conscious understanding of exactly what it is that they need. They also need us to find that joy and to come back for more. So they come with their big eyes and their powerful lungs, to plug right into our brains.

A major focus of research on perinatal mood and anxiety disorders is what happens when the normative changes that are part of the adaptation to new parenthood don't occur or are disrupted. Repeated studies have identified blunted responses in key parts of the motivation and salience networks in mothers with postpartum depression, though one research group reported increased responsiveness in the amygdala to certain stimuli. Those differing results likely are at least in part due to just how much we have to learn about the heterogeneity of perinatal mood and anxiety disorders. They also point to the idea that the neurobiological adjustment to parenting depends on a just-right kind of tuning, with allowance for variability. A balance between pleasure and drive, joy and threat, quick subconscious reaction and top-down decision-making.

For all the ways that human parenting is different from that of rodents, this one might be most important: human parents are not as dependent on hormones to begin the task. Babies may be cared for by anyone who chooses to do so. But those who do make that choice also go through their own transition to a parental brain, driven—just as in gestational parents, and in male or virgin rats turned parental through exposure—by hormonal shifts and experience.

Researchers at Bar-Ilan University in Israel and their colleagues found greater activation of the amygdala in mothers who have primary responsibility for caring for their babies than in fathers who are secondary caregivers. But that's not the case when looking at fathers who are primary caregivers. In those fathers, the amygdala activation was comparable to mothers, and the amygdala showed particularly strong functional connectivity with a region called the superior temporal sulcus. In fact, across all fathers in that study, the more time a father spent caring for his child, the greater the connection between those two brain regions, which is thought to facilitate better detection of social cues. One could imagine how that detection might be particularly important for a parent whose alert systems were not intensely primed by pregnancy.

There's much more to say about fathers and nongestational parents, but for now the point is that there is more than one path to a responsive parental brain. And to that point, let's go back to oxytocin and vaginal delivery. Pregnant people hear a lot about the importance of vaginal births and breastfeeding as the ways to give their baby the best possible start in the world. I will forever be in awe of the body in birth, and I have written elsewhere about the challenges and joys I experienced breastfeeding. Childbirth and feeding, and particularly the degree of trauma or support a person feels through those processes, do affect the postpartum experience and the parental brain. However, neither factor is strictly definitive of a person's development as a parent.

Remember that difference in neural activity between mothers who delivered vaginally and mothers who delivered by C-section? It disappeared. By three or four months postpartum, researchers found no significant functional difference in brain circuitry between the two groups. The same researchers saw a very similar gap in brain activity between exclusively breastfeeding mothers and exclusively formula-feeding mothers within the first month postpartum, but no data has been published on what happens to that difference. Again, these studies are quite small, so it's frankly hard to know how their findings would hold up at a population level. A separate study looking at structural changes in the maternal brain found no measurable differences according to type of delivery or lactation, though there, too, the sample sizes were small.

For these factors that are loaded with such moral weight for pregnant and postpartum people, small studies are almost all we've got to gauge the impact on parental brain development. That's a problem I hope institutions funding parental brain research are looking at more closely. For now, let me say it again: as far as we can tell, there is *no one right way* to get to the responsive, flexible state that a baby and a parent require.

Perhaps the most important thing we can do for our children is to really take them in. Hear them and smell them and watch them. Engage with them. Hormones lay the groundwork, but it is this interaction that ultimately wires a parent's brain in ways that are necessary to care for their own particular child.

* * *

ON ONE OF THE LAST days of 2019, I was on my way to meet my sister for lunch and a movie—*Little Women*—and I had what public radio fans call a "driveway moment," though in my case it was a parking meter moment. I texted my sister that I'd be a few minutes late and sat in my car listening to Wendy Wood, an expert on the psychology of habit making, talk with *Hidden Brain* host Shankar Vedantam about why so many people struggle to stick with their New Year's resolutions—it was that time of year.

Wood explained that habits are forged not through willpower, or the "just do it" attitude many people bring to the task. Rather, they require a slow shift in subconscious processes through the association of particular cues with particular rewards. Those processes are driven largely by dopamine, through its role in detecting rewards and coding those rewards to the environmental cues that prompted them. Good habits typically are formed not so much by controlling our thoughts or behaviors themselves as by changing the cues in our environment, she said. Big life events, like a move or a marriage, change lots of cues at once, creating what scientists call habit discontinuity. "They shake everything up," Wood writes in her book *Good Habits, Bad Habits: The Science of Making Positive Changes That Stick*, "and for a moment, all of your behaviors—habitual and otherwise—are in the air, waiting for you to direct their placement."

New parenthood is a big disruption, but it also comes with a tiny air traffic controller, giving precise, powerful cues on how to land those habits. I started thinking about those early months as a period of rapid habit reformation. It only makes sense that the process can be painful and disorienting. Forming even one new habit is hard. But there's something about parenthood that makes it a fundamentally distinct form of discontinuity.

Having a baby doesn't require just one big wave of habit change. It throws a parent into perpetual change. Babies require us to quickly form lots of new habits and then to change them just as quickly. They need us to become competent *and* remain highly responsive as they grow. They need efficient, consistent care, but they need it to be flexible. That's a big ask. It requires a kind of readiness that might be entirely novel to parents.

Researchers studying motivation often talk about it in terms of "appetitive" and "consummatory" responses, the first being seeking or searching behaviors and the second being the actions taken in achieving the goal, in achieving satiation. About a decade ago, Mariana Pereira and a colleague organized a workshop for researchers to talk about their investigation of maternal motivation and settle a dispute. Some of the researchers were using that breakdown—appetitive versus consummatory—to talk about maternal motivation and others were not. It was a technical point, a bit of inside baseball, but they ultimately came to a consensus that, I think, has real meaning for the rest of us.

A person's urge to check their smartphone or to eat a basket of French fries or even to use a particular drug is satiated once those goals are achieved. It may come back again soon after, so that there is a cycle between seeking and satiation. But maternal motivation is different. It is a complex *state of being* that is maintained "without a decline, for long periods of time, as long as the appropriate stimuli are provided," the workshop participants wrote. The goals of that motivation may shift or even rest into a passive readiness—feed, burp, play, change, swaddle, shush, check, write a to-do list, drink tea, feed again. The motivation remains. It is not really ever satiated, Pereira told me, perhaps because the drive is not toward one's own satisfaction but toward the baby's, and that baby's needs are perpetually changing. "The energy that is involved to remain always there, always ready—it's fascinating," she said.

Consider S5, the mother rat who couldn't stop. She was part of a study, published in 1969, in which she and a group of other pregnant rats had been trained to press a small lever near their nesting boxes to receive a pellet of food down a short chute. One day after S5 delivered a litter, she pressed the lever and received her usual allotment of food: six presses and six pellets. Then she pressed the lever again, and a pup slid down the chute. Her own.

Imagine her surprise, a blink of joy in encountering her child, and then the terror. What was the pup doing here, on this chute, cold and alone? Her body responded even before such a question could form. She carried the pup three feet to the safety of her nest and went back to the lever. Another press, another pup to gather. She continued like this—press, pup, press, pup—until all six of her own pups were at home in the nest. Then she returned again to the lever.

Before she became a mother, S5 would have been averse to pups. Now she was indiscriminately drawn to them. Rats will care for any pups, not only their own. So S5 kept pressing the lever and retrieving pups who were not her own, gathering tiny foster rats to her nest. One baby and then another and another, until perhaps they morphed into a river of babies, a current of need. For three hours, the mother rat worked, retrieving a total of 684 rats, at a furious rate of one every fifteen seconds, traveling more than two thousand feet with pups in her mouth and an equal distance on return to the chute, in search of another. To say she never tired would be a lie. Surely, she was exhausted by the gargantuan task and just one day postpartum. But she didn't stop. The human experimenters quit first, tired of delivering pups to the chute.

S5 was the "best performer" in the study, but the four other mother rats tested were similarly motivated: all bar-pressed to retrieve hundreds of pups each. In 1999, a group of researchers in Alison Fleming's lab expanded on the results in a study that proved foundational in understanding how the brain adjusts the specific value of pups to be a powerful rewarding and reinforcing stimulus, and the role the MPOA and the amygdala play in that process. "Just think about it," Pereira told me. "If you bar-press and you get your son and then you bar-press again and you get your son—you would not stop bar-pressing."

* * *

IN THE WEEKS AFTER MY first son was born, I felt possessed by worry.

My husband and I had moved into our first home, with just a few weeks left before Hartley was due. The kitchen was still being renovated, so our moving boxes were sitting there amid construction dust when we learned that the old kitchen had high levels of lead paint on the walls and cabinets, an issue neither we nor our contractor had tested for or properly mitigated. We learned there was lead paint on the house's doors and on the chipping floor of the back porch. It was on the windowsills, inside and out. This house was supposed to be the home in which our son began his life. Instead it suddenly felt like a hazard zone. I sobbed to my sister on the phone: *I've already failed him,* I told her.

With about two weeks left until my due date, I developed high blood pressure and was induced. Hartley was born small, at less than six pounds, a wide-eyed little guy with plenty of hair. I was in complete awe of him. And I was afraid.

In a March 2020 interview, Chelsea Clinton described the "cellular explosion level" love she felt when her daughter was born, and the intense protectiveness that came with it. She recalled telling her husband this after the delivery, in a nod to the History Channel show they'd been watching in the final days of her pregnancy: "If the Vikings come marauding through this hospital, I'm going to get up and defend my newborn child." He looked at her and responded, "What are you talking about? We're in Manhattan."

I, for one, don't doubt that Clinton would have stood up to the Vikings. For me, though, there was no outside marauder. The threat was much closer: What if *I* make the wrong choices? What if *I* can't feed him or protect him? What if *I* really do fail him?

In those first days and weeks at home, I squandered precious hours leaning over Hartley's bassinet to check that he was still breathing. I did not heed the advice I had been given over and over to sleep when the baby slept. Instead, I Googled, researching the particular magic required to gauge whether a newborn is eating enough, or to interpret the color schemes of an infant's poop. I read about potential toxins in baby wipes, in toys, in the food I ate that became the food he ate, in the air around us and the water piped into our home. Then there was the lead paint. It was a real but manageable risk. In my mind, however, it grew to cartoonish proportions. I cleaned our floors incessantly but still imagined a cloud of poison dust following us as I carried my baby, so tiny and fragile, from room to room.

Outwardly, I was managing OK. With help from my husband and our extended family, I was eating well, showering enough, and occasionally getting out into the late Maine winter for fresh air and a walk, though for a while leaving the house with Hartley sent me into a full-body sweat. I fielded work calls while on leave from my job as an editor at a daily newspaper. I wrote thank-you notes, in a timely fashion even, for the baby gifts we received. I began researching lead mitigation companies. Hartley was growing steadily, though he sometimes spent whole afternoons cluster feeding.

At my six-week checkup, my ob-gyn screened for postpartum depression. She noted that my responses to the standard questionnaire were somewhat mixed, though my score was well within the normal range. She asked whether I had thoughts about harming myself or my child, and when I said no, she moved on. But anxiety had become a constant companion. It was an unrelenting static in my mind. A current of need.

I worried about the worry. I worried that it was crowding out all the things I should feel, like warmth and contentment. Gratitude. Presence. I worried because I had felt this way before.

As a kid, I struggled with obsessive-compulsive-like symptoms. I washed my hands until they were raw and cracked. Numbers took on unreasonable meaning. And I obsessed about the safety of my family members. I lived with that constant static of worry, from the time I flicked the bathroom light switches repeatedly in the morning until I counted the footsteps from the door of my bedroom to my bed at night. At some point, I decided I was tired of it and that I would start grabbing door handles and not washing my hands right after, to prove to myself that nothing bad would happen, that the fate of the people I loved was not somehow controlled by the minute workings of my own mind. Bit by bit, I devised what I now see as a kind of self-directed exposure therapy, though I didn't know that term then. I found a way to manage my unreasonable thoughts.

What I felt after Hartley was born was familiar. And that was deeply unsettling to me. Now, my son's fate truly was in my hands. It relied on the competence of my mind and my actions. My obsessiveness was back. Motherhood had made me feel this way again, I thought, and

I would be a mother forevermore. Would I always be this anxious? Would my baby suffer for it?

* * *

I LOOK BACK ON THAT time with the perspective of someone who now goes to therapy regularly, and I realize that I could have benefited from some professional support. I wish I had sought it out sooner. But there's something else that would have helped, too, that eventually did help: knowing that at least some of the worry I experienced in early motherhood was normal.

More than sixty years ago, pediatrician and psychoanalyst Donald Winnicott described the period after childbirth, when a woman becomes intensely focused on her baby, as a state of "primary maternal preoccupation." He characterized the time from the end of pregnancy to a few weeks after birth as one of heightened sensitivity. Perhaps the women Winnicott observed obsessed over their babies' eating and sleeping patterns, too, or refused to be apart from them. Maybe they fretted over their own competence as a parent but were reluctant to allow others to help, or they expressed guilt when their thoughts strayed from their baby for even a few moments.

In Winnicott's thinking, this sensitivity was not a side effect to be endured, but a necessity of caregiving and the very path by which a person becomes able to respond appropriately to an infant's complex needs. Winnicott wrote that this preoccupation was extreme enough that it "would be an illness were it not for the fact of the pregnancy." He called it a "normal illness," in line with a "dissociated state" or a "fugue," and one "not easily remembered by mothers once they have recovered from it."

To be sure, there is more than a touch of patriarchal thinking in Winnicott's analysis. Women with "a strong male identification"—by which I assume he was referring to ambition or interest outside of domestic life—may have a hard time reaching this state of sensitivity, he said, and much of the woes of children and families lay at their feet. Still, I found his words weirdly comforting. Researchers at the Yale Child Study Center found them to be prescient.

James Leckman was already a well-known researcher studying

Tourette's syndrome and obsessive-compulsive disorder when, in the 1990s, postdoctoral researcher Ruth Feldman—now herself a renowned neuroscientist—introduced him to Winnicott's idea of preoccupation. Leckman remembered what it was like when his own daughter was born in 1974, the drive he and his wife both felt to prepare their apartment before her arrival. He repainted rooms and lugged wood up three flights of stairs to build a cradle for her. His wife asked him to pull the fridge out from the wall to clean under it. Things needed to be just so.

Leckman thought it possible that the preoccupation he had felt and that so many other parents describe could be similar to obsessive-compulsive disorder in its symptoms and maybe even in the neural substrate underlying those thoughts and behaviors. He set out with Feldman and other colleagues to measure the degree and nature of preoccupation among parents. In 1999, they published an analysis of a series of interviews with forty-one mother-father pairs, conducted near the end of pregnancy, a couple weeks after their babies arrived, and again at about three months out. The questions homed in on the parents' behaviors, state of mind, and emotional states.

Almost universally, they found, parents worried about their children. What was striking, though, was the degree of preoccupation across the board. At two weeks postpartum, mothers *on average* reported thinking about their baby for fourteen hours a day. For fathers, it was half that. More than three-quarters of all parents described the need to check on their babies even when they knew everything was OK, and some did this compulsively. Parents talked about how they regularly worried they would drop their baby, or that the baby would be attacked by the family pet, or that their own negligence would somehow cause the baby to be hurt or sickened. Worse, what if they lost control, especially in their own state of exhaustion, and hit or shook their baby?

It is not uncommon for parenting researchers to screen participants for depression and anxiety, even if their study is not explicitly related to those symptoms, and to find that a large majority have subclinical levels of either, or both, and that a smaller group meet clinical diagnostic criteria. Rutherford told me it is rare for a mother not to endorse any anxiety symptoms. That poses a challenge for researchers trying to tease out what those symptoms mean in a parenting context, to determine when they are truly adaptive and when they are problematic, given how common they are.

"Parents are beset with worries about their new infant, the safety of their home environment, their own health and well-being, as well as their fundamental adequacy as parents," Leckman and his colleagues wrote in the 1999 paper. "The worries about the infant have a characteristic content that is shared across families."

Mia Edidin hears these worries, to some degree, from most of the parents she works with. Edidin is a social worker and clinical director at Perinatal Support Washington, a nonprofit in Washington state that runs parent-support groups, offers therapy, and operates a "warm line" that struggling parents can call into for peer support. She keeps a short list of topics that come up with nearly every family. On it is the Big One, the massive earthquake due, someday, from the Cascadia subduction zone. It's a risk people in the Pacific Northwest live with daily. But for new parents it becomes a real and present danger. They think, "I have actually threatened the safety of this being that I am so intricately tied to that it hurts," Edidin said. And for a new parent, that sense of having put your child in danger "is the worst feeling ever."

Edidin tries to help parents identify anxious thoughts about their baby's well-being that may be irrational. When I interviewed her for a piece published in the *Boston Globe* in May 2020, she told me the coronavirus pandemic made that harder to do. The whole world had entered a state of vigilance. But it was still possible. "We can use the data that we have right in front of us," she said. "In new motherhood, regardless of COVID, we can look at our baby to determine if our baby is OK."

That strategy is something Leckman and his coauthors noted, too. Being physically close to the baby, even if worrisome thoughts persist, can lessen the distress. "With the child in arms," they wrote, "parents can dispel, at least for a moment, the worries by checking on the infant or by making sure that the baby is safe through some other action." The researchers concluded that parents of newborns experience an "altered mental state" that has value, propelling them in their transition to parenthood—and that also can make them more vulnerable to mental illness.

Many birth parents do develop perinatal mood or anxiety disorders.

The figure commonly quoted in the United States is one in five mothers, though it's hard to gauge precisely, given the inadequacy of postpartum care, the stigma still often attached to postpartum depression, and the fact that anxiety disorders or childbirth-related post-traumatic stress disorder are generally less recognized and less often screened for by health care providers.

As it stands, postpartum depression is a wretchedly unspecific diagnosis. One researcher told me it is a "garbage bag" term, a diagnostic category into which many misunderstood or little-understood postpartum disorders get placed. Leckman said it is likely that some portion of postpartum disorders occur when this evolutionarily conserved sensitivity in parenthood gets off course. "The way in which the brain is organized and built, there's also a vulnerability that you can go too far down that road," he said. "There's still a lot that we don't know and understand. We have these words that we use to describe these realities, but words have their limitations."

The weeks when birth parents commonly experience the most intense parental preoccupation—when even walking through a doorway becomes a treacherous act, lest the baby's head accidentally bump the jamb—overlap with the period in which researchers have documented activation of brain circuits that essentially amplify the baby. In this sense, parental motivation seems to be deliberately colored by worry. The lens of a parent's attention fixates on their child just as the potential threat of the objects that cross that plane seems to grow. The result can feel like a cruel trick, or a sometimes-burdensome, bewildering superpower.

Over time, the act of caring for a baby becomes a kind of exposure therapy. You take your baby out into the world—for a trip to the grocery store, a long weekend to see family, or eventually into the wild terrain of solid foods—and he is OK. You are OK. You do it again. Meanwhile there is joy, too, and that joy grows and, hopefully, the worry eases. Ideally, the waters begin to settle. You realize that the ache and the sweetness have the same source, and so perhaps you negotiate to accept some of one for more of the other.

For most parents, the intense preoccupation of the first weeks begins to diminish by about the fourth month postpartum, when parents report an increase in positive thoughts, including about their own ability to parent a baby who can now smile and coo back at them. And parents generally report less preoccupation and worry the second time around. It's not only that they are experienced and have a clearer, conscious understanding of what to expect with subsequent children, though certainly that is a factor. But the neurobiology of parenting subsequent children is different.

For one thing, it's thought that just as the parenting experience is shifting toward something more pleasant, birthing parents' neural activity is shifting, too—from the amygdala and other regions implicated in feelings of alarm and vigilance, to areas involved in emotion regulation, including the medial prefrontal cortex. Pereira, who is now based at the University of Massachusetts, and Joan Morrell have found that, in rat mothers, maternal responses become "more distributed" in the brain as the postpartum period progresses, with more brain regions becoming involved. Among other changes, the goal of the MPOA seems to shift over time. Or rather, the goal stays the same: to make a mother respond flexibly. But the means are different. Instead of being the intense organizer and distributor of infant signals to motivational circuits, the MPOA becomes a kind of blocker, inhibiting overexpression of maternal behavior so that the mother can be responsive to what older pups need, including more independence and a different learning environment as they grow.

Plus, in both rodents and humans, changes to the parental brain stick. In a pair of studies, Rutherford and colleagues at Yale used an electroencephalogram, or EEG, to measure specific electrical activity in the cortex, thought to indicate attentional processing, in fifty-nine women as they viewed infant faces. The women were tested at two months and seven months postpartum. About half of them had prior pregnancies. Compared to the first-time mothers, the more experienced ones showed activity of a lower average amplitude to infant faces, which the researchers said could be interpreted as a more efficient processing or a less intensely reactive one.

Rutherford said she often hears from study participants about just how anxious they were with their first child and how different it was the second time around. She thinks it's helpful to be able to tell them that's a reflection of the neural reorganization they experienced as new parents. "We think that first-time parenting is so important, because it really sets the foundation for thinking about second-time parenting and beyond that, too," she said.

My husband and I got lucky when Hartley was born in 2015. Dr. Steven Blumenthal, a beloved, longtime pediatrician, was on duty at the hospital. When he first came to examine our tiny son, my body buzzed with anxiety. He handled Hartley expertly, of course, and listened to our concerns: I was struggling to breastfeed. Hartley didn't seem to be able to suck quite like he should, and my milk hadn't come in. Plus, he was so small. Dr. Blumenthal gently rolled our baby from one palm to the other, looking him over from all sides. He paused and looked at us, smiling. "There's nothing that you can say," he told us, "that will make me worry about this baby." Over and over in the months that followed I heard his voice in my head and willed myself to have faith that he was right.

Dr. Blumenthal retired soon after our second son, Ashley, was born in 2017. Still, I heard his voice. And this time, I believed him.

*   *   *

IT REALLY WOULD BE A cruel trick if new parenthood opened parents to the flood of infant stimuli without offering any way to control the spigot. Thankfully—for parents, babies, and the future of our species, which depends on people's willingness to have children—there is a flip side to all the hypersensitivity of those early weeks.

An infant's cry stirs a parent to act, and cortical regions respond to help them put that cry into context. Studies have found structural and functional changes in parts of the maternal brain involved in self-regulation. Those include the prefrontal cortex and cingulate cortex, where researchers have documented long-lasting changes in the volume of gray matter and heightened responses to own-baby cues.

Rutherford and her colleagues have suggested that the way the brain regulates emotions in the postpartum period may be distinct from how it does so in any other time of life, because of the intense emotional demands and the fact that babies have virtually no capacity for regulating themselves. She thinks of the parent as the baby's "external prefrontal cortex." A baby cries because she is hungry and a parent feeds her and burps her and helps her to feel regulated again. A baby cries because he is tired and a parent swaddles him and rocks him and holds him close until he is calm. It can take a lot of energy to do those things while muting one's own exhaustion or frustration or worry. And, Rutherford said, parents generally aren't very good at this to start. It might begin as a kind of conscious awareness, a reminder: *I can do this. Take a deep breath.* Over time, though, the capacity to self-regulate while paying attention and addressing a child's need may become more habitual.

To be clear, that does not mean parents should never get upset or feel dysregulated themselves. Rather, it's a matter of building their capacity to deal with their own emotions while tending to another, often wildly dysregulated being. And that could be important for the life of a parent in the long term. Helping a baby to regulate their emotions is different from helping a grade-schooler or a teenager. But doing so may draw on the same skills, Rutherford said. "You need to have those skills built up," she told me, to create a "lifelong capacity to be able to advance those and sculpt those in different ways."

In her writing on addiction and parenting, Rutherford explains that truly addressing the nature of drug use or relapse in parents won't be possible without recognizing the life stage they've entered, one that differentiates them from nonparents at "behavioral, cognitive, and neurobiological levels." Understanding and addressing postpartum mood and anxiety disorders depends on that knowledge, too. So does grappling with what parenthood means for a person's own life and their sense of self. Rutherford told me she often gets pushback on the idea that parents are different, occasionally when applying for grants for her work and more often when talking, for example, with colleagues outside her field who respond with disbelief. "Parenting is a big change in life," she said, "whether you are willing to admit it or not."

I met Rutherford in her "before" days, about four months before her daughter, Amelia, was born. Struggling through those early weeks postpartum, particularly while an ocean away from her family in England and distanced from local social support because of the pandemic, made Rutherford think about new approaches to her work. How can the lab capture the particular changes in quality of sleep, not just quantity, that comes with parenthood and analyze how that affects the brain? What

about a baby's changing temperament? She also learned from the pleasure of parenting, from the drive she felt to engage with Amelia when
she woke up in the morning, the joy she felt while playing together, and
the reinforcement that brought.

The neural reorganization of pregnancy and the postpartum period
is aimed in large part at helping just such a drive to develop. "It doesn't
have to always be this young love affair," Rutherford said. "But your baby
needs to eat or your baby needs to be held, and just being able to offer
that is enough. Then anything else on top of that is going to be amazing."
Maybe doing enough—holding and listening and responding—*is* love.

The great poet Mary Oliver urged us to bring children to the woods
and "stand them in the stream," to plant in them a love of nature. "Attention," she wrote, "is the beginning of devotion." This is true in parenthood, too. Attention is the first task. Before all else. The rush of hormones
during pregnancy and childbirth and the persuasiveness of babies make
sure we provide it. We become hooked, so that our infants can go to work
as the master manipulators they are, armed with smiles and coos and
chubby cheeks. What happens next is a kind of entwining. Our sense of
self grows. It extends to include more than it did before.

If I could go back and change one thing about my own transition
to parenthood, it might be this: I would make Oliver's sentiment my
motto. *Attention is the beginning of devotion.* Frame those words. Hang
them over the bassinet.

CHAPTER 4

Our Babies, Our Selves

Elizabeth could tell when her daughter was struggling. Claire's mouth would begin to quiver just slightly. The air in her room on the neonatal intensive care unit seemed to shift, as the baby's congested breathing quieted. Elizabeth knew her daughter was about to "spell." Moments later, alarms would buzz when Claire's heart rate or blood oxygen level dropped precipitously, sometimes to life-threatening levels, and staff would rush in to suction out the baby's airways or otherwise stabilize her.

Claire had arrived by emergency C-section at a Boston hospital, a month or so after a routine ultrasound had detected excess amniotic fluid. The fluid grew in volume, and then Elizabeth's water broke as she turned over in bed on a Sunday morning, at thirty-three weeks and four days—early but not *so* early. Elizabeth had been encouraged by that. But it quickly became clear that her baby wasn't only born prematurely.

Claire often had bubbles or froth around her mouth, and her care team suspected that she had a swallowing problem, something Elizabeth remembered a doctor citing as a possible cause of excess amniotic fluid. But no one could offer a clear diagnosis or even a sense of whether her swallowing was an isolated physiological challenge or part of a broader developmental concern. "From early on, there were just these sort of question marks hovering around her," Elizabeth told me.

The uncertainty was terrifying. Paralyzing, really. Elizabeth struggled to talk to the NICU providers, worried that any question she asked about a potential diagnosis or treatment would be met only with a heart-splitting response. She dropped her gaze when she walked in the hallways of the hospital, afraid to meet their eyes. She would spend a long day at the hospital, still recovering from major surgery herself, then go home and eat oatmeal for dinner, crawl into bed by 8 p.m., and be up again at 2 a.m., awake and worried, in the dark.

Soon, her sister came from New York, bearing fortitude. Bring a Boppy pillow to the hospital, she told Elizabeth, and a mobile. Make the space your own. Hold your baby. "This is *your* baby," Elizabeth recalled her sister saying with a growl in her voice. The two left the hospital for breaks, to get pizza and for walks. Elizabeth started taking an anti-depressant.

Things shifted, not all at once and not evenly. Claire would spend six months in the hospital, transferring between three NICUs and a rehab hospital as providers tried to find a diagnosis and give her the care and therapy she needed in order to go home. On leave from her job as a teacher, Elizabeth would pack her lunch and something to read—typically a celebrity memoir, nothing too heavy—and spend hours on end holding her baby. Her sweet baby. Often, she or her husband would stay with Claire through much of the night. Other families would be discharged, their babies catching up to expected developmental milestones, seemingly "fixed," Elizabeth said. New ones would arrive. Claire remained. But her family's time in those hospitals began to feel less fearful.

Sometimes Elizabeth would alert a nurse or a doctor that a spell was coming, even before the alarms sounded. After hospital staff had stabilized Claire, someone would turn to Elizabeth with a look of congratulations, for her accurate prediction. For being faster than the monitors. More sensitive. More intuitive. "Nice job, Mom," they'd say.

Elizabeth *was* more. More of all those things than the machines were. More attuned to her baby than she even fully knew at the time. But, Elizabeth told me emphatically, this was not the result of a mystical link between mother and child, not some connection kept intact from the womb to a beeping isolation bassinet. She knows better than that. "It's not some divine relationship that we have," she said. "Or, maybe it is divine, but it's because I spent the hours to know." To see the patterned behaviors and the particularities of her own daughter, she said. To figure out how to respond to them. To be changed, herself, by her baby.

Babies capture the attention of the adults in their lives, and then they use it. They shape those adults, at a fundamental level, into parents. They make them into people who will direct the resources of their own brains and bodies to meet the needs of the brains and bodies of someone else—needs that can vary wildly from baby to baby, or from day to day. This takes knowing. Parents must be able to identify their child's needs, long before that child can ask for another snack, discuss the ups and downs of the school day, argue about the necessity of socks, or maintain eye contact—and even if their child's development limits their ability to do any of those things. Parents rely intensely on brain networks involved in perceiving and responding to another person's mental state, networks that are changed through pregnancy and through the work of caregiving.

Donald Winnicott, the psychoanalyst who described "primary maternal preoccupation," surmised that the initial hypersensitivity a new mother experiences allows her "to feel herself into her infant's place." Since then, researchers have found that the parental brain changes in ways suited precisely to that purpose. Circuitry involved in social cognition—how we read, interpret, and respond to cues from the people around us and from our broader social context—seems to strengthen and become highly responsive to the deluge of cues a baby provides. Researchers have theorized that this is the result of a kind of neurobiological linkage, an association of our own bodies to our babies'—whether or not we've birthed that baby—and that this link may be the foundation for human affiliation.

The connection between parent and child often is portrayed as something that happens in a particular sequence, with a particular feel, and almost always with a supreme emphasis on the mother-infant dyad, to the exclusion of all others. It is a closeness or an all-knowingness, an attachment grounded in preserving what is natural or primal. A forgotten magic. I do not doubt that's how it feels for some mothers. But that idea has never felt to me like it accurately represents the nature of family or of this stage of life, which is full of unexpected turns and hard days or months or years. Which is characterized as much by disconnect—the uncrossable chasm between one person's inner life and another's—as it is by connection. The parental brain, and not just the maternal brain, accounts for all this. Through its inherent flexibility, it expands our capacity to stretch beyond ourselves, to get a little closer, at least, to the other side.

For parents like Elizabeth and her husband, connecting with a newborn comes with particular challenges. Claire didn't come home after delivery. Elizabeth didn't have the chance to breastfeed as she might have. And Claire spent her days connected to monitors and a feeding tube. Then there's the fact that babies born prematurely are generally much less able to send the cues that other newborns might, through coos or cries, grasping or turning their heads, or developing even somewhat recognizable eating and sleeping patterns.

A few years ago, a group of researchers in Italy analyzed the brains of ten mothers of very preterm infants, all born before thirty-two weeks or who weighed less than about 3.3 pounds. The mothers' brains were scanned while they viewed images of their own baby and an unknown baby, in states of happiness or distress or with neutral expressions. The researchers compared those brain-scan images to the scans of mothers of full-term infants and found distinct differences in the patterns of brain activity between the two groups. The study was small and limited by the fact that the preterm infants were all relatively healthy, without other clinical complications. Still, the findings were fascinating.

For both sets of mothers, the brain scans showed stronger responses to their own infant than to a stranger's, but the mothers of preterm infants showed even higher activation in areas related to emotion processing and social cognition. In that group, the researchers found heightened activity in the inferior frontal gyrus, a region of the prefrontal cortex thought to be involved in decoding facial expressions or socially relevant cues. That was true when that group looked at all infants, but especially when viewing their own and even more when seeing images of their baby in distress. The NICU mothers also showed higher activity in the left supramarginal gyrus while viewing their own babies, no matter the expression. That's a part of the parietal lobe that previously had been implicated in perception of infant faces and cries.

The mothers of preterm babies were responding to their conditions of parenthood by effectively working harder to read their vulnerable baby's limited cues, "to successfully respond to the infant's needs and to promote their survival," the researchers concluded.

The findings hint at what leaders of neonatal intensive care units around the world have recognized in recent years. Even in the NICU, where babies are surrounded by professionals who have dedicated their lives to understanding and caring for tiny people just like them, parents are key. Thirty years ago, babies in the NICU were typically kept in one large room, and parents were invited to visit during limited hours. Over time, those visiting hours were expanded and eventually eliminated, and parents were seen in a whole new light. "They're not visitors," said Dr. Carmina Erdei, a neonatologist and pediatrician who directs the Growth and Development Unit within the NICU at Brigham and Women's Hospital and who cared for Claire. "They are parents. They're caregivers. They're family. They're the most important people in the baby's life at that time."

Hospitals are reimagining the role for parents in different ways. In one model, called Family Integrated Care, parents become active, present members of their baby's NICU team. They participate in daily rounds with the providers, give oral medications themselves, monitor and chart their baby's progress, and discuss what they see with the nursing staff. They receive coaching from nurses on how to bathe or dress or position their babies, and they participate in educational sessions about child development, parenting a preterm infant, or coping with stress. A large study compared that model with standard NICU care across twenty-six hospitals in Canada, Australia, and New Zealand and found that infants whose parents were closely involved in their care saw significantly higher weight gain day by day. After three weeks, those parents also scored better on measures of stress and anxiety.

Instituting such a model, which requires parents to be in the NICU at least six hours a day, is challenging in the United States, Erdei said. Unlike in the three countries included in the study above, the United States has no national paid parental leave program. Many parents have to go back to work while their child is in the NICU because they do not have leave from work or because their jobs allow so little leave that they must reserve it for after the baby is discharged. Still, the Brigham and many other hospitals are finding ways to involve families in care more and more.

Parents in the Brigham NICU are encouraged to lead the daily check-in with their baby's care team—a job that otherwise is done by a resident or another clinician-in-training, Erdei explained. Babies often are cared for in single-family rooms with couches that fold out for parents who are able to stay overnight. And the NICU staff works closely with a team of perinatal mental health providers to get parents who are struggling with the trauma and stress of having a preterm infant the help they need, so they can be engaged in their own development as parents, she said.

"It's the concept that really, the parent is and should be the primary caregiver for the baby, and that they really know their baby the best," Erdei said. "They often are able to understand [the baby's] cues and respond better than any provider, no matter how good we are."

When Elizabeth and her husband brought Claire home for the first time in January 2020, they had no diagnosis. When I spoke with her again nearly a year later, they still didn't have one. At nineteen months, Claire was a cheerful toddler making progress in therapy, but she could not crawl or talk or eat by mouth. If her daughter had been born full-term and healthy, Elizabeth suspects she would have been the kind of mother who reads parenting books, closely watching her baby's development and comparing it with what's expected for a typical baby. She might have sleep trained at some point. Now, she said, none of that industry advice seems relevant to her or to her family.

"I continue *not* to look at milestones or developmental resources online, because I know that is not her trajectory," Elizabeth said. "I know that now, and it took me awhile to understand it. . . . Maybe my daughter won't be able to walk, and I will, and that will be a profound difference between us, and I can't change that, but I can also be very OK with it. And that will be helpful to her."

The list of things that Elizabeth worries about, now and for the future, is long. But, she said, there's also a certain freedom in recognizing who her child is and what her challenges may be, in having already begun a process that is inherent to parenthood, of consciously grappling with the idea that her child is a separate person whose life is affixed to her own but whose trajectory is, in many important ways, beyond her control. It's a process she's watched other parent friends go through as their child struggles in school or with emotional challenges or through adolescence. Claire was just twelve hours old when Elizabeth learned that her daughter would be different from the baby she had expected her to be. From that point on, all Elizabeth's parenting has been about meeting Claire where she is.

* * *

THERE IS A CENTRAL CHARACTERISTIC of the brain that seems to crystallize in parenthood: it is predictive. I feel this most viscerally when it comes to the physical safety of my two rambunctious sons. I turn from a conversation with a friend at a playground, barely breaking my sentence, and catch my two-year-old midair as he leaps from a too-high platform. Or, as my boys grapple in the living room, transformed into lion cubs or hyenas, I feel my muscles primed and ready to intervene in the moment just before they slip too far into the wildness.

This is not a characteristic particular to parenting, of course. The brain is predictive by design. In 1988, neurobiologist Peter Sterling and epidemiologist Joseph Eyer outlined their concept of allostasis, or "stability through change," by which the brain anticipates the demands on the body, regulates its various organs and systems to meet them, then uses success or failure to adjust future predictions. The fact that our bodies contain limited resources but must respond efficiently to the ever-changing circumstances of our lives (and the ever-evolving nature of our species—of all species) depends on this fact. But the concept of allostasis was a challenge to the dominant idea of homeostasis, which long assumed that a person's organs were controlled more or less locally, through negative feedback loops that corrected errors in order to stay within set parameters of optimal operation. The goal of homeostasis was constancy, not change.

Sterling is a lifelong activist, and he explained in his book *What Is Health? Allostasis and the Evolution of Human Design* how his thinking on allostasis stemmed in part from his own internal conflict between spending time in the laboratory as a student of neuroanatomy and spending time in the streets, working on social justice and anti-war campaigns. When he joined the faculty at the University of Pennsylvania, his colleagues, including Eyer, encouraged him to look for the places where his interests overlapped. He had noticed a higher prevalence of stroke in the poor, mostly Black neighborhood of Cleveland he often canvassed while at Western Reserve University. Textbooks would tell him that stroke and underlying chronic hypertension were caused by too much salt intake and a person's inherited intolerance to salt—lifestyle choices and bad genes. "No role for the brain; no role for racism," Sterling wrote.

The dominant model of medicine might take measurements of a person's blood pressure, label high values "inappropriate," and assign a treatment, typically a drug or a combination of drugs, to bring those values back within an optimal range. Allostasis suggests that high blood pressure may be the result of poverty or systemic racism, and the chronic stress they induce is a perfectly "appropriate" response, though not a healthy one. Treatment could include both encouraging individuals to reduce stress, through rest, play, or exercise, and changing society.

That latter goal is hard, and allostasis has been a somewhat controversial idea. Some have argued that a new concept is unnecessary, because the modern notion of homeostasis has evolved to include the regulatory role of the brain. Others have proposed models of their own, recasting or weaving together the two. No matter what you call it, the idea that our brains are constantly adjusting to try to make better predictions in the future has changed—or should change—how we look at health. It's given researchers better insight into how environmental and systemic factors, particularly the stresses of trauma or poverty in early childhood, can affect a person's lifelong health, for example. It has a lot to tell us about parenthood, too.

Sterling wrote that the brain keeps a kind of "shopping list" of basic needs, which are constantly updated—water, salt, glucose, temperature regulation, and so on. A person is driven toward fulfilling those needs through a carrot-and-stick system. The stick is the anxiety that comes in anticipating those needs, with the salience-detecting amygdala playing a key role. The carrot is the release of dopamine to the nucleus accumbens and prefrontal cortex, when that need is met. The balance between the two, anxiety (or effort) and pleasure (or satisfaction)—and sometimes the imbalance between them—allows the brain to learn from experience and adjust its future predictions.

Neuroscientist Lisa Feldman Barrett describes allostasis as "body budgeting." All organisms have limited resources that can be drawn down quickly and that may require sleep or food for renewal. The availability of those things (a new parent knows well) is not always guaranteed. So even single-celled organisms make predictions to determine whether a given activity is worth the resources it requires. In more complex creatures, the brain developed as the "command center" for those calculations. Human brains have evolved to make predictions not only about our bodies' internal needs but also about our needs in relation to members of the social species to which we belong. "Your body budget is like thousands of financial accounts in a giant, multinational corporation, and you have a brain that's up to the task," Barrett wrote in *Seven and a Half Lessons about the Brain*. "And all your body budgeting takes place in a massively complicated world made even more challenging by the other brains-in-bodies that you share it with."

We're up to the task. That's comforting. Yet new parenthood—to extend the corporate metaphor—is a time of disruption. It is a major acquisition, finalized before anyone has seen the target company's books. Babies arrive as mostly unknown entities. Their resources—those pleasure-inducing sounds and smells, those heavy-lidded marbles of wonder—become your resources. Their needs become your needs.

Before I ever was pregnant, my brain's shopping list included the basics of food and water and shelter and connection, and I had a routine for meeting them, a path I'd walk at the grocery store, an order for checking items off my list, and a predictable temptation or two from off-list items that would make it into my cart. When my first son was born, his needs somewhat abruptly took the top spot on my shopping list. All of his needs. All of mine. Now it was as if I were clumsily pushing two shopping carts through the aisle, one with a wiggly wheel and piled high with sustenance, the other carrying a tiny baby in a car seat who could do little more than track the fluorescent lights on the grocery store ceiling as they rolled by overhead. Still, my brain worked to predict his needs, driven by the push-pull of anxiety and reward, refining those predictions through dopamine-driven learning. Parents become the orchestrators of allostasis on behalf of their baby's body while also maintaining their own regulation. But *how*? How can the parental brain understand the needs of a baby, communicated through what often seems like a previously undiscovered language?

* * *

EVERY PERSON HAS AN INTERNAL system for prediction, for gauging the current and future needs of the body and determining which resources are required to meet those needs. A broad network of brain regions coordinates to sense a person's internal state and to make sense of it, a process referred to as interoception. This is about far more than taking inventory of the physical body. It's thought that the brain creates a kind of mental representation of bodily sensations, attaches concepts of emotion and abstraction to it, and uses that representation like a barometer to anticipate potential future conditions, based on past experiences. This process also provides a sense of self in space and time—separate from and in relation to other people—what neuroscientist A. D. Craig called "the fundamental image of the physical self as a feeling (sentient) entity."

Barrett and her colleagues have proposed that this process of prediction is carried out through a distributed system in the brain made up of the salience network, discussed in chapter 3, and what's known as the default mode network. Together, these networks form what the researchers called "a high-capacity backbone for integrating information across the entire brain."

In the default mode network, we have yet another case of a brain system that has outgrown its name. When researchers collect images of people's brains engaged in particular tasks, they often also look at the brain before or after those tasks as an experimental control, when the test subjects are essentially at rest. By the mid-1990s, researchers had noticed a web of brain regions that were more active at rest and that showed a relative decline in activity when a person began a task. This, they thought, represented the brain's passive baseline state, or default mode. For years, researchers either ignored the brain's resting state entirely or figured it had very little value in terms of controlling the function of the brain. This was simply the brain at rest, in a drifting daydream. In 2001, a group of researchers from Washington University in Missouri challenged that idea, by pointing out that brain regions that were more active at rest were the same ones associated with self-referential processing. They suggested the default network was essential to how the brain constructs the narrative of the "multifaceted 'self.'"

The default mode network—with hubs generally in the medial prefrontal cortex, the inferior parietal lobule, the precuneus, and the posterior cingulate cortex—is not a do-little default system at all. It plays a key role in our internal life, in how we recall memories about ourselves and use them to build an ongoing autobiography, to solve problems (including moral dilemmas), and to simulate alternate outcomes and future needs. A fundamental characteristic of the default mode is that understanding the self goes hand in hand with understanding others. The default mode network repeatedly has been shown to encompass people's "theory of mind" and mentalization: their capacity to perceive another person's beliefs, emotions, and mental states. One seminal paper described its function as a "'life simulator'—a set of interacting subsystems that can use past experiences to explore and anticipate social and event scenarios." In parenthood, research suggests, this network changes.

Several studies have linked motherhood to altered activity in components of the default mode network, or to overlapping regions generally thought to support mentalization. In one, mothers and nonmothers were asked to carry out a goal-oriented task (counting syllables) that would typically be expected to deactivate the default mode network, while also listening to a baby's cry and other emotional sounds. In the mothers—but not the nonmothers—hubs of that network remained partially active during the task. Researchers suggested this may reflect a redistribution of mothers' cognitive resources toward the infant cry and other sounds, as socially salient and potentially self-relevant cues. These findings might make sense to any parent who has rushed to meet a deadline before the end of nap time, engaged in the work at hand *and* entirely aware of the sounds of a stirring baby. Other studies have compared mothers with postpartum depression to those without and found differences in resting state connectivity in ways thought to underline the importance of those brain regions to a healthy adaptation to parenthood.

In one remarkable study, researchers based in Spain and the Netherlands looked at the anatomy of the brains of women before they were pregnant, after childbirth, and two years postpartum. After pregnancy, the women showed significant loss in gray matter volume spanning the midline of the brain, including the medial frontal cortex, precuneus, and the posterior cingulate cortex. Loss in this case is thought to represent an adaptive fine-tuning, and the changes overlapped significantly with the theory-of-mind network. The research group then followed up with a subset of those women and found that most changes persisted at least six years postpartum. These studies are worth spending more time on, which we'll do in the next chapter. But for now, the point is that having a baby seems to restructure parts of the brain involved in processing social interactions and our sense of ourselves within a social context, and many of those changes may be permanent.

The body of evidence in fathers is smaller, but researchers have found that brain regions involved in mentalizing activate when fathers are exposed to infant cues. Among them is the superior temporal sulcus, discussed in chapter 3 for its activation in primary- and secondary-caregiving fathers—a brain region implicated in social cognition and prediction making. When researchers looked at the brains of fathers and nonfathers as they viewed images of children (not their own), they found a bunch of differences in regions related to reading the emotional cues of others and interpreting their mental states. The areas of heightened activation in fathers lined up with the default mode hubs, and the researchers noted that it's possible fathers find even the faces of children unknown to them to be more "self-relevant" than nonfathers do, because they draw connections to their own child.

If these social and self-referential brain networks are changed by pregnancy and parenthood, then what does that mean exactly about parents' sense of self—how we experience our internal lives as part of the world around us? The research to date is a long way from answering that question. And really, it's not a question science will ever fully answer for us at an individual level. Still, it's a fascinating one to consider.

Winnie Orchard, a researcher based in Australia whose work also explores the long-term structural effects of parenthood, told me that she sees the changes in the default mode network as reflective of how a person's "self extends a little further" in parenthood, to encompass the child. All that daydreaming and rumination, all that work of interoception, the capturing of our internal selves and the stories we build from that information and use to anticipate whatever may come next—our kids become central characters in that narrative, and the future we plan for is theirs, too.

* * *

IT MAKES SENSE THAT A brain network so involved in interpreting our body's internal state is changed by having a baby. After all, for the forty weeks or so of gestation, a baby is a literal part of a birthing parent—and in many ways remains so. The birthing body becomes a body that has carried a child. In its incredible capacity for lactation, and as a result of the hormonal and metabolic changes that requires. In its shifting weight and shape. In separated abdominal muscles or an altered pelvic floor. In the trauma and healing of pregnancy and childbirth, layered over the trauma and healing of life before. In the very common experience of phantom fetal kicks, which many people report feeling for years after pregnancy. Or in the fetal cells that cross the placenta and can set up long-term residency in a birthing parent's body—and in the bodies of people who have had a miscarriage or an abortion—including in the brain, a little-understood phenomenon known as microchimerism.

Out of the womb, babies shape their caregivers' body budgets. They dramatically alter sleeping, eating, and exercising habits. They dominate the waking hours, reshape the family's social life, require near-constant physical contact, and so change their caregivers' subconscious existence in the world that the adults find themselves rocking back and forth on the balls of their feet as if to calm a sleepy baby even when standing alone in a grocery line. As one group of researchers put it, the boundary between self and other is "as permeable as the umbilical cord" during gestation. After birth, babies require so much from their parents that the line "is further blurred, extending the enmeshment that occurs in the womb into the realm of daily life." Babies depend on it. They depend on their parents to take care of them, to help them to survive and thrive, of course. They also depend on their caregivers to show them how to be a human among other humans, to be part of a social species.

That may sound like a high-minded goal, a divine one even. But the mother-infant bond is the most common and most enduring social bond across mammalian species. Maternal behavior is "the most primordial caregiving system" among mammals, wrote Michael Numan and Larry Young, whose work has been fundamental to understanding the neuroscience of parenting in other animals and in finding the parts most relevant to humans. The neural circuitry involved in maternal behavior likely provided the "neural scaffold" upon which other bonds were built, including those between mating pairs and within broader kinship structures. Maternal motivation, they wrote, may have been the evolutionary foundation for empathy, altruism, trust, and cooperation—so many of the characteristics by which we define human nature.

We might think about the complete dependence of newborns on their parents as a limitation that allowed for the primate brain to grow and the pelvis to change shape so that humans could walk on two legs. But that vulnerability also was an opportunity. It created a dynamic in which the basic architecture of a baby's brain is developing when the baby is out in the world, living in tandem with at least one other human being. The brain development that occurs in that context supports the complex web of relationships that stretches across a person's lifetime. Babies' basic bodily needs must be met. Parents must meet those needs by adjusting their own. The human brain enables this by making baby and parent reliant on one another.

Different models have been proposed to explain this co-regulation. Ruth Feldman, the Simms-Mann professor of developmental social neuroscience at the Interdisciplinary Center in Herzliya, Israel, describes this as "biobehavioral synchrony." A mother-infant pair coordinates biological responses (heart rate, oxytocin levels, and neural activity), while also matching behaviors (gaze, affectionate touch, and vocalizations). Think of the quiet euphoria when a baby with a full belly falls asleep on her parent's chest. Or the rhythmic exchange of reactions in a game of peekaboo. The brains of parent and infant become tuned to one another, particularly during moments of social engagement.

When we connect with friends, romantic partners, and colleagues, and even as we view ourselves as a member of a sports team or as part of a nation—in moments that are often less quiet but perhaps also euphoric—we "repurpose the basic machinery" established in the connection between parent and baby, Feldman wrote. For the role it plays in species survival and its ability to teach the sociality that is so much a part of human nature, she called the parental brain "a peak expression of human evolution."

Neurobiologist Shir Atzil and her colleagues, including Barrett, relate this connection to allostasis. There are all sorts of ways parents tend to their newborns and regulate their body budgets. They feed them. They fret over the right number of layers in winter and the right sun protection in summer. They nurse and sing and shush and stroke their cheeks to calm them. A baby has a need and learns that, whenever that need is met, a parent is there, said Atzil, who leads the Bonding Neuroscience Laboratory at the Hebrew University of Jerusalem. That cycle repeats over and over, every day and through the night. By the time the baby is one week old, Atzil told me, "they've already had hundreds of trials, learning that mommy equals reward. Daddy equals reward. Human equals reward."

The brain circuitry that supports a baby's allostasis and social processing—the salience network and the default mode network, plus the information superhighways that connect them—is still very much under development. It takes years to develop, during which these interactions with the adults who care for him are wiring his brain to understand that other humans are essential to getting his own needs met. Humans aren't born with a predetermined "social brain," the researchers proposed, "but rather biologically adapt to become social as a result of allostasis dependency."

This idea highlights the flexibility of parenting in a couple of important and exciting ways. First, if social affiliation is essentially a skill that babies acquire through their parents—and the broader social context around them—then parenting is clearly a powerful evolutionary tool for transferring the cultural knowledge and behaviors necessary to thrive within a particular community or social niche, far more quickly than natural selection would allow. And, it seems, the role of a parent in this case can be filled by any adult capable of lovingly meeting a baby's needs.

(It's worth noting that this social dependency model is not limited to mammals. Most birds are social, and their babies can't survive without a committed parent. They've formed various caregiving structures, often involving both mothers and fathers and sometimes other adults, through which complex social behaviors are passed.)

Then there is this fundamental point about allostasis that is also a fundamental point about parenting: it is life or death. It's not ultimately about regulating a person's emotions or arousal. It's about regulating their basic physiology, Atzil told me. What new parent doesn't feel the weight of this truth in their first hours and days at home with a newborn? "I mean, this is it," Atzil said. "This is a mind-blowing experience. You have to take care of this infant. . . . You have to be super attentive. You have to be super motivated. You have to pay attention, and then you become a caregiver. This neurocircuitry is strengthened."

In 2017, Atzil and Barrett published a paper, with a group of researchers, that further clarified the circuitry in human mothers. Using a scanner that combines fMRI and positron emission tomography, or PET, they studied the brains of nineteen women as they observed videos of their own children and unfamiliar children. The women had babies aged four months to two years old, and none were breastfeeding. With the help of a tracer injected into the mother's arm that binds to unoccupied dopamine receptors in the brain, the researchers could compare the mothers' dopamine responses when viewing the infants. Simultaneously, they used fMRI to examine connectivity between brain regions that make up what is referred to as the medial amygdala network, including hubs in the nucleus accumbens, hypothalamus, medial prefrontal cortex, and posterior cingulate cortex. The researchers also observed the women in their homes, coding the degree to which they responded to their infants' cues for social engagement, through their vocalizations and broader behavior.

The study found that mothers who showed more synchronous behaviors, meaning they were more sensitive and responsive to their baby's cues, had a greater dopamine response to their own babies than to others. Mothers who showed low synchrony had a stronger dopamine response to the novel unknown infants. The more synchronous mothers also showed stronger intrinsic connectivity in the medial amygdala network. Network connectivity and dopamine were linked, too—those with stronger connectivity also had increased dopamine in key network hubs when they viewed their own children. The researchers concluded that, just as animal studies have suggested, maternal bonding in humans relies on dopamine responses, particularly within this network important for social processing.

The medial amygdala network is like a multi-span bridge between salience detection and mentalization. Atzil told me this network, and the dopamine that acts on it, seems to be central to how the brain processes all those urgent social and allostatic cues and attaches ideas about *self* and *other*, those abstract ideas that form the basis for future predictions.

Just as babies are creating mental models of the people who care for them, parents create predictive models of their babies. They have to, because taking care of a baby requires so much energy. "When you're hungry, your brain gets a notice from your body that you're hungry. When your infant is hungry, you don't have a receptor in your body that signals that," Atzil said. "You have to be so attentive, so immersed in your infant's very subtle cues in order to realize that they're going to be hungry." And parents don't typically wait until a baby is screaming to feed her. Instead, they learn from her cues and build a concept that helps them to anticipate that hunger, so they might even stir from their sleep before she ever utters a sound, knowing that the time is coming. That model is built from brain systems that process anxiety and reward, our sense of ourselves over time and our sense of others.

Atzil and her colleagues made another interesting finding in the same paper. They collected the mothers' blood to measure circulating, or peripheral, oxytocin, and found that oxytocin level was inversely related to the network connectivity and dopamine responses. Stronger connectivity in the medial amygdala network meant *lower* circulating oxytocin. Peripheral oxytocin is used as a very loose proxy for central oxytocin secreted in the brain, though there's no clear link between the two in humans. Scientists don't yet have a way to closely study the neuropeptide's activity in the brain. They're still figuring out exactly where oxytocin receptors reside; while they have made great strides in recent years, they lack the minimally invasive techniques necessary to track it. This finding suggests that bonding-related activity in the brain is not dependent on an increased level of oxytocin in the plasma. Just the opposite, in fact.

We often are told a story about the all-powerful nature of oxytocin, the "love hormone," about how it washes over birthing parents in the moments after their child arrives and during breastfeeding to make them fall in love, or how it fills a partner's cup the first time they hold their child. That story is "just not true," Atzil told me. "It doesn't work like that." It's not that oxytocin doesn't play a critical role. It does. It stimulates contractions and promotes labor. It enables milk letdown. Oxytocin is a driver of the dopaminergic system that shapes human maternal motivation. Stronger spikes in circulating oxytocin have been correlated with more affectionate behavior by mothers and more stimulatory interactions by fathers. Higher baseline plasma oxytocin has been linked to greater activation of the nucleus accumbens and more synchronous behavior between mother and baby. But it's the linear or even mystical nature of that story, the notion that a surge in oxytocin acts like pixie dust to fuse the maternal-infant bond, that's so problematic, or what Atzil called a "wrongful simplification."

For one thing, baseline plasma oxytocin does not generally differ between breastfeeding and formula-feeding parents. Or between men and women. Oxytocin is not a love hormone. It does not even seem to be explicitly "prosocial." For example, it may play a role in processing fear signals in social contexts for humans, and in rodents it's been linked to maternal aggression toward intruders. Increasingly, it is thought of even more broadly as a regulatory agent that facilitates survival and adaptation through flexibility.

Oxytocin is involved in all sorts of processes that keep the human body operating efficiently, including in the cardiovascular and gastrointestinal systems. Its role in energy metabolism seems to have really ancient roots, predating the evolution of vertebrates. Biological psychiatry researchers Daniel Quintana and Adam Guastella have proposed that oxytocin evolved to have a central role in learning and behavior responses to better predict and manage the body's energy needs. It's not that oxytocin is all about love or bonding. Oxytocin is all about allostasis. In fact, Quintana and Guastella write, it should be called an "allostatic hormone."

The finding by Atzil and her colleagues points to how much we have to learn about oxytocin's allostatic role in the context of bonding. What is clear is that it does not happen all at once or through a single mechanism. It is continuous, and it's also reciprocal.

It has to be. Humans are wildly diverse. And while babies continue to develop in the arms of their caregivers, they also arrive with their own genetic makeup, their own temperaments, their own distinct needs. As the study of NICU mothers indicates, the parental brain seems to adjust to predict and meet those needs—the needs of one's own particular baby.

In a separate study, researchers in Mexico City looked at how groups of mothers processed infant faces. They scanned the brains of mothers whose children were developing typically and mothers of children who were autistic. Their children were older—preschool or early school aged—so the mothers viewed babies who weren't their own. Still, the researchers found what they called "an adaptive neural specialization" among the mothers of children with autism, with a lateralized cortical response (stronger activity on the right side, linked to emotion processing) that was more pronounced the more sensitive and responsive a mother was observed to be toward her own child. The researchers couldn't say whether this difference was innate to the mother's biology or the result of her experience as a parent. But, once again, they suggested that having a child with particular needs, in this case a developmental difference that can affect a child's own social processing and communication, prompted the brain to respond differently, to better identify and react to the child's emotions.

Animal research could offer some clues as to just how the parental brain adjusts in this way. University of Massachusetts behavioral neuroscientist Mariana Pereira and her colleagues, who have made important findings about the flexibility of the maternal brain in rats and the changing function of the medial preoptic area, or MPOA, now are taking a closer look at *how* rat mothers adjust. Recall that the MPOA acts like a kind of receiver, taking in a lot of pup stimuli and initiating a response. In research not yet published as of the writing of this book (and therefore not yet vetted through peer review), the researchers deactivated the MPOA in experienced mother rats and then presented them with pups with varying needs. Some were newborn or slightly older, well-cared-for pups. Others were made extremely needy by being separated from maternal care for half a day. The mothers cared for all the pups. But compared to a typical response by a mother rat with a functional MPOA, they did not lick and groom the demanding pups as much and they spent less time in contact with them in general, despite the pups' urgent cues for warmth, food, and attention. In other words, they couldn't efficiently read the pups' needs and adjust accordingly.

Next, the researchers planned to present experienced mother rats with demanding or nondemanding pups and then map the specific differences in the MPOA response and its projections to other key brain regions. This is the basic science of the parental brain, but it could have real-world applications.

When mother rats who are bred to have qualities similar to depression are given pups with varying needs, they also struggle to match their care to the pups' demands. Pereira said the ultimate goal of this research is to gain insight into how best to support struggling parents, to create drugs that promote parental sensitivity in people with postpartum depression, for example, or to make promising interventions, such as mindfulness programs, more targeted to parental care. That is very important and worthwhile, and at the same time I'm interested in simply knowing more about how the parental brain adjusts to babies for whom there is no factory model, or to the changing dynamics of a growing family in which each child arrives with their own quirks and needs. "That's the beauty of the parental brain," Pereira told me, "that it has to remain very open and flexible so that you can actually see your kids."

Researchers have a long way to go in understanding the interplay between a parent's brain and a baby's, let alone siblings and other family members. Some have called for more studies of the transactive nature of brains, to include examining parent-child interactions in real time. That work is limited in humans by the challenges of safely studying the brains of infants and by the fact that bonding likely begins when the child is still a fetus in the womb. But the questions scientists are pursuing will undoubtedly take them in that direction, toward examining parent and child at once. In reality, you can't disentangle the two.

Before I ever was pregnant, I loved to swim. I've never been very good at it. But I grew up spending my summers splashing around a lake in northern Maine or floating on its surface, watching the clouds drift over the forested ridge at the water's edge. In the winter, I would lie on the living room carpet, hundreds of miles from that lake, and imagine myself there, seeing my hands pull my body through the glassy water, pale oars moving between layers of reflected sky and dark abyss. In the water, I could lose myself in the weightlessness, in the everything.

When I became pregnant, I didn't want to swim. I thought it was the coldness of the water and the change in my body—that body within my body, and all the extra blood to keep warm. Then Hartley was a toddler, and the water still didn't appeal to me. When my boys were three and five, I swam out a bit from the dock on a blue-sky day, looking for that chance to lose myself. I couldn't, and I knew why. Part of me was tied to the shore, where two boys in swim trunks and neon-colored floats were calling me back, to catch them when they jumped.

* * *

I THINK THIS PART OF the parental brain research—the enmeshment—is beautiful. It's also terrifying and troublesome. Terrifying because of the high stakes of being responsible for another human's development. Troublesome because of the long history of blaming mothers for every possible thing that can go wrong in the trajectory of human life. Troublesome, too, because of the way that a mother's connection to her child is so often cast as something determinate and absolute.

Mothers have long been seen as the hinge upon which their child's future swings, with problems in a child's development considered a direct consequence of a mother's sins. Centuries of folklore, superstition, and popular opinion encouraged the idea that an expectant mother's internal life—her desires and her fears, big or small—could manifest in the body and brain of her future child. Among the things physician and midwife instructor John Maubray cautioned against in 1724 were anger, passion, "perturbations of the mind," and serious thought. By the late nineteenth century, these ideas had congealed into a theory of "maternal impressions." A mother's transgressions were deemed the direct cause of epilepsy, blindness, intellectual disability, mental illness, delinquency, and more. Meanwhile, child prodigies also were linked to a mother's prenatal influence, her attentiveness and purity of mind.

In his 1897 book on the topic, C. J. Bayer wrote that a mother who visits a home for the blind and finds her sympathies stirred might render her own child blind. If she develops a distaste for certain foods, she will arrest her child's development of a taste for those same foods. Any desire not to be pregnant would produce a "murderous brain." Mothers, Bayer wrote, are the "sole arbiters" of their child's destiny: "Make the tree good, and the fruit will be, must be, good."

I texted bits of Bayer's writing to friends: *Look at this—how absurd! Does he know just how many little murderers there would be if his theory were true?* It's funny, now. Or it would be, if it weren't a precursor to the maternal guilt so many of us carry today.

Many medical professionals in Bayer's day were already quite critical of these claims, particularly as the study of embryology grew. One speaking before the Obstetrical Society of Boston the year before Bayer's book was published said there was "no proof that maternal impressions can have any effect on the developing embryo." The United States Children's Bureau would later print a pamphlet for new mothers officially refuting the idea. Yet changes were underway—in medicine and in households across the United States—that in some ways affirmed Bayer's basic premise: good mothers produce good children. Bad mothers produce bad children.

The field of child development was just beginning to blossom, sparked in part by Charles Darwin's observations of his own son's development, published in 1877, and by similar diaries printed around the same time. A movement took hold among mothers to observe their own children's growth and to share what they learned with other women through child study societies. Many women saw themselves as partners to the psychologists of their day, but their efforts were overshadowed and discounted by the work of male experts. One of them, James Sully, wrote in 1881 that a woman's maternal instinct—though not a man's paternity—"unfits her" from the scientific study of children, making her incapable of objective analysis. (Sully seems to have softened on this point slightly, later calling on parents to help him with his own data collection, but it's not clear whether he, in fact, meant for mothers to respond.) Women were broadly excluded from the field, their perspective dismissed by the men whose work would be the measure of their success as mothers.

Leaders in child development would go on to make remarkable progress that would shape education, public health, parenting, and the fundamental ways we think about childhood. But as they charted the "milestones" of a typical child's development, they simultaneously laid down "major nodes of anxiety for mothers," as writer Sarah Menkedick described. "Suddenly there was a prototypical 'normal' infant who hit all of these targets, an exceptional one who surpassed them, and a dysfunctional or damaged one who missed one or several," she wrote in *Ordinary Insanity: Fear and the Silent Crisis of Motherhood in America.*

Those measures took on outsized meaning to generations of women who were told that their children's well-being required them to educate themselves about the latest scientific findings and to follow the dictates of medical professionals. The practice of mothering was changed from one learned from other mothers and through experience to one dictated by doctors and other medical experts. Rima Apple documented the rise of scientific motherhood and its persistence in her book, *Perfect Motherhood: Science and Childrearing in America.* For much of the twentieth century, mothers were told, quite explicitly, to do as the doctor ordered or risk their child's well-being. Physicians were king, held up as mothers' educators and children's saviors, a view promoted by physician organizations that were fast accumulating power. But, Apple wrote, mothers in the first half of the century also were eager to embrace physician guidance at a time when advances in medicine and public health were shrinking infant and child mortality rates. The global economy was changing quickly. People were more likely than in past generations to live apart from their extended family. And family size was shrinking, too. The relative preciousness of each child seemed to grow, and women were less likely to have experience caring for younger siblings to tap into once they became mothers themselves.

Much of the formal parenting advice women received in the first part of the twentieth century today reads like a parody of itself. In his 1928 book, *Psychological Care of Infant and Child*, John B. Watson took a tack similar to Bayer's, proposing that mothers bear almost complete responsibility for how their children turn out. Humans are conditioned and, in that context, a mother's love and affection are a "dangerous instrument" that breeds "invalidism." Better to leave the baby in a fenced backyard for much of the day, unattended but with a sandpile and small holes to crawl in and out of. "Do this from the time it is born," Watson wrote. Despite criticism from some peers and the fact that anyone who had actually raised children could have pointed out the error of Watson's thinking, his book sold tens of thousands of copies in the first months of publication and shaped parenting ideals through the 1930s. Once again, it's funny. And it's not.

It's no wonder that the first words of Dr. Benjamin Spock's 1946 classic, *The Common Sense Book of Baby and Child Care*, felt like a breath of fresh air to so many women: "Trust yourself." Spock offered a gentler approach, and Apple wrote that he and his peers changed the tide. Scientific motherhood still reigned, but now mothers had permission to use their own brains. They could weigh expert advice—and there was plenty of it, still—but then make decisions for themselves.

Yet even in Spock's welcome rethinking, a mother was measured by her ability to complete the many necessary tasks of parenting and, now, by the degree of fulfillment that she felt in doing so. Spock and the architects of the modern parenting advice industry that grew up in his image constructed the idea of a "good" mother as one who is tireless, self-sacrificing, relentlessly empathetic, and ever-present, who with a little help embraces her role as sole arbiter of her child's well-being with confidence, according to Shari Thurer, the psychologist and feminist scholar. The "how-to-raise-baby" industry boomed and mothers were the subject of a piling on. The baby advisers reminded mothers that they possessed enormous power to nurture or to shatter their children's mental health. "While they reassured mother of her natural ability to carry out her tasks, their assurances rang hollow, rather like a coach telling his or her team before the big game not to be nervous," Thurer wrote in *The Myths of Motherhood*. "Perhaps their aim was to reduce tension, but their effect was to create a degree of anxiety and guilt in mothers that is unparalleled in history."

The narrow if/then thinking central to Bayer's theories persists. It's there in how we talk about breastfeeding, for example, as supremely and unconditionally consequential for maternal development and child health outcomes, even when its exact causality for those outcomes cannot be separated from other neurobiological factors and parental behaviors, or from a family's financial security, education level, or other measures of support.

It's there in attachment parenting, the parenting philosophy based on John Bowlby's work that surged in popularity in the 1990s, promoted by William and Martha Sears. Attachment parenting approaches remain common today, though they are often discussed in looser terms, as natural parenting, and promoted by experts or influencers on social media. A lot has been written about the Searses' version of attachment parenting and whether it is restrictive or empowering to mothers, and about whether the parenting culture that has grown up around it is true to the philosophy that the Searses proposed. I believe families should choose the parenting styles that suit them best. The point I want to make here is about promised outcomes.

On page 4 of *The Attachment Parenting Book: A Commonsense Guide to Understanding and Nurturing Your Baby*, published in 2001, the Searses lay out the philosophy in a simple graphic. It lists the essential Bs of attachment parenting: birth bonding, breastfeeding, baby wearing, bed sharing, belief in baby's cry, balance and boundaries, and "beware of baby trainers." Practice the Bs, the Searses wrote, and your child is more likely to grow up to fit the adjectives listed in columns A and C: accomplished, admirable, affectionate, and assured; caring, communicative, considerate, and curious. Good mothers produce good children.

Sometimes when I read the parental brain literature, I start to feel the way I feel when I look at those columns: nauseated. Researchers categorize the people or the animals they study in terms related to the type of caregiving or degree of pathology they demonstrate. Mothers are sorted into securely attached or insecurely attached. They are anxious or well adapted. Synchronous or intrusive. Depressed or healthy.

Often these categorizations are based on brief observations of a mother and her baby, just a few minutes at a time. Attachment may be coded by watching how a baby responds when his mother leaves a room and then returns. Sometimes those families are followed over time, their early categorizations compared with their child's development even years later in life. Those categories are often important to the mechanisms of the research, for evaluating differences in neural activity or connectivity in the brain and for characterizing brain responses that correlate to adaptive or maladaptive parental behavior. They are important because loving, attentive parental care really does matter for a newborn's health and future.

But often I read these papers and I think, what about real life? Can the researchers' observations account for whether baby and mother slept enough the night before or whether they're hungry? If a baby is frequently cared for by other loving adults, including other parents, family members, or day care professionals, will that change how he responds to his mother's brief absence? What about individual differences in the expression of behavior, emotion, or attentiveness? What about neurodivergent mothers or babies, or differences in the cultural context in which they live?

Researchers characterize a mother-infant dyad, but babies exist in families with other parents, siblings, neighbors, grandparents, teachers, and childcare providers. They exist together in an often asynchronous world, in which poverty and climate change are intrusive. A global pandemic is intrusive. Racism is intrusive. Our own family members can be intrusive. How are we to remain synchronous—sensitive and appropriately responsive—despite it all? And do any of us ever fit into just one category consistently, throughout our children's lives, through difficult developmental stages, through any given morning? What about the constant seesawing of demands in a family of multiple children, where the moments in which everyone's needs are met at once are few and far between?

I know that my children are deeply connected to me and to my husband, as I am to them. But there are many days I feel the frustration of those competing needs in my chest like a water line, threatening to rise and drown me out. Sometimes I yell or cry, or feel a kind of paralysis characterized not by disengagement but by overengagement, an inability to stop fretting. After one particularly hard morning, I sat at my desk reading a 2011 paper coauthored by Atzil about how natural variations in the maternal brain and behavior "shape the infant's lifetime capacities for stress regulation and social affiliation." The paper outlines differences in brain activations between mothers whose behavior was coded as synchronous and those coded as intrusive, or demonstrating excessive parenting behavior. "Well-adapted parenting appears to be [underlaid] by reward-related motivational mechanisms, temporal organization, and affiliation hormones, whereas anxious parenting is likely mediated by stress-related mechanisms and greater neural disorganization," it read. My chest tightened.

Months later, I interviewed Atzil. She told me about her three children, how she had one during each phase of her postgraduate career: the first while getting her graduate degree, the second during her doctoral work, and the last during her postdoc. At each stage, she said, she collected data on mothers while holding an infant in her arms. When I told her about how I got started on this project, about the worry I felt during my transition to parenthood and my need to understand it, she said her story was similar. "It was very hard," she said. "A lot like you describe. A lot of anxiety. Very overwhelming. Very different from my fantasy about motherhood." She had been on track to study neuroimmunology, but the neuroscience of parenting captivated her.

We talked for a while about the maternal circuitry and the nature of allostasis, and then she said something that felt to me like the *big reveal*. Biological processes, including those that shape parenting behavior, are not binary, she said. They exist on a spectrum, with no categorical cutoffs. "A secure attachment or a nonsecure attachment—you cannot find any neural process that can differentiate these categories," she said. "You can think about the continuum where very complex behavior by the mother interacts with the very complex behavior by the infant."

She used to believe synchrony was the goal of well-adapted motherhood. It's not, she said. She began to change how she writes and talks about this topic to reflect this, to emphasize the biological process of allostasis in attachment. "The endpoint is, we need to keep our infants alive," she said. To do that, a parent must be attentive and responsive to a baby's needs.

Synchrony is a powerful tool. A parent can hold a baby close and regulate his temperature. A parent can babble and sing to a baby and regulate his mood. But there are other tools, too. Sometimes space is the thing that a parent needs to regulate themselves and be better prepared to help their child. Allostasis requires help from other people, including family members and trusted caregivers who are also quite capable of paying attention to and responding to a baby's needs—and, as we'll see in the next chapter, essential to meeting those needs. One researcher told me that asynchrony might be an important part of a baby's regulation, because the sense of being out of sorts also provides important information about how the world works. Life doesn't always match one's predictions.

The whole process, Atzil said, is plastic. That's why an adoptive parent and child can develop a very close bond that serves that child's allostasis. It's why a birthing parent who has postpartum depression can also raise a healthy child and develop a deep connection. It's also why those decisions that can feel so very consequential when caring for an infant, such as whether to continue breastfeeding or to try sleep training, should be made in the context of what will allow a baby and her caregiver to maintain their overall well-being, their mutual allostasis. This plasticity is the quality that allows bonds to develop between children and the people who care for them across a whole range of cultural contexts and family structures, within many differing parenting philosophies.

* * *

THE CIRCUITRY FOR SOCIAL PROCESSING is important to parenting, but it is not dedicated to parenting. The brain regions that help parents read, interpret, and respond to their children's cues are the same ones they use to read, interpret, and respond to social and emotional information from other people in their lives and from the world around them. If we think about that circuitry as being refined or strengthened through parenthood, then what does that mean for how we use it in the rest of our lives?

"Does it mean that after we have a baby, we become experts in reading other people's allostasis, and being very sensitive and responsive to that?" Atzil said. "I think, yes." She hasn't tested this, and I haven't found any research that does that exactly. But, she said, the intensive social processing that parenting requires could logically result in enhancement of the social mechanisms that support the connections we make with other people. Of course, the parental brain is quite selective. A parent's motivation is related to how they respond to *their* child, not to all children everywhere. So any kind of social enhancement might also be selective, affecting our closest, most intimate bonds. But it's interesting to think about parenthood as a kind of social training, giving us skills that improve with use.

In fact, there is a thread in the parental brain research comparing parenting to music training, in the sense that music training builds over time. The effects are cumulative. Playing music requires so many of the things that parenting does: close attention and interpretation of nonverbal cues; high-level thinking plus intense motor control; synchronization with fellow performers in such a way that the music not only presents as a whole but also captures the emotional context that each musician, with their own separate brain, intends it to. The performances that audiences hear are so often the result of lifetimes of practice and expertise grown over time.

In one key paper, a group of researchers based mostly in Denmark and the United Kingdom tested how first-time mothers' brains responded to the sound of unknown infants crying; they found that key brain regions, including the orbitofrontal cortex and the amygdala, were activated more strongly the longer a person had been a mother, or the older her baby. This makes sense, the researchers wrote. In the first months of life, a baby cries for a total of about 121 minutes per day. As the days go by, mothers accumulate experience listening and reacting, which shapes their neural responses, "as musical training shapes responses to music stimuli." (The same researchers have published work that found, among parents who were depressed, prior music training protected their ability to interpret infants' sounds of distress.)

This got me wondering about professional musicians who are parents, and whether they experience the training ground of new parenthood any differently than the rest of us. Did they see parallels between their musical mind and their developing parenting mind? Between their art and their child? A mutual acquaintance introduced me to Aoife O'Donovan and Eric Jacobsen, and I somewhat sheepishly sent them these questions by email. They were interested, which I took as a sign that my thinking wasn't entirely off-base, so we set up a time to talk. O'Donovan and Jacobsen are married with a daughter, Ivy Jo, who was three when we spoke and a big fan of the music from Sergei Prokofiev's *Romeo and Juliet* ballet. Both parents are extremely accomplished in their musical careers, which are quite different from each other.

A cellist and conductor, Jacobsen is the music director of the Orlando Philharmonic Orchestra, so his work can involve leading dozens of musicians who have come together from around the world. Synchrony is a particular kind of challenge in orchestral music, he said, with so many people and so many factors at play. "When you feel you're in collaboration, when you're truly in sync with someone, you're both leading the same way," he said. "But obviously, it's lead-follow. It's the birds in the sky. How do they stay together?" Sometimes as a parent, he said, he's very aware of his conductor-like role. When, for example, Ivy Jo is having a meltdown, is it going to help to engage her and try to make her laugh, or to give her space?

O'Donovan's practice of synchrony onstage is different. She is a singer and songwriter and part of the folk trio I'm With Her, with Sarah Jarosz and Sara Watkins. NPR's *Tiny Desk* series rightly described the three women as sounding like sisters, as if they've been playing together their whole lives. When Ivy Jo was eight weeks old, O'Donovan took her along on the band's tour. Watkins had an infant, too, and a nanny helped to care for both. The two mothers both would wake when either baby stirred, each tucked in a travel cot on the tour bus, and marvel at the fact that the cries didn't seem to bother anyone else in their very tight quarters.

Onstage, O'Donovan and her bandmates watch one another so closely. They move together. They breathe together. You can see it happen, watch them take off, wing tip to wing tip. O'Donovan told me about a moment when the trio was at Tanglewood, in the Berkshires of western Massachusetts. They were playing and singing an old gospel song, "Don't You Hear Jerusalem Moan," and toward the end of the song, their voices broke into a round, layered over one another. The instruments dropped off, and then the lyrics met again—"and my soul's set free . . ."—and, in a chill-inducing moment, the strings returned. The women walked off the stage, O'Donovan recalled, and Jarosz turned to the others and said, "It was like the whole earth cracked open when we hit that one note."

It's such a powerful moment precisely because of the way the musicians, by design, sound "out of whack" and then come back together, O'Donovan explained. "That's all you're ever trying to do is get to that point," she said. "Even if you're playing by yourself—it's having fluidity with your right hand and your left hand, or your voice and your instrument." You strive for the ability to get off "the path" of the music and return to it, to know where it is. "That's something that's definitely applicable in parenting, and then really in all relationships," she said. "Sometimes your paths have diverged, but the goal is to be aware of really where the other person is and to be able to . . . know that you will meet up again."

I think about what O'Donovan said and what I've learned from Atzil, and I decide that, perhaps in place of a single parenting philosophy, I will adopt a mascot of sorts. I've read Maurice Sendak's *Where the Wild Things Are* to my children countless times. It is a favorite in our house, as it is in so many. In it, Max is a mischief-maker who is sent to bed without dinner, then transported "through night and day and in and out of weeks" to an imaginary world in which he becomes king of the wild things. My boys are drawn to Max's wolf suit, the yellow eyes of the creatures he meets, and the odd human feet on the one who otherwise looks most like a bull. I linger on the last page, empty but for the five words that describe the supper Max's mother left for him after all: "and it was still hot."

Max's mother is out of view. But I can feel her. My Maxes are now six and four, ever in costume or launching themselves off the furniture, moving through the world half inside stories of their own making that almost always involve monsters with terrible gnashing teeth. I have never sent my boys to bed hungry, but I know the feeling of anger rising at the end of a long day and overflowing. I can feel how hers drains away to show the steady tenderness that is always there, for her boy full of vim and vigor and still in his wolf suit upstairs. I can almost see her test the soup—still hot—cut a slice of cake, and carry a tray to her son's room. She sweeps the hair across his forehead and pulls back his hood so he doesn't get sweaty in his slumber.

This, it seems to me, is the whole point. Know their hungers. Tend their bodies. Soften to their spirits. The work is in the reaching, not in arriving at the other side of the chasm or in pulling it closed. It's there, in knowing that we *can* meet in that impossible space between and feel the whole world beneath us fall away.

CHAPTER 5

The Ancient Family Tree

My great-aunt and great-uncle had twelve children within thirteen years, and none were twins. As a kid, I thought about those numbers with awe and a touch of jealousy. This was superhuman effort, resulting in a family that was revered by my own not so much for its size as for its volume of love and intellect. My great-uncle was a federal judge and his wife a loving matriarch to a family that remained close, was stacked with lawyers and medical professionals, and grew to include four dozen grandchildren. Once I had my own two boys, those numbers came to represent a mathematical impossibility.

How did she do it? A dozen pregnancies are hard to fathom. But then, what about twelve childhoods full of breakfast? Or Sunday Mass? Or bath time? What about potty training and school supplies and the task of tending hurts, big and small? What about laundry and birthdays and the job of guiding her own children into parenthood? Like me, Aunt Marion was a woman with two hands. And somehow she managed a brood six times the size of mine.

The answer of course is that she had help—from her devoted husband, from extended family members, from older children who cared for younger siblings, and likely from hands that were hired or traded in kind with other families in the big Irish Catholic community where she had deep roots.

Babies and parents grow in tandem, their social circuitry changing in response to one another, and one might interpret that as confirmation of the absolute importance of the maternal-infant bond. Doesn't it follow that a baby belongs in the arms of his mother, and therefore a mother belongs with her baby? There is a fundamental problem with that logic, one thrown into sharp relief by the basic math of Aunt Marion's motherhood and one that exists today for just about every parent I know struggling to make a living and raise a family: a parent's attention is divided. This has been true through all of human evolution. It may even be central to human nature.

Mammal babies are born mostly helpless, so they became really good at hooking the adults on whom their survival depends. As we've seen, their sweet features and siren calls are powerful stimuli that activate and alter circuitry driving motivation, responsiveness, and one's sense of self. *Don't look away*, they say. *Take care of us. Our survival is your survival.*

In most but certainly not all mammals, babies have tethered themselves entirely to the adults who birthed them. Among nonhuman primates, adults in about 20 percent of species will help a mother by holding or sometimes providing food to her baby. Apart from some especially cooperative monkeys, though, that help represents relatively little direct support of the baby's survival. Maternal care dominates.

Somewhere around two million years ago, in the early Pleistocene era or perhaps sooner, human ancestors diverged from their primate relatives in an important way. They began having babies with shorter intervals between them, becoming pregnant with a second child—or third or fourth—years before the first could feed or protect themselves. As a result, anthropologist Kristen Hawkes wrote, "human babies are without full maternal engagement as a birthright." Those babies relied on help from other adults. They had to. They couldn't have survived without it. Or maybe it's the other way around. Ancestral human mothers couldn't have had babies so close together, in a way that dramatically increased their reproductive success and made their species the dominant and most distinctively social primate on the planet, without substantial child-rearing support.

To early humans, mothers mattered in a big way. *And* they were not nearly enough. Natural selection favored families in which babies were good at capturing the attention of their caregivers and in which adults—not just female ones, but all adults—were drawn to the catch.

Lots of primates are social, but some prominent anthropologists believe that the very thing that propelled the evolution of humans into such cooperative creatures was the dramatic dependence of babies on other adults.

That dependence swung open the door to what E. O. Wilson first called "alloparenting"—"allo-" from the Greek word for "other." It made possible the wide diversity of family structures that exists today and drove the patterns of neurobiological changes that parental brain researchers are discovering as they piece together what researchers call a global parental caregiving network. Their findings highlight the neurobiological commonalities across parents—mothers, fathers, or others, birthing or not.

All human adults have the capacity to develop as caregivers. All human adults, not only birth parents, are fundamentally changed by the act of parenting. This chapter and the next one will explore research highlighting that fact—and how many of these changes seem to last, in part because these parental behaviors could someday benefit other children, including later offspring, nieces, nephews, neighbors, or, importantly, grandchildren. And we'll consider whether this new story about the long history of human parenting could fundamentally change how we think about the people who parent and the categories we try to fit them into.

This isn't just some "Mr. Mom" party trick, an add-on feature that evolution gave to fathers to make them feel the whole child-rearing experience is relatable to them. Nor is it an attempt at shoehorning families that include babies born with the help of a surrogate or donor or those raised by same-sex, nonbinary, or adoptive parents into a new biological truth. It's true that humans today have mechanisms for reproduction that have never been available to any other creature in the history of our planet. But the capacity for adults to be deeply involved in rearing children who were carried by another adult, regardless of whether the birthing parent was a mate or a biological relation, is not new at all. It was there from the start. It may even be the fundamental characteristic that set humans apart.

Affiliation, or the capacity to connect with other people in deep and lasting ways, to associate our own internal states with theirs, to predict and plan alongside them, to share a state of mind or to understand where our mindsets diverge—these things are fundamental to human society. And they may be rooted in the particular neediness of an ancient human child who has just become an older brother—imagine, number eleven in a family of twelve—and in the commitment of someone nearby to watch out for him.

* * *

I KEEP COMING BACK TO this point because it matters: a lot of popular thinking about parenthood and especially motherhood comes from what we see as "natural," or our sense of how things have *always* worked, back through evolutionary history and as evidenced today in the ways human behavior lines up with that of other mammals. Yet our understanding of other species, and of our own, often is based on observations made by male scientists of yore who applied their own moral judgment in place of science and created a record that is erroneous or incomplete.

Prominent naturalists writing near the turn of the twentieth century documented what they saw as a "distinctive psychology" within females of all species, one that extended to women and affirmed motherhood as their essential role, as science historian Marion Thomas has described. Here, the naturalists said, notice the sacrifice of the crab spider, who expends all her physical resources to lay and protect her eggs and then "gently lets herself die." Or consider the tirelessness with which a female wasp nourishes offspring that will never know her as their mother, just as human mothers engage in "heroic acts" of caring for children whose affection is not guaranteed. But what about the many examples, across taxa, of mothers who eat or abandon their children or simply have little involvement in rearing them? What about the relatively small but diverse group of species in which males are intimately involved in or even primarily responsible for child-rearing?

There, too, were Konrad Lorenz's repeated representations of himself as a mother figure to his geese, particularly as he told and retold the story of his "goose child" Martina. Historian Marga Vicedo argues that this characterization made it easier for psychologists of his day to adopt imprinting as a basis for the mother-child connection. It also allowed Lorenz to present as an expert on the topic of human bonding. Yet Lorenz knew that, when the geese imprinted on him, they weren't looking up at the face of a man with a broad white goatee and a pipe in his hand and thinking, *Mama.* They were associating themselves with the human species more generally, not with a specific maternal figure.

And there was John Bowlby's analysis of the maternal behavior in four species of primates—chimpanzees, gorillas, baboons, and rhesus macaques—when building his theory of attachment in humans. In his landmark book, first published in 1969, Bowlby explained that he chose these species because they were terrestrial, like early humans, and because there were ample field studies on them at the time. These species also happen to engage in intensive maternal care. Mothers hold their infants constantly, never putting them down for months on end. Anthropologist Sarah Blaffer Hrdy argued another factor may have been at play when Bowlby selected these primates over others who don't follow the "continuous-care-and-contact" model. "Each of these species conformed to preconceived Western ideals of how a mother *should* care for her infant," she wrote in *Mothers and Others: The Evolutionary Origins of Mutual Understanding.*

Bowlby found affirmation in modern hunter-gatherer societies, where mothers were thought to follow a similar constant-contact model, with babies held continuously or worn in a sling. "Only in more economically developed human societies, and especially in Western ones, are infants commonly out of contact with mother for many hours a day and often during the night as well," he wrote. The primate way, as he saw it, was the natural way.

Except there was more to this story. In the wild, it's true that ape infants are cared for exclusively by their mothers. Chimpanzee mothers don't let their babies out of their grasp for the first three and a half months. In orangutans, it's at least five months. But across primates, the parenting picture is far more diverse.

In many species, fathers, older siblings, and other females hold a mother's baby and sometimes provide food. South American titi monkey mothers hold their babies to feed them a few times a day, while the fathers or other offspring care for the infants *most* of the time. Among marmosets and tamarins—also New World monkeys, whose ancestors split from African monkeys around forty million years ago—the norm is cooperative rearing involving fathers and other adults. These species are fast breeders, producing twins and triplets in short order, and Hrdy argues that such reproductive success is enabled by the help mothers receive from other family members. That's a resource often lacking for ape mothers, who most often move from their troop of origin to another group to find a mate. A subfamily of monkeys called colobine demonstrates the influence of trusted alloparents—"family daycare," Hrdy calls it—quite clearly. Among the colobine, those species in which females move away from their own kin to breed within another troop follow practices of exclusive maternal care. But in most species, females typically stay near their own parents and siblings, and then alloparents play a central role. Hrdy wrote that "there is no one, universal pattern of infant care among primates." And exclusive maternal care seems to be a method of "last resort."

The picture among modern hunter-gatherer communities also is far more nuanced than the psychologists of Bowlby's day thought. These communities have long been viewed as a window into how human societies worked before much of the globe transitioned to agricultural societies, somewhere around twelve thousand years ago. Researchers often look for evidence of early human food traditions, reproductive patterns, and various other characteristics that persist in hunter-gatherer peoples today. But it's important to note that almost none of the research on those societies includes an equal native voice, and, until relatively recently, researchers rarely considered the ways in which hunter-gatherers flexibly adapted to the modern world themselves, in quite diverse ways.

One of the first systematic studies of infant care among modern hunter-gatherer communities, published in 1972, focused on the !Kung people of southern Africa and described how !Kung infants were rarely put down and often carried on a mother's back or in a sling. But, Hrdy noted, later analyses made an important distinction. !Kung babies were held almost continuously, but as much as 25 percent of the time, people other than their mothers were holding them. Among the Hadza of northern Tanzania, brand-new babies are held by relatives and neighbors as much as 85 percent of the time in the first days after birth, which in some ways sounds quite ideal for a recovering birth parent.

Of course, today, parents around the world regularly let other people hold their babies, sometimes passing them around to adults who marvel at their tiny toes, snap first photos, and wonder whom they will look like as they grow. And we know that, despite the ongoing idealization of mothers who follow something like a continuous-care-and-contact model, that style of child-rearing has simply not been the reality for any but the smallest minority of people throughout modern history. "Human mothers are just as hypervigilant" as other ape mothers, Hrdy wrote, "they are just not so hyperpossessive."

Why? Humans are much more closely related to chimpanzees than to marmosets, so how did human parenting chart a different path than in other great apes? One answer to that question seems to be grandparents. Grandmothers, specifically.

* * *

ANTHROPOLOGISTS LONG ASSUMED THAT, IN ancestral families, the men hunted and the women foraged and tended to the children. The food a father caught was at the center of a family unit. It was the currency that kept a pair bonded. Habitual food sharing at home (or at a home base, in the case of nomadic people) formed the foundation of family life. The hunting male was added on to the mother-offspring social groups seen in other apes. The hunting hypothesis provided the origin story for the modern nuclear family.

In the early 1980s, some researchers studying the Hadza and !Kung people, along with the Aché foragers of eastern Paraguay, started noticing behaviors that did not fit that theory. When men hunted, they didn't bring the bounty home to their partners and offspring. They shared it. Careful observation of food sharing among the Aché found that, for any given person in that community, as much as three-quarters of daily calories were provided by someone outside their nuclear family. Hadza men prioritized hunting big game, even though their success rates were quite low. The meat they brought in was a major part of the community's diet, but it was not reliable enough to sustain the daily needs of their partners and children.

A group of anthropologists, including Kristen Hawkes, James O'Connell, and Nicholas Blurton Jones, concluded that this kind of food sharing couldn't really be considered "paternal effort." The men in these cases were providing a public good in exchange for social capital, for the benefit of the whole group of which their own offspring were one part.

Hawkes and her colleagues started looking more closely at women's food collection strategies and made some remarkable observations. This one stood out most of all: among the Hadza, older women past their own reproductive years were the most productive foragers, by *a lot*. Older girls who hadn't had a pregnancy foraged for less than three hours a day, and childbearing women foraged for about four and a half hours per day. But the older women averaged more than seven hours a day. They worked at about the same rate as other women and often were doing the hardest work of all, digging up deeply buried tubers. The researchers realized that not only was the idea of men provisioning their own nuclear families wrong, but it seemed there was a provider no one in their field had fully accounted for: hardworking grandmothers.

Hawkes and her colleagues synthesized their work with observations that dated back to the 1930s and 1950s to propose the "grandmother hypothesis," linking longevity among ancestral grandmothers to the health and development of their daughters' offspring. Hadza kids were active foragers, too, but they weren't very good at digging the deep tubers that were a staple of their diet. When young children were weaned, their weight gain tracked with their own mother's foraging efforts. But that changed once she had another baby. Her foraging efforts fell off with a newborn to care for. Then, the older children's weight gain was linked to their grandmother's foraging efforts.

Nonhuman ape mothers stop reproducing at about the same age as human mothers do, but those apes typically don't outlive their fertility. If ancestral human grandmothers aged even a tiny bit slower—meaning they outlived their reproductive years slightly—they could have provided essential help to their daughters in gathering food and tending to dependent grandchildren. And that would have left their daughters more available to have another baby more quickly.

Having a baby is costly. It's generally thought that, across species, the bigger and needier the baby is, the longer it takes for a mother to recover and breed again. Among the apes, Hrdy notes, humans produce the largest and slowest-maturing babies, yet we breed fastest of all. Perhaps that's because, when ancient human mothers needed the help, their own mothers were there.

Helpful grandmothers, the hypothesis goes, gave their descendants a better chance of survival and of carrying their own slower-aging genes forward. Natural selection favored a longer-lived grandmother, then, and menopause was born. Mathematical modeling found that even if very few ancestral women lived past reproduction, those "subsidizing grandmothers" could increase the success of their descendants enough over time to leave a big mark on the human population. Overall longevity, in both males and females, would increase significantly, leading eventually to populations like those in modern hunter-gatherer communities, where a third of adult females are beyond their reproductive years.

By this thinking, of course, that trajectory also produced longer-living males, who remained fertile into old age. The ratio of available reproductive men to reproductive women increased. More males meant more competition, which could have strengthened bonds between mates, as ancestral men—who were likewise growing in their capacity to read and connect with the minds of others—aimed to stick with a woman lest they be outcompeted elsewhere.

There's good evidence of the importance of grandmothers in more recent history, too. Researchers in London analyzed data on family structure and child mortality from forty-five research papers, representing populations from around the globe and across the past four centuries, mostly those without access to modern contraception. Specifically, the researchers looked at correlations between child survival and kin survival. Almost universally, mothers' survival was linked to child survival in the first two years of life. But the "mother effect" declined or even disappeared by about age two, suggesting that others were there to provide competent care if a mother died. The effects of a father on child mortality were much less consistent, depending on the social context. But the presence of a maternal grandmother was rather consistently protective.

When researchers combed through detailed church records from preindustrial Finland—from 1731 to 1895, a time when tuberculosis, smallpox, measles, diarrhea, and other as-yet-unidentified infectious diseases were of particular risk to young children—they found that the proximity of maternal grandmothers (but not paternal ones) significantly boosted survival rates of children after weaning, between ages two and five. That benefit fell off once grandmothers themselves reached about age seventy, when their own needs may have directed family resources away from the youngest children. And within the first French families to settle in Canada's St. Lawrence Valley in the seventeenth and eighteenth centuries, women who lived close to their own mothers started having children earlier than their sisters who lived farther away, and they had more children, with lower rates of mortality.

The grandmother hypothesis is no settled matter. In fact, some of the very researchers Hawkes has worked alongside studying hunter-gatherer communities disagree with her conclusions. Critics say the hypothesis unnecessarily minimizes the contributions of fathers in caregiving and food provisioning, that nutrient-dense kills were an essential factor that allowed mothers to reduce their own foraging efforts and increase the pace of baby making. Ancestral humans may not have followed a clear sex-based division of labor, and fathers may have played a significant role in feeding and carrying young, reducing the energetic demands on mothers and supporting earlier weaning. Male "helpers," or men without children of their own, may have been even more important than post-fertile women in providing food to others' offspring. Some contend it was hunting and the "skill-intensive" learning it requires that drove human longevity, and there is no evidence that grandmothers ever became the dominant "breadwinners" of a family.

But that last point is not at all what Hawkes and her colleagues put forward. The spoils from hunts *were* nutritionally important, without a doubt. But what grandmothers offered, really, was their presence. They filled in the gaps with nutritional staples, day in and day out, whether or not the men returned with the meat. And, as important, they occupied toddlers and older children while their mother nursed a newborn, teaching them how to dig for the best tubers or entertaining the many whimsies of their imaginations. They learned their grandchildren's minds, and they let theirs be known, too.

The reality is that probably all the factors mentioned above shaped human evolution to varying degrees. But the contributions of trusted grandmothers point to something important. It's not that a grandmother-supported family is the standard human family or even the "human way." But rather, human mothers couldn't, and most often didn't, do it alone.

The nuclear family, subsidized and glorified through much of the twentieth century and especially in the United States after World War II, may never truly have been the basic family unit. Maternal grandmothers were perhaps the helpers most often available in early human families, and their inclination to help could have led to an ever-stronger predisposition in generations that followed to read the needs of children and to meet them. Alloparents have long taken various forms, as aunts and uncles, grandfathers, older siblings, and close friends. No matter who gets the credit or why, it is clear that cooperative child-rearing played an essential role in human evolution. "Without alloparents," Hrdy wrote, "there never would have been a human species."

I recognize my own bias in reading the work of Hawkes and Hrdy. The grandmother hypothesis *feels* right to me. Maybe that's because I know the ache of not having a close grandparent nearby, not only to drop in for holidays but to support my husband and me in the intimate, everyday moments of raising a family. Maybe it's that, when I read Hawkes's description of the possible cooking patterns of ancestral savanna-dwelling people who lit a fire and engaged in "mutual batch processing," I think of the double batches of belly-warming casseroles I've made through the years, half to feed my kids and half to deliver to a friend with a new baby. For sure, when I read Hrdy's writing about the origins of maternal ambivalence, I recognized myself.

Hrdy suggested that ambivalence may be derived from alloparenting. It grew, she wrote, as ancestral mothers considered questions like, "*Shall I ask my mother to hold the baby while I crack these nuts?*" Or, "*Should I carry my baby with me on a long trek to gather food, or leave him with auntie?*" Human parents have always been simultaneously protective of their babies and dependent on support from others to raise them, which naturally leads to internal tension. Love and ambivalence both are part of motherhood, Hrdy told me. "They are built into it."

Maternal ambivalence is not some quagmire women suddenly found themselves in when they entered the modern workforce, not some stain on the true nature of motherhood introduced by a woman unwilling to attend fully to her biological destiny. One could argue that, precisely by grappling with their own emotional tumult, early mothers shaped the path of human nature. The trajectory Hawkes describes required not only a grandmother willing to help, but also a mother willing to let her.

Hawkes has argued, along with neuroscientist Barbara Finlay, that the grandmother hypothesis could explain far more than human life span and menopause. Across mammalian species, longevity is consistently linked to the duration of development in childhood. Longer development is linked to a bigger brain. Support from grandmothers (and others like them) may have driven a pattern in human life history that not only allowed brains to grow bigger but also, because ancestral babies were weaned earlier than other primates, ensured that more of their brain development would occur in a supersocial context. Hawkes and Finlay point specifically to the plasticity of the brain's motivation and reward systems, and suggest that early human infants may have developed to be particularly responsive to social rewards because of their efforts to connect with alloparents.

When early human babies were passed around by family and group members, they had to develop skills not needed to the same degree by other ape babies. They had to work hard to read the faces of the people who held them, to determine their mental states, and to vocalize in ways that would attract their affection and also the attention of their mothers. This effort drove development of "a new kind of ape equipped with differently sensitized neural systems, alert from a very early age to the intentions of others," Hrdy wrote. Natural selection favored babies who could monitor and influence the minds of others—and adults who, no matter whether they had birthed the babies themselves, would be receptive to their calls. Hrdy told me babies began working hard to connect with adults with one simple message in mind: *choose us.*

*   *   *

ONE SPRING DAY AFTER SCHOOL pickup, I chatted with Meredith McCabe, whose eldest grandson, Oscar, was in kindergarten with my son and whose daughter is a friend and fellow journalist. McCabe asked me how my book was coming along and what I'd learned so far, and I offered my standard line about how changes in the parental brain are very different from the "mommy brain" story we're fed—the changes are flexible and adaptive, priming us for the challenges of parenthood. And perhaps grandparenthood, I added. She was quiet for a moment as we watched the boys gathering acorns under a line of towering oaks, her granddaughter sitting on her hip. The thing that had struck her most of all, she said, was just how bonded she felt to her grandchildren. She hadn't expected it.

She would tell me later, when we talked in depth about her life as a mother and grandmother, that she was a worrier who had suffered two miscarriages herself, and because of that she had been so focused on helping her daughter get to Oscar's delivery day that she hadn't really thought too much about what it would feel like to be a grandmother. Then she received a text at around 2 a.m. from her son-in-law, in New York City, saying the baby was on the way.

McCabe drove through the early morning hours from Maine to the city—an anxious drive, with no updates from the hospital. Eventually one came: Oscar was here. "I just said, 'Is she OK?'" McCabe said. "I wanted to know if my baby was OK." She was, but it was a hard delivery. And Oscar, who was hypoglycemic, spent a few days in the NICU. Then they were home and well, and McCabe could sit with her grandson in her arms—and marvel at him.

She had been around newborns since she'd had her own, of course, and she knew that babies were special, but this was something different, she said. Something visceral. "I could just feel it internally—something, some kind of connection that came over me in such a way that you have to notice it," McCabe said. "It wasn't just my daughter's baby, my son-in-law's baby, and he's not my baby, but he is my grandbaby."

Changes in the parental brain seem to last, long past the postpartum period and long past a person's reproductive years. That may be because human children are dependent for so very long. It wouldn't make sense, after all, for a birthing parent's brain to change during pregnancy and the postpartum months only to *snap back* to its prepregnancy shape once a child was weaned or cut his first tooth. It is an absurd idea that any part of us (bellies, breasts, or brain) would be made to do that, and anyway it would be a big waste of energy. After all, that baby still needs a responsive and caring parent, for many years to come. And after him and his siblings, there may be others.

It's possible that these changes remain because survival favors them. It may be, Elseline Hoekzema told me, that if parents are "still in this caregiving mode, if it's still active when the grandchildren arrive," those grandchildren have an evolutionary advantage—or, at least, they did in early human days.

Hoekzema is a neuroscientist and director of the recently established Hoekzema Lab at Amsterdam University Medical Center. She spent time as a doctoral student studying different aspects of neuroplasticity in Barcelona, where she worked with two other women, Erika Barba-Müller and Susanna Carmona, who, like her, were beginning to think about becoming mothers themselves. Out of curiosity for what motherhood could mean for their own brains, the women designed a study to look at the anatomy of the brain before and after pregnancy.

They recruited couples, men and women, who were not yet pregnant but hoped to be, ultimately ending up with a study group of twenty-five first-time mothers and slightly smaller groups of first-time fathers and of men and women without children. The process took more than five years, as the researchers fit the work in around other projects, which in Hoekzema's case were focused mostly on the aging rat brain and neurodevelopment disorders in humans. At least at first, they had no funding for their maternal brain project.

When their results were first published in 2016 in the journal *Nature Neuroscience*, Hoekzema was pregnant with her second child and overwhelmed with the hundreds of requests for interviews that poured in from journalists around the globe. For the first time, the group had found evidence that pregnancy changes the brain in ways that last, not only through those intense sleep-deprived first months, but for years.

Comparing brain scans before and after pregnancy, the researchers found significant reduction in gray matter volume in new mothers' brains, particularly in regions involved in social cognition. The volume changes were distinct enough that a computer algorithm could clearly sort the women according to whether they'd had a baby.

The researchers also measured the new mothers' neural responses when viewing pictures of babies—their own and others—and found that several areas that showed the strongest neural activity when the women viewed their own babies also had lost the most gray matter volume during pregnancy. The researchers suggested the volume losses represented not a decline of function in those brain regions but rather "a further maturation or specialization" of the network involved in social cognition. Among the new mothers, greater volume change also correlated with higher scores on a questionnaire meant to measure attachment. And when the researchers specifically analyzed changes in the ventral striatum, which includes the nucleus accumbens and is part of the reward network, they found that women who had greater volume loss also showed a stronger response within this brain region to pictures of their own babies. The authors wrote, "Our findings provide preliminary support for an adaptive refinement of social brain structures that benefits the transition into motherhood." (The group's initial analysis found no volume changes in fathers' brains, scanned before and soon after their partner's pregnancy. Notably, the men were not scanned at two years postpartum. A later analysis of the same data from before and after a partner's pregnancy found reductions in volume and cortical thickness in fathers' precuneus, a default-mode hub important for theory of mind.)

Most interesting of all, those possible refinements in mothers seemed to stick. Among a smaller number of mothers who returned for a scan two years into parenthood, the gray matter reduction mostly remained. The researchers followed up at six years postpartum, too. Again, most of the volume reductions persisted, and again they correlated with measures of attachment. "These findings open the possibility that pregnancy-induced brain changes are permanent," the authors wrote.

At first glance, it seems as though the team's findings directly contradict another group's results, which found *increases* in gray matter volume in mothers' brains between the first month postpartum and four months postpartum. The study designs and especially the time frames are quite different. That 2010 paper, by Pilyoung Kim, James Swain, and colleagues then at the Yale Child Study Center, focused on postpartum months in a mixed group of first-time and experienced mothers and did not measure prepregnancy volumes. It correlated increases in mid-brain regions with a mother's positive perceptions of her baby. A 2020 study found comparable results when analyzing a similar, small group of mothers at one or two days postpartum and again within six weeks postpartum. Both Hoekzema and Kim have suggested the difference in their findings might be because the brain doesn't change in a linear fashion. Rather, gray matter might decline in volume during pregnancy but rebound some, depending on the brain region, afterward.

Hoekzema's team found a partial volume recovery in the hippocampus, from the early postpartum scan to the two-year scan. The hippocampus is a highly plastic part of the brain that is important for learning and memory. It's also where there is greatest evidence that adult humans experience neurogenesis, meaning the creation of new neurons from neural stem cells or the descendants of stem cells called progenitor cells—a process shown in animal models to be affected by changes in hormones.

The proliferation of new cells in the hippocampus repeatedly has been found to be reduced in postpartum rat mothers, whether they have just birthed their first litter or their fifth. Researchers often describe this as a cost to the lactating mother, as her body and brain direct energy resources elsewhere. For mother rats, hippocampal cell proliferation returns around weaning. The prospects of studying whether this holds true in humans are complicated for lots of reasons, though researchers often hypothesize that a similar dip in production could be behind subtle deficits in certain types of memory during pregnancy and the early postpartum months. (More on this in chapter 8.)

Hoekzema and her team wrote that it's possible—though, as yet, unproven—that their results reflect a similar pattern in humans, with a drop in the creation of new neurons during pregnancy and later recovery. She told me it's unlikely that the significant brain changes that occur with pregnancy and the postpartum period always would be entirely adaptive. "There might be a cost, which could be for instance memory loss, which could be a sensitivity for the development of mood disorders, or could be other things as well," she said.

It is easy to jump to the conclusion that loss of brain matter must be bad, because those costs are what people most often think of—if they think of anything at all—in relation to the brain and parenting. Memory loss was all Hoekzema and her colleagues heard about when they first began sharing their results, she said. "People around us were immediately like, 'Oh, volume loss! Oh, it's horrible! I can't remember anything!'" Hoekzema said she heard this even from colleagues working in the field of adolescent imaging, which was surprising. The teenage brain is far more studied that the maternal brain, and it is generally accepted that a reduction of gray matter in adolescence represents a fine-tuning of networks, through synaptic pruning and changes in myelination, meant to help teens adapt to life as adults—not a loss in brain function.

So the researchers, with Carmona leading the analysis, decided to compare the data they had on twenty-five mothers' brains, before and after pregnancy, to data from twenty-five teenage girls—girls who were going through a life stage also characterized by a spike in hormones, significant behavioral shifts, and an increased risk for mental health disorders. Between the two groups, the structural changes in the brain looked the same, strikingly so. Both displayed a very similar flattening of the cortex and a widening of the grooves on the surface of the brain, along with a nearly identical reduction in total brain volume that tracked along the same morphometric pattern.

The similarities between the mothers and the teens don't mean that the life stages are directly analogous. But they point to the idea that the changes accompanying pregnancy, though complex, are adaptive and almost certainly *not* part of a distinctly neurodegenerative process.

* * *

THE SAMPLE SIZES OF THE studies published by Hoekzema and colleagues, like those by the Yale group, are somewhat small, partly because of the challenges inherent in recruiting people who are not pregnant at the start of the study and who become pregnant and carry a baby to term by the study's end. But the findings are strengthened by the fact that the study is longitudinal, tracking each person's brain change over time, rather than comparing groups at different time points. The results need to be replicated and expanded, with larger sample sizes, and that work is underway. But already the group's studies are considered by many in the field to be seminal. They certainly raised public awareness of the long-term effects of pregnancy and parenthood in humans and seem to have inspired more researchers to pursue prospective studies imaging parents' brains over time.

When I spoke with Hoekzema in spring 2021, she was preparing for a larger study, with funding from the European Research Council. There are still so many unanswered questions, she said: How does pregnancy affect the brain's white matter, dense with myelin-coated axons connecting brain regions? How exactly do changes in the parental brain structure and activity affect the way a person functions? How do these changes unfold over time? Which hormones are triggering them? How does little sleep and excess stress affect the brains of birthing parents? And what happens to the brain during second or third pregnancies?

Hoekzema was able to work full-time on the maternal brain research after pilot data helped her secure grant funding, and she continued work on the project at Leiden University, where she analyzed the data. Now she is directing several studies on the topic from her lab in Amsterdam. "I find a lot of things very interesting," Hoekzema said, "but now that I've found this topic, I don't think there's any I find more fascinating. As a mother and also as a scientist, it's just so fundamental."

Some researchers are beginning to examine the long-term effects of this fundamental life stage by looking at the fingerprint parenthood leaves on the brains of older adults, whose own children are long grown. Similar to the "mommy brain" story of new parenthood, the story we most often hear relating parenting and brain health in later life is limited and disheartening: women have a significantly higher risk than men of developing Alzheimer's disease, and having children has been associated with earlier age of onset and greater cognitive decline, though the evidence for this is somewhat mixed. In other words, child-rearing *could* ultimately have a neurodegenerative effect for some mothers. But recent research suggests that the full picture is quite a bit more complex than that and perhaps less dire.

Using new techniques that combine neuroimaging data with machine learning, researchers in Oslo and Oxford have published a series of papers looking for patterns across thousands of brain scans. The scans are part of a massive database of biomedical information called the UK Biobank. By assessing scans from 19,787 women, between ages forty-five and eighty-two, the researchers found that those with children had "younger-looking" brains. A computer system analyzed hundreds of brain features related to volume in cortical and subcortical areas and estimated the mothers' "brain age" to be younger than expected given their actual age.

This effect was stronger the more children one had (though the results for women who had more than five children were less clear). The researchers, led by Ann-Marie G. de Lange, who now directs the FemiLab on women's brain health at the University of Lausanne in Switzerland, identified brain regions where the effect was most prominent, including the hippocampus, the thalamus, the amygdala, and especially the nucleus accumbens, which is part of the reward and motivation system discussed at length in chapter 3. In 2021, the authors published new findings specifically about white matter, the loss of which is thought to be a factor in age-related cognitive decline. More childbirths, again, were linked with a "younger" pattern of white matter.

For now, these are somewhat distant correlations between pregnancies and the status of the brain in later life. The analysis didn't include measures of cognitive function or other metrics of brain health. Brain age is used as a proxy for those things, with older brain age linked to Alzheimer's disease, schizophrenia, and cognitive impairment. It's not entirely clear whether the protective effects, if that's what they are, identified by de Lange's group come from a physiological response to pregnancy, from the act of parenting over time, or from some important social and economic differences between people who have multiple children and those who don't—differences that might even have existed before a person became pregnant. Large studies that follow the same people over time, starting before pregnancy and continuing into late life, are needed to get closer to cause and effect. In the meantime, the researchers wrote, their findings indicate that the brain changes a person goes through during pregnancy and the postpartum period "may be traceable decades after childbirth."

Other researchers have tried to link those traceable effects to cognitive function. Pulling from a large database of health information that was collected to test whether regularly taking a low dose of aspirin could prevent disability or dementia, researchers at Monash University in Melbourne examined the brain scans of nearly 550 Australians in their seventies and eighties, about half men and half women, who had parented at least one child. They also looked at a small group of nonparents and collected results from cognitive tests taken by the study participants.

Motherhood, they found, was associated with a "dose" effect in cortical thickness in specific regions of the brain: an increase in the parahippocampal gyrus, which is associated with memory consolidation and cohesion, and a decrease in three regions generally involved with complex sensory processing, among other things. The differences were more significant the more children a woman had. The researchers found differences between fathers and nonfathers, but not the same dose effect. Mothers of multiple children also scored slightly better on a verbal memory test.

Starting with the same sample of older adults, the Monash group then looked at a different measure of preserved brain function, this time evaluating only parents and looking at data collected during a resting state. The researchers found that the more children a woman had, the more segregation she showed between brain networks, between hemispheres, and between anterior and posterior regions. Lead author Winnie Orchard explained that segregation in this case is a positive thing, reflecting less effects of aging.

In a typical healthy, aging brain—one that is nonetheless declining—brain regions that are losing function will connect more strongly to others, essentially recruiting help to get a given job done. "To do that same task," Orchard told me, "they need more support." But mothers showed less of that other-region recruitment than expected, and again this effect was linear. More children meant less recruitment. "The results are consistent with a more flexible and resilient late-life maternal brain," the researchers wrote. No such effect was seen in fathers.

The study database collected only the most basic information about parents—whether they had children and how many. It didn't include hormonal data, or information on how a person parented, how long they parented, or their family structure. Nor did it include birth or feeding methods, whether a participant's reproductive history included pregnancy loss or abortion, or whether a parent's children were biological or adopted. So it's hard to determine whether the effects the group tracked were related to pregnancies directly or to the "environmental complexity" of parenthood, the researchers wrote. While the hormonal changes of pregnancy and the postpartum period may have gotten things started for mothers, these women were scanned three decades or more later. Parenthood, they said, presents lifelong challenges that are amplified by each subsequent child and that demand "rapid behavioural change and skill acquisition."

Then how do we explain the lesser effects, or the absence of impact (depending on the study), found in fathers' brains? Orchard's group wrote that participants in the database they used were from a generation that overwhelmingly followed "traditional" parenting arrangements, with fathers as breadwinners and mothers as primary caregivers. So those men may have spent far less time immersed in that complex environment kids create, resulting in less parenting-specific changes in their brains.

As we know, experience matters, and experience comes only from time and proximity. The brain of a person who leaves the house before the kids wake up and returns after bedtime, or who sees his children only intermittently, or who simply views babies as not his business, does not have the time or proximity necessary to be transformed—at a neurobiological level, at least—by his status as a father. Certainly not compared to fathers among the foraging Aka in the Central African Republic who, according to the work of anthropologist Barry Hewlett in the 1980s and 1990s, spend as much as 47 percent of their time either holding or within arm's reach of their infants. And also not compared to my own husband—and many parents like him—who learned early on what it meant to calm a newborn with his body by rocking and shushing and holding. Who took responsibility for the job of helping our first son learn to drink from a bottle when I returned to work, reading and responding to the baby's cues in the process. And who almost single-handedly kept our children, then two and five, engaged in games and homespun science lessons in the first weeks of the COVID-19 pandemic. Paternal experience varies widely. Which may be why other studies *have* found significant structural changes in fathers, in the immediate postpartum period and much later in life.

The same group of Yale researchers who documented gray matter increases in postpartum women later conducted the first study of structural plasticity in fathers. They scanned the brains of sixteen men in the first weeks of fatherhood and again between three and four months out. This was a mixed group of first-time and experienced fathers. The researchers found changes over that time period in the volume of brain regions key to parental care. Among them were decreases in hubs of the default mode network and increases in the lateral prefrontal cortex and superior temporal gyrus, which elsewhere have been found to be active in fathers, more so than in mothers, when they viewed their own babies versus others.

Separately, researchers at the University of Southern California in Los Angeles used data from the big UK Biobank, but this time looked at both men and women in midlife. They analyzed data on 303,196 people, mostly in their fifties and sixties, comparing the number of children that participants had and their performance on two cognitive tests measuring response time and visual memory. Parenthood was associated with faster response times and fewer errors in memory. The difference in performance was greatest for those who had two or three children, compared to those who were not parents, and the effect was strongest in fathers.

The researchers also took data from a smaller group—13,584 people— and analyzed their brain age relative to peers. They found that parenthood was linked with younger-looking brains, with slight reductions in relative brain age with each additional child. In men specifically, having two or three children was linked with the most significantly reduced brain age. The fact that the patterns were different between sexes but significant for men as well as women means that it is important to study the effects of parenthood in the context of sex, the researchers wrote. But it seems "lifestyle and environmental factors"—meaning the life of a parent and not only pregnancy history—affect the long-term health of the brain.

Of course, animal models have repeatedly confirmed this very common-sense finding: an individual's environment shapes their brain, throughout life. Rats who are raised in a large cage with toys, other rats, and daily time to explore a maze develop greater cortical depth, compared with their own littermates who are raised alone, with no toys and no maze. But in one fascinating paper from 1971, researchers found that, after a female rat raised in that impoverished environment became a mother, her cortex was comparable to that of a virgin rat raised in an enriched environment.

It may be that parenthood, for humans too, is a particular kind of enriching environment. That's not at all meant to imply that the lives of people without children are impoverished. But parenting comes with particular "lifetime cognitive and social demands." Many of these demands are, I would argue, physiologically distinct from enriching demands unrelated to parenting, because of the intensity of children as stimuli, because of the particular allostatic connection between baby and parent, and because of the relentlessness of parenting. "You're constantly learning and growing with the child and you have to parent differently at each life stage," Orchard told me. "Or maybe you have to parent, you know, two or three different children at two or three different life stages. And that involves this set shifting of, 'OK, well, I need to give this child this, and I need to give that child that'—at the same time. You know, it's difficult and it evolves. It changes. It's never stable. You can never get complacent."

Yet Orchard stops short of saying that having children is outright good for the brain. While parenthood seems to have enduring effects, those effects are too complicated to characterize as clearly beneficial. The study of this topic is complicated by the huge number of variables within a person's reproductive life that can shape their hormonal trajectory and life experience.

Some studies—but not all—have found that having no children or few children is linked with better cognitive function later in life than having many children. A person's cumulative estrogen exposure is thought to be an important factor in later brain function, and reproductive history can influence that exposure in confounding ways. Estrogen increases during pregnancy, but women generally have lower estrogen levels after having children, so pregnancy can lead to lower cumulative levels. Many other factors, including contraceptive use, time spent breastfeeding, and a person's age at their first or last pregnancy, shape estrogen exposure.

The links among pregnancy, parenthood, and Alzheimer's disease specifically are nuanced. Having five or more children, what is sometimes called "grand multiparity," has been linked not only to greater risk of the disease but also to increased severity of symptoms. Yet in a small study of older British women that collected detailed medical histories, higher cumulative estrogen exposure, including from *more* months spent in pregnancy, was found to be protective against the disease. Certain genotypes that carry a risk for Alzheimer's—but not all—are thought to interact with reproductive history to result in worse outcomes, including earlier onset. But there again, researchers have identified a need for much more information about how the diversity of parenting experiences affects risk and disease progression.

Parenthood affects a person's health in complex ways across the life span. It is not a homogenous experience, so it makes sense that its late-life effects on the brain would be variable across a population. What is clear is that those effects last, so a person's reproductive history is an important, formative component of their physical and mental health over time, certainly for mothers and likely for all engaged parents.

We can't draw a direct line between the long-term effects of parenthood and the evolutionary role of grandmothers. After all, rat mothers enjoy clearer long-term benefits of motherhood, including better cognition after weaning than nonmother rats and some protection from age-related decline in spatial memory and hippocampal neurogenesis. It's not that the effects of motherhood endured only after human grandmothers evolved to need them. But in my mind, they are related in the way Hoekzema implied earlier. When grandmothers (and other experienced alloparents) are needed by their kin, even long after they are done raising their own children, they may have a conserved capacity to think about those babies' needs and to connect with them.

So far, only one study that I know of has looked at how a grandmother's brain responds to her grandchildren as stimuli. The study included fifty grandmothers who had at least one grandchild between ages three and twelve; many of the grandmothers were highly involved in their grandchildren's lives, and ten of the fifty lived with their grandchildren. Researchers at Emory University compared fMRI data when the women viewed pictures of their own grandchildren, unknown children, the child's parent (often the grandparent's own biological child), and an unknown adult. If the grandmother hypothesis is true and a grandmother's care for her descendants drove human longevity, the study authors wrote, then a grandchild should be "a particularly salient stimulus to the brain of post-reproductive women."

The grandmothers—perhaps unsurprisingly—showed similar or even greater activation in some brain regions when viewing their grandchild's adult parent, compared with viewing their grandchild. That was especially true in the precuneus and might reflect a greater capacity for taking the perspective of the other familiar adult. But regions involved in emotional empathy, including the insula and secondary somatosensory cortex, were more strongly activated by the grandchild. The researchers used data from a previous study in fathers and found that, compared with fathers viewing their own child, the image of a grandchild prompted stronger activation in grandmothers' empathy-related regions as well as in key subcortical areas involved in motivation and reward.

McCabe, the grandmother I chatted with outside school, is retired from her work as a clinical social worker in schools and now offers therapy to adults one or two days a week. "The rest of the days I'm watching grandchildren, for the most part," she said. She had long helped her daughter and son and their spouses with childcare support, taking care of Oscar and the three grandchildren who arrived after him. Then the pandemic hit, and her home, an old farmhouse about thirty minutes outside Portland, Maine, became the center of their extended family life. The parents would work inside and McCabe would lead the grandchildren on adventures outside, looking for frogs in the pond or tromping around her four acres of land in search of new species to add to their "critter list."

McCabe is remarkably conscious of the fact that her grandchildren are growing and changing, and so is she. When she feels worn out, she said, she reminds herself that they won't always need her in the same way, and she won't always be able to give them quite so much. For now, she cherishes the moments when she can recognize how much they get from their time with her. "I see it in their little faces whenever I arrive or they arrive," she said. "It's pretty precious. It's an amazing gift for me."

* * *

PUZZLING OUT THE DETAILS OF early human development excites Hawkes, forty years in. Questions about ancient families are very present for her today. She is obsessed with how we got to be "this animal," she told me over Zoom, pointing with her index fingers emphatically at her own face. When I asked her whether she thinks the work of ancient grandmothers made alloparenting across the species possible, she answered with a detailed dive into the intellectual history of her field, before arriving back at a simpler response. "I do," she said.

Parental care does not follow a set pattern across species. It is not dictated by a gendered "distinctive psychology" at all, but by an individual species' changing context. It is an incredibly flexible and potent tool of evolution, what E. O. Wilson considered a group-level mechanism for adaptation. Ancient humans followed a pattern that has emerged as needed in mammals and beyond, wherever a species fills an ecological niche in which expansive social bonds allowed them to survive and thrive, often when facing the pressures of predation or an unstable environment, like the receding forestlands and growing savannas that early humans experienced.

Cooperative breeding involves helpers outside of the breeding pair and is what one group of researchers called "an extreme form of cooperation." It occurs in only about 3 percent of mammals. It's typical for certain mice and meerkats, porcupines and beavers, wild dogs and those fast-breeding monkeys. That tally does not include "plural" breeders, in which groups of females work together, mostly apart from males, to raise their children (think elephants and lions). It's notable that the only animals other than humans known to experience menopause are certain toothed whales, including orcas and beluga whales, who also have complex social structures and rely on alloparental care.

Many, many more birds are cooperative breeders. Researchers are still figuring out why species, even closely related ones, differ in their approach, though there is some good evidence for what Wilson proposed back in 1975: families trend toward more cooperation in environments with variable productivity, as a buffer against the hard years.

Soon after we moved into our home abutting a pocket of trees in an otherwise densely built neighborhood, we realized we had company. A group of resident crows—a flock of crows is called a "murder"—would wake with the sun, and we would rush to close the windows in our infant son's room lest they wake him with their noisy greetings. At first, they were annoying. I grew to love them. In the evenings, as we came home from work and day care and started settling into our nighttime routines, I'd look for them, flying home from the horizon line and settling into the treetops.

In the spring of 2021, a pair of crows began building a nest in a maple tree at the edge of our yard. My sons and I would watch them as they carried sticks and grass to the nest and set them into place. We watched as the father, I assumed, carried food to the brooding mother and sometimes swapped places with her, so that she could weave off through the trees in search of food and a change of scenery.

One day, one crow was sitting on the nest and another was very close by, when a third crow approached. We had seen other crows near the nest during the building process, and I had interpreted the pair's interactions with them as confrontational, a vying for territory. So I expected this interloper to be chased off as well. Instead, the bird on the nest stood up and moved to the side, and the third bird calmly hopped onto the edge of the nest to get a closer look, presumably, at the hatchlings that had just emerged.

I instantly assumed this was an aunt, come to check on her sister and the babies—the bias of my own mind, missing visits with my sister and her family, stymied by the pandemic. But it made me reconsider the whole scene we had been witnessing. Was it two crows who had built the nest, or more, a rotating cast whose members I couldn't differentiate? In the weeks that followed, as the adults worked together to deliver food to the nest, I'd wonder how many were provisioning those hungry, growing chicks.

It turns out that birds in the corvid family, which includes crows, ravens, jays, and magpies, are remarkably cooperative. They are thought to be cognitively complex, highly social, long-lived, and loyal. About 40 percent of corvids are cooperative breeders, some assisted by older offspring and some by unrelated group members. Some species breed "colonially," with various nests in close proximity. Most likely, the helpers at the nest in our yard were siblings born last year and not yet breeding themselves.

Parenting does not follow a set pattern. How can we account for such variability across species and settings? Across time? The answer lies partly at the heart of a much broader cultural debate raging right now, about the nature of sex differences and the brain.

As I write, the United States seems to be cresting the latest wave of political rhetoric about gender and family, fueled partly by panic over the falling birth rate and partly by outrage among mothers who have realized the degree to which their own suffering during the pandemic was exacerbated by elected officials and employers who, for decades—and still—flatly refused to acknowledge the real needs of families. "Covid took a crowbar into gender gaps and pried them open," economist Betsey Stevenson told the *New York Times* in February 2021. Blame political apathy, or the contingent of conservatives who have decried efforts to create paid leave or accessible childcare as "lefty social engineering" and who have fallen back on the entrenched idea that the need for childcare represents a failure of the American family—something required by poor, broken families but certainly not a universal good.

People who hold that view often seem to believe that human children were meant to be cared for by one committed mother at home, provisioned by a father at the hunt—that this is the family structure human biology dictates. That this is how it has always been.

They are wrong.

CHAPTER 6

Inclined to Care

For a long time, Catherine Dulac wasn't interested in parental behavior as a research focus. She studied sensory influences on social behavior in mice. "Parenting was absolutely not on my radar screen," the Harvard professor of molecular and cellular biology told me. "I was more thinking about interaction between adults—male/male, male/female, fighting and mating, which are more classical-type social interactions that people work on." Classical, she said, as in those deemed most important by the men who have dominated science and to whom fighting and mating were more fundamental than caregiving, which was seen as a distinctly female behavior.

In the early 2000s, Dulac and her colleagues were investigating the role that a mouse's vomeronasal organ, a tubelike organ that opens into the nasal cavity, plays in detecting pheromones and triggering sex-specific social behaviors. They found that females with genetically impaired vomeronasal signaling displayed male-typical behaviors, such as mounting and pelvic thrusting. When the researchers later looked at males that also had impaired signaling, they found the mice were less aggressive toward pups and instead would build nests and groom and crouch over the pups as if to nurse. In other words, the researchers said, the brains of the male mice seemed to contain functional circuitry for female-typical behavior, which normally was masked by vomeronasal control. And vice versa.

Those findings were published over multiple papers in the prestigious journal *Nature* and received a lot of attention, but they have been somewhat controversial. Some researchers have presented contradictory findings and questioned the lab's methods. But it is interesting to me because of how it led Dulac to parenting.

The field of neuroendocrinology had long considered caregiving as a classical social behavior worthy of study and one for which there was shared capacity across species. But a general sense had hung on—in other corners of science and through much of the second half of the twentieth century—that testosterone (and its metabolite estradiol) shaped the male brain in such a way that male and female brains contained different sex-specific neural networks, and that those very different circuits naturally produced different behaviors related to mating and caregiving. (Men are from Mars and all that.) "The brain between males and females had to be as different as the genital organs of the male and the female—so, you know, structurally different," Dulac told me. "And, I think, structurally they're just not different."

For one thing, she said, "the brain is difficult to build." Creating different versions for different sexes would be inefficient. Instead, Dulac came to see the brain as something that is generally shared and that incorporates regulatory switches. Those switches may be moderated by a number of factors, including biological sex and social context.

This is a simple way of describing something complex. The brain is complicated and made more so by the meaning we make out of each new finding. We know that humans (and other mammals) possess the capacity to care for children they did not birth or to whom they are not biologically related. We see that all around us in engaged biological fathers, loving adoptive parents, and other committed caregivers. The science of sex differences in the brain that has evolved in the past two decades or so shows a much more nuanced and layered picture, with average differences throughout the brain that can nevertheless vary quite widely from person to person and that are shaped by factors related to *or* separate from sex hormones. Yet we also have seen that our cultural understanding of parenthood is rooted deeply in our cultural understanding of sex and gender. The research on the parental brain is upending both, showing that the neural capacity for parenting behaviors is shared across the species and, at the same time, calling into question the rigid bounds of gender.

The question of how similar or different male and female brains are is a tricky one that seems often to be distilled down to troubling stereotypes. The first time I published something about the maternal brain, I received an email from Larry Cahill, a neuroscientist at the University of California, Irvine, and a prominent sex-difference researcher. He more or less congratulated me for my interest in the topic (though I had written about motherhood, not about womanhood) and pointed me to his research.

For a very long time, researchers maintained that females were harder to study because they are more "variable" due to the fluctuation of their reproductive hormones, despite the fact that males' hormones fluctuate, too. Females were simply ignored, in animal models and human studies alike. If females were included, data was not sorted by sex in a meaningful way (and often isn't, still today, after funding agencies have taken steps to close this gap). The result has been widespread sex disparities in diagnoses and treatment outcomes, including failures to identify heart attacks, stroke, or neurobiological differences in women, and more adverse reactions to prescription drugs. Plus there has been a broad underappreciation of sex as a biological variable in the processes of neuroplasticity, or in the prevalence and progression of mental illness.

Cahill has been an influential advocate for the inclusion of females in studies of humans and other animals in neuroscience. And he's been a controversial voice for the idea that sex differences in the brain underpin stereotypical differences in men's and women's behavior. Consider, he told me by phone, why there are so few women plumbers. He suggested this disparity may be linked to women's stronger average sense of smell, resulting in higher reactions of disgust toward stinky things, while I wondered about the generations of men who have guarded the gates to the trade through male-dominated apprenticeship programs.

Others take what I consider to be a far more nuanced view, which acknowledges that studying sex differences is essential because biological sex is an important factor in every person's development. But when it comes to shaping the brain and behavior, it is one factor among many, including gender identity and the ongoing, complex experience of being a body in the world. As Catherine Woolley, a neuroscientist at Northwestern University, wrote in January 2021, "Sex differences in the brain are real, but they are not what you might think."

Woolley's lab has made important findings about sex-based differences in molecular activity in the brain, including in a mechanism for adjusting synapse strength in the hippocampus. Understanding such differences is critical, she wrote, because drugs designed around those mechanisms could work one way for a male and another way in a female. But she also wrote that, just because a difference exists at a molecular level, it doesn't mean it produces a fundamental difference in how people live their lives. In fact, researchers are learning more about specific "latent sex differences," which exist in the brain without producing differences in functional outcomes. "There are two routes to the same result," she wrote. Or, perhaps, many.

Understanding those routes—where they overlap and where they diverge—is important, of course, which is why research that includes females and analyzes for potential sex differences is so important—a point that Dulac emphasizes, too. But so is rigorous critique of that analysis, lest we once again find ourselves cloaking old ideas about a woman's essential nature in new science.

Sometimes research into sex differences offers a whole new way of seeing things. Recall that Dulac and her colleagues found that particular pools of galanin neurons in the medial preoptic area (MPOA) were essential to the execution of parenting behaviors in the mice. Activating them prompted parenting, including in virgin females and males. Without them, caregiving behaviors were dramatically reduced. The number of galanin neurons in the mouse MPOA was *not* sexually dimorphic, or different in males and females. The sexes shared a circuitry for parenting—a species-based, rather than sex-based, "parenting instinct," though one that is "both hardwired and plastic," Dulac told me. She and colleagues at the Harvard Center for Brain Science wrote that this finding added evidence to the idea of "bipotential male and female brains," with core parental circuitry that is active, or not, depending on an individual's physiological state, environment, and exposure to offspring cues.

Mice are not humans. We don't know whether a similar set of galanin neurons is present in the human MPOA. But the anatomy and function of the hypothalamus, where those neurons live, is highly conserved across vertebrates, meaning that creatures evolved but the hypothalamus remained much the same. Dulac offers lots of qualifications to this statement—"we don't have the proof yet"—but she believes the likelihood that there is a set of neurons in the human MPOA that "express galanin-controlled parenting" is "pretty high."

The more interesting point, to me, is the broader one. There could very well be sex-based differences in precisely how those pools of galanin neurons work. Yet, at a very fundamental level, the parenting circuitry may be something that exists *universally* and is regulated differently across sexes, from individual to individual, and depending on the social context of the species. It is not written only into the brains of females.

This, of course, was not an entirely new idea. The early work of Jay Rosenblatt and colleagues pointed to the universality of caregiving behaviors in rodents decades ago. Later, in 1996, they found that the MPOA stimulated "maternal behavior" in males as it did in females and that male rat caregiving was impaired by lesions to the MPOA. Dulac's work added important details about the commonality of caregiving and the diversity of its expression.

As she and Harvard colleagues Lauren O'Connell and Zheng Wu wrote, variation in parenting styles between species and within them may be possible precisely because this parenting circuitry—as well as an opposing circuitry controlling aggressive behavior—is shared. This may seem counterintuitive at first, a sameness driving difference. But these circuits might be like levers, adjusted "across large evolutionary distances." That's because, Dulac told me, from an evolutionary perspective, parenting is very useful. And, clearly, not only for mothers.

* * *

JAKE ROBERTS NEVER PLANNED ON being a father. He had almost no experience with babies or little kids. And he had no model for fatherhood. Growing up in Biddeford, Maine, his own father was distant. The way he saw it, he told me, "I don't want to be a dad, and I shouldn't be a dad." At least, that's how he saw it right up until the moment on April Fools' Day 2011, when his wife told him she was pregnant. ("Is this a joke?" he asked.)

A friend encouraged Roberts to go to Boot Camp for New Dads, a nationally licensed program run out of regional hospitals by the non-profit Maine Boys to Men. It brings together expectant fathers and new fathers, with their babies. "He was like, 'You gotta go. There's real, live babies. You get to change diapers, and they're pooping and peeing and crying, but it's just cool to do it. And it's just guys, man. It's just guys,'" Roberts recalled. He was in. After all, he said, he had a lot of ground to make up.

Roberts told me boot camp might have been the first time he *ever* saw a man out on his own with his baby. "It was cool to see—hey, here's this guy. The baby's crying. He stopped the baby from crying. He changed the diaper and he fed them. I was just like, 'Alright. Well, you know, they can do it. I can do it.'"

After that, Roberts said, "I was kind of hooked."

He was hooked on being a dad—baby Luc's arrival began just as he was taking a turkey out of the oven on a Sunday night—and he was hooked on talking about fatherhood. Roberts returned to boot camp with his son, as a coach this time, and later became a facilitator helping to run the program. "That old stereotypical, traditional outlook for men, as far as being a dad and fatherhood—it's like you got to wait until they're toddlers and you can roughhouse with them, which is so wrong, when you read the science" about babies and bonding, he said. "Why would you not want to be involved? There's so much magic that happens when they're younger."

I knew about Roberts because my husband attended one of his boot camps and also became a coach. Like Roberts, Yoon also had very little prior baby experience and no direct paternal role model. Boot camp changed things for him. It gave him—us, really—a whole new language for talking about the kind of father he wanted to be in those early months, about how to support me during labor and while breastfeeding and how to cope when a baby is crying and you can't figure out why. It gave him a sense of agency in the role he wanted to play as the father of a newborn and an awareness of the very common phenomenon of

gatekeeping, when birthing parents directly or indirectly prevent others
from being true partners in caregiving by not giving them a chance to
learn how to do it (see: maternal vigilance and the social pressure to do
it all).

When our oldest son was about a year and a half old, Yoon quit his
job at the newspaper where we both worked to start his own business
as a freelance photographer and video producer and to stay home part-
time. It was a change that felt right to us in large part because of all the
ways he had chosen to be present during our son's first months. Those
choices had shaped his relationship with Hartley, our relationship, and
the balance of our home. And, very likely—for Yoon and Jake alike—
they had shaped the development of his parental brain.

For many birthing parents, aspects of pregnancy and delivery, the
flood of hormones, the life-and-death intensity of feeding and caring for a
newborn, and the social expectations that accompany it all can feel non-
negotiable. For many nongestational parents, full entry into parenthood
is more of a conscious choice. But it is also a transformative one, on a
biological level.

In this area of the parental brain field, most of the research is on
cisgender, heterosexual, biological fathers. The lack of research on any
parents but these and gestational mothers is glaring and an obvious
obstacle to really understanding the mechanisms of parental care in
humans. We will come back to this point. First, let's look at the studies
on those fathers who make up the bulk of the research and consider
how these findings might apply more broadly.

We really don't know how or when paternal care came into the picture for humans. In mammals, fathering has evolved many times, along
different evolutionary pathways. In ancestral humans, it likely came
along with the development of pair-bonding, or longer-term mating.
But the question is complicated, to some degree, by the fact that paternal care is far from universal. In formal terms, it is "facultative rather
than obligate." A father is not always present. Rather, a whole lot is left
to circumstance. For ancient families and modern ones, the degree of
paternal involvement has hinged on proximity, resources, the strength
and sustainability of the relationship between parents, or the availability of other caregivers to help.

Sarah Blaffer Hrdy wrote that "human males may nurture young a little, a lot, or not at all." Human patterns for conceiving kids and raising them are remarkably diverse. Yet a father's physiology changes when he spends time with pregnant people and babies. "To me," Hrdy wrote, "this implies that care by males has been an integral part of human adaptations for a long time."

In the most extreme cases, expectant fathers experience pregnancy-like symptoms. The phenomenon is known as *couvade* syndrome, from the French word for to brood or to hatch, and is sometimes called phantom or sympathetic pregnancy. Ariel Ramchandani, writing for *The Atlantic*, looked at case studies and other research to date and found "the symptom list has seemed to include almost everything: diarrhea, constipation, leg cramps, a sore throat, depression, insomnia, weight gain, weight loss, tiredness, toothaches, sore gums." Also, morning sickness.

The syndrome is well documented though often dismissed as purely psychological and derided, including by expectant fathers' actually pregnant partners. It's hard to say just how common it is. Prevalence estimates vary widely, and self-reporting of symptoms likely depends largely on cultural expectations. (It is, however, entirely expected in those cooperative breeding New World monkeys, with males gaining up to 15 percent of their body weight when their mates are pregnant.) But the syndrome seems symptomatic of something much more common: a major shift in hormones as fatherhood approaches.

A study published in 2000 analyzed concentrations of prolactin and cortisol in the blood of thirty-four couples during at least one of four stages: in the middle of pregnancy, just before childbirth, days after baby's arrival, or a few months in. The researchers also looked at estradiol in women and testosterone in men. They found that, on average, the men and women fit a similar hormonal pattern. Both groups showed increases in prolactin and cortisol as childbirth approached and decreases in estradiol or testosterone in the first weeks postpartum. It may seem obvious at this point that those hormonal shifts in women are important mechanisms for preparing her body and mind for the transition to parenthood. But, the researchers suggested, hormonal shifts do something similar for fathers, "priming" them for paternal care.

In the two decades since that paper was published, there's been increased interest in the hormones of new fathers, with attention seemingly tracking the growth in hands-on fatherhood. The studies to date, many of which have focused on fathers' decrease in testosterone, have provided some clarity and many new questions.

Testosterone is thought to regulate a person's physiological commitment to mating or caregiving, and the trade-offs between competition and cooperation that those two things require. This idea, referred to as the challenge hypothesis, is derived from seasonal patterns in male birds who first compete for mates and then cooperate in chick rearing. With some variability, the birds experience a drop in testosterone from the early breeding season to their offspring's arrival. The pattern holds up in some mammals, including paternal primates, like marmosets who experience a drop in testosterone with exposure to offspring. The 2000 paper and others have pointed to a similar pattern in humans, but these studies often have relied on cross-sectional data that compared groups of men in different stages, rather than following the same men over time.

Some of the strongest data to date on fathers and testosterone comes from a study led by anthropologists Lee Gettler and Christopher Kuzawa, who followed hundreds of young men living in and around Cebu City, in the Philippines, for four and a half years, starting in 2005. The men provided saliva samples in the morning and evening when they were twenty-one years old and again when they were twenty-six years old. Out of a larger study group, 465 men were single and without children at the start. The researchers later found that those men who had higher morning testosterone at the outset were more likely to find partners during the study period. Among men who became partnered and had children, they saw a median decline in morning testosterone of 26 percent and in evening testosterone of 34 percent, while the median age-related declines in men who remained single and childless were 12 percent in the morning and 14 percent in the evening.

At the end of the study, fathers of newborns had greater declines, compared to their levels at the beginning of the study, than fathers with slightly older children. And those who reported spending at least three hours a day on childcare had lower testosterone than those who reported little or no involvement with their children. Notably, the involved fathers and the uninvolved fathers had shown no significant differences at baseline, suggesting that it was the act of caring for children that lowered testosterone, rather than a particular hormonal predisposition that led to caregiving.

It's not only interaction with a baby that changes fathers but also, if they're in a relationship, interaction with their partner. A group of researchers led by Darby Saxbe, a developmental psychologist and founder of the University of Southern California Center for the Changing Family, followed twenty-seven heterosexual couples throughout pregnancy, measuring their salivary testosterone levels about every eight weeks. When their babies were about three and a half months old, the fathers answered questionnaires meant to assess their own levels of investment, commitment, and satisfaction with their partner specifically (not with parenthood).

The study found that fathers' testosterone levels decreased during pregnancy and mothers' levels increased, but it's how they changed that's notable. In later pregnancy, those levels changed together, with the degree of decrease in the father correlated with the degree of increase in the mother. For fathers, both the overall decline in testosterone during pregnancy and how much their hormonal change tracked with their partner's predicted how positively they responded to the postpartum questionnaire about their relationship.

Scientists don't know exactly how a pregnant woman influences an expectant father's biology in this way. They point to proximity, time, and intimacy in a general sense—synchrony. Hormonal synchrony isn't always positive. Saxbe's research also has found that partners' cortisol levels can change together, and that correlation was strongest when women reported experiencing physical or verbal aggression or controlling behaviors from their partners. Saxbe told me that she thinks about that as a kind of "stress contagion." But the research indicates that, with testosterone, synchrony is adaptive. The testosterone paper was limited by the small number of couples included and by the fact that no postpartum samples were collected. Still, the authors suggest that changes in testosterone "may underlie fathers' dedication" to their partners, especially at a time of stress during the transition to parenthood, when a person's satisfaction in their relationship often dips.

Two recent meta-analyses look at the big picture of testosterone research in fatherhood. In one, the authors reviewed dozens of studies that, taken together, assessed testosterone in thousands of straight men. On average, men in committed heterosexual relationships had lower concentrations of testosterone than single men, and that difference held up across ages and when comparing samples from what are sometimes called WEIRD countries (Western, Educated, Rich, Industrialized, and Democratic) with others. Overall, the researchers found, fathers have lower concentrations of testosterone than men without children. Testosterone was lower still in those fathers categorized as being active or experienced parents, though the authors noted uncertainty around the evidence for this conclusion.

In a separate meta-analysis, researchers also found lower testosterone linked to fatherhood, but the authors emphasized that the effect size, or the degree of difference, was small—so small that, if applied to a population, it would be nonexistent for most men. The authors offered several explanations for this, related to the nature of neuroscience and the nature of testosterone.

Many studies on the challenge hypothesis in humans are "underpowered," meaning they include too few fathers to result in strong statistical outcomes. The downregulation of testosterone likely depends on a wide variety of factors that relate to social context. Those factors are not always accounted for, and so the researchers wrote that they couldn't examine their effects in a detailed way. These social factors may include how committed a father feels toward his partner before pregnancy and over time, how mentally prepared he is for children, his prior caregiving experience, and how hands-on he is as a parent. To the latter point, the authors wrote, biological fatherhood—basic procreation—seems to have far less influence on a man's physiology than "social fatherhood."

* * *

TESTOSTERONE IS A TRICKY THING. Just as oxytocin is dubbed the "love hormone," testosterone is the star of another cultural narrative that stretches the facts. It is cast as the driver of masculinity, the maker of male genitals *and* the male mind, the fuel for male competitiveness, male sexual appetite, male dominance, and male risk-taking. That narrative can shape researchers' bias, sometimes leading to study designs that affirm stereotypes instead of exploring the nuances of the biology behind human behavior. For one thing, a fuller understanding of hormones is hampered by the fact that researchers often study particular hormones only in the sex to which those hormones are deemed most influential— testosterone in males, and estradiol or progesterone in females—though they are present in all humans and are part of a complex neuroendocrine system.

Testosterone does shape the development of male-typical genitals. After puberty, the average circulating testosterone in males is many times higher than the average in females, and it underlies secondary sex characteristics in men such as denser muscle mass and greater upper-body strength. But those averages are two pinpoints in a broader range in which there may be overlap between males and females—a range that could look different if people who are intersex or nonbinary were included. The same can be said for many identified sex differences in brain structure. There is overlap between sexes and variability across elements so that an individual's brain anatomy might be female-typical in one region but more male-typical in another. As the authors of a recent multidisciplinary review titled "Future of Sex and Gender in Psychology" put it, "most brains are gender/sex mosaics."

Some prominent scientists dispute this idea. One review that has been held out as clear evidence of the gender binary and "the most recent, comprehensive, and rigorous study" on adult testosterone levels was written by researchers who are paid consultants for, or received financial support from, World Athletics, the international governing body of running and track and field. They determined that testosterone "has a strikingly nonoverlapping bimodal distribution with wide and complete separation between men and women." That sounds convincing. But consider that the paper is specific to sports competition and funded by organizations interested in determining the line between male and female competitors, whom to exclude, and how. The study explicitly excluded women with high testosterone as abnormal.

Sari van Anders, a professor of psychology, gender studies, and neuroscience at Queen's University in Kingston, Ontario, told me that this line of thinking makes for a "just-so story: women with T higher than X are abnormal. How do we know? Because of this distribution of women, from whom we've excluded any women with high T." High testosterone in women is pathologized, van Anders said, even when women with high levels are healthy. And the occurrence of very low testosterone in men, including in healthy elite athletes, is explained away.

Testosterone is quite variable between individuals and across a person's life span, even within a given day. It generally peaks in males after puberty and declines with age, and concentrations vary greatly between societies and within them, across socioeconomic conditions. Quantifying those differences has proven quite difficult.

Moreover, although we think about testosterone as a driver of gendered behavior, it's possible that gendered behavior is a driver of testosterone levels. In one study, led by van Anders, researchers measured salivary testosterone of trained actors before and after they performed a monologue that required them to wield power, specifically to fire a subordinate. The actors, men and women, performed twice, once in a stereotypically male way that involved taking up space, smiling little, posturing in a dominant style, and interrupting, and once in a stereotypically female way, with less-frequent eye contact, hesitancy, higher voice register, and a general goal of "trying to be nice." Women, but not men, showed significant increases in testosterone after both performance styles, suggesting that the very act of possessing and wielding power, apart from gendered presentations of that power, may propel testosterone increases.

It's possible, the authors wrote, that men's average testosterone is higher than women's not only because of heritable factors but also because they receive a lifetime of encouragement toward competition, agency, and power attainment. In other words, the perceived biological basis for a gender binary may have been created in part by the socially constructed gender binary. It is self-affirming.

We can't weave a new story unless we unravel the old one. What is considered "normal" in parenthood is fundamentally linked to what is considered "normal" in our perceptions of gender. And those are informed by the way the science investigating sex and gender is performed and how its findings are framed. The way van Anders, who also studies parenting, put it, hormones are biochemical substances that move around in our bodies and form a "cultural narrative that circulates in our societies." This is "hormones as rhetoric."

The rhetoric says masculinity is created by testosterone and the competition and aggression it promotes, and testosterone is innate and the very factor that determines what some see as the wide and complete separation between men and women. The rhetoric says mothers, with their itty-bitty bit of testosterone and overwhelming amounts of "love hormone," possess their own sex-specific, innate mechanism for nurturance.

The reality is that the capacity to bond with children is flexible, possessed by all, and regulated differently depending on the individual. Testosterone is not a unilateral driver of masculinity, fixed and certain. It is an important, malleable component of the hormonal system that influences the human brain and behavior, especially our orientation toward social bonds, in all genders.

A central theme of van Anders's work is asking fundamental questions about social behaviors. Questions such as—in the context of her work on sexuality—what is desire? And what is parenting? Parenting is often seen as a set of warm, caring behaviors. But it also may involve protective aggression, a kind of vigilance, which increases testosterone. Fathers' circulating testosterone has been found to increase when listening to audio of infant cries, which researchers associate with a motivation to care. (Experienced fathers listening to a baby cry also had a notable rise in prolactin, a hormone typically associated with mammalian milk production, that also has been linked to paternal care, with some mixed results.) In the context of the challenge hypothesis, this is referred to as the "offspring defense paradox," an exception to the parenting-equals-low-testosterone rule.

Van Anders and two colleagues, Katherine Goldey and Patty Kuo, have proposed a more nuanced model for how testosterone behaves, particularly in relation to the neuropeptides oxytocin and vasopressin, that takes into consideration social goals. It also attempts to separate those goals from ideas about masculinity and femininity, but the authors wrote that it's hard to do so completely because the very study of those hormones has been so gendered. There are lots of studies on testosterone in fathers, for example, and very few on testosterone in mothers (or on women and aggression). This, despite the fact that women see major spikes in testosterone in the prenatal period—one 2014 study of twenty-nine pregnant women found a sixfold increase in testosterone in salivary samples across pregnancy—followed by a decline in the postpartum period to levels lower than in women without children. "How do you know [change in testosterone] has anything to do with fathering," van Anders told me, "as opposed to mothering, as opposed to parenting, as opposed to grand-parenting or caregiving in any way?"

The idea that hormonal changes facilitate engaged parenthood, in men as in women, has implications that go beyond helping men understand their transition to fatherhood—a worthy goal itself. It could serve as a new lens through which to consider men's health and to view the health of families more broadly.

Fatherhood affects many men's lives in myriad and ever-changing ways, contributing stress and joy, emotional stability or uncertainty. The research to date—what little of it there is—suggests that fatherhood has a protective effect on men's health. Researchers studying the neurobiological effects of fatherhood say it should be considered a major event for men, too, worthy of study. "Men's health is not really seen as being shaped by paternity," Saxbe said. That may be partly the result of the variability in active fathering. But, she said, the gap in the research obscures the bigger picture for men and for families.

Saxbe, USC colleague Diane Goldenberg, and Maya Rossin-Slater of Stanford University School of Medicine have written about new parenthood as a critical transition period in adult health, from which developing patterns of weight gain and mental illness can be retained over the long term. The perinatal period may represent "an inflection point" for health disparities by race and socioeconomic status, they write, and they suggest this may be linked in part to unequal access to paid family leave policies. An important factor in that argument and in Saxbe's work overall is the idea of family health, in which parents and children influence one another.

In a 2017 study, Saxbe and colleagues looked at testosterone levels and symptoms of postpartum depression in fathers, and how they related to postpartum depression in their partners. Among 149 couples, fathers who had low testosterone levels (sampled at nine months postpartum) reported more depressive symptoms. Fathers with high testosterone seemed to be protected, but in those couples with higher-testosterone fathers, the mothers were more likely to report depressive symptoms and aggression from their partners.

As I read that paper, I thought, this makes sense. If men engage in fatherhood, they experience neurobiological changes that adapt them to their new role and—as with mothers—those changes convey risk. And, in fact, as many as 10 percent of men may develop postpartum depression, and some may experience other related mood disorders, including anxiety or obsessive-compulsive disorder. Saxbe and her coauthors wrote that paper partly in response to suggestions among doctors that men be treated for postpartum depression with testosterone supplementation. What if that intervention effectively blunts a father's transition to parenthood or even puts the mother at greater risk?

Instead, they wrote, clinicians should "take a more nuanced view" of the role of testosterone and a family's needs. "Taking care of a baby is isolating and stressful and boring, and it's undervalued by our society. It's not seen as worthy employment," Saxbe told me. "When you put men in that role, they are going to maybe pay the same psychological price that women do." That doesn't mean men shouldn't do it, she said. In fact, society needs more men in caregiving so that more people can see that the best answer is to provide the infrastructure, like paid leave and supportive workplaces, to protect "the whole-family system."

Imagine that.

*　*　*

IN 2008, BIOLOGICAL ANTHROPOLOGIST JAMES Rilling was teaching a course on social neuroscience and decided to add a unit on love and attachment. He was searching through the literature and thinking about just how imbalanced it was, with so much about mothers and so little about fathers. This is true today and it was especially true then, before the few studies on brain structure and function in fathers had been published and before Lee Gettler's group published the data from the Philippines. Rilling, who now directs the Laboratory for Darwinian Neuroscience at Emory University, knew of the evidence that children with positively engaged fathers have better developmental outcomes, and he knew that paternal care is variable from family to family. "I became interested in the question of, why is it that there's so much variability among men and the degree of their commitment to caregiving and why do some men get more involved than others?" Rilling said. Certainly cultural and social factors were at play. But what about hormonal and neurobiological ones?

He and colleagues designed a study, one touched on in chapter 4, that was in part an investigation of whether the challenge hypothesis held up in human fathers. It analyzed plasma hormone levels in sixty-three fathers with children between ages one and two, and in thirty men without children, and assessed the men's neural response when viewing images of unrelated children and of sexually provocative women, also unfamiliar to them. The study was cross-sectional, comparing groups of men rather than following the same men over time, and it assessed only parental status, not relationship status, which is important given that men experience hormone changes upon becoming partners, too.

Among the study participants, fathers' testosterone levels were on average 20.5 percent lower than nonfathers'. Their oxytocin levels were 33 percent higher. I've spent a lot of time thinking about the hormonal storm of pregnancy, but it is also true that a persistent rain can reshape the landscape. The hormonal shifts that accompany fatherhood may not be as predictable or as dramatic as the endocrine roller coaster that birthing parents experience, but they are real, and they likely have long-lasting effects on the paternal brain, too.

Of course, as we've seen, testosterone is not everything, and it's really hard to isolate the effects of one hormone from another, particularly in the context of social relationships. Testosterone and oxytocin work in concert with one another, or perhaps in opposition, depending on the situation. Oxytocin influences the neuropeptide vasopressin, which may have a role in paternal care. Testosterone can be converted to estrogen, including in males. And testosterone interacts in important ways with cortisol. Yet most studies look only at one or two hormones at a time.

Rilling and colleagues found differences in brain activity between fathers and nonfathers, but those differences were only partly correlated to differences in hormones. When viewing pictures of children, fathers had stronger neural responses in hubs of the reward system and in brain regions involved in processing facial expressions and theory of mind. Specifically, the fathers' reward and motivation responses were stronger than the nonfathers' when viewing sad and neutral child faces, which the researchers hypothesized could be linked to fathers' propensity to sustain motivation to interact with their own children even in "times of distress or ambiguity." Nonfathers had stronger neural responses in areas of reward and motivation when viewing sexually provocative images.

Only in one brain region linked to face processing and empathy—the caudal middle frontal gyrus—were both fatherhood and lower testosterone correlated with greater activation in response to images of kids, prompting the authors to write that a testosterone decrease in fatherhood "may function to enhance empathy." Interestingly, there was no clear pattern associating either testosterone or oxytocin with response to sexual stimuli. This might have reflected challenges in hormone measurements, they wrote, or it might be that sexual responses are more steady and less responsive to the more acute changes in hormones that occur in the postpartum period.

These findings seem, to me, to affirm two things seen throughout the literature on fathers: men's neural responses are changed by fatherhood, especially around motivation and empathy. And we still don't have a great handle on how hormones shape behavior, in humans generally or in parenthood specifically. When I put that idea to Rilling, he responded, "I think there is considerable evidence that high testosterone biases men toward mating effort and away from direct caregiving." He also said those findings—the lack of correlation between testosterone and neural responses to sexual stimuli, which on some level challenges the challenge hypothesis—still surprise him.

Those findings also point to something that might seem obvious, something clearly not lost on researchers but that sometimes feels missing in the distilled findings they publish. Parents in these studies are people, in all their diversity, defined by far more than their parental status, and whose behaviors are not always readily categorized.

Of course, categorization is an important tool of research, and I appreciate the ways that Rilling's group has tried to tease out nuances of paternal care. They went on to explore how fathers of daughters and fathers of sons interact differently with their children and how those differences correlate with differences in the fathers' neural responses. They've looked at how a first-time father's reaction to newborn cries could vary with his age, with older fathers describing those cries as less aversive and showing more muted neural responses. And, in a small study of twenty new fathers who engaged in a video game in which they had to soothe a crying infant, the researchers added evidence to the idea of a global parental caregiving system and, with mixed results, identified lower activation in key parts of the system involved in motivation and emotion regulation for fathers who reported more frustration.

In one of his first papers on parenting, a review of the literature, Rilling wrote something that stuck with me. One important lesson to take from what we know so far "is that parenting might be thought of along a continuum with under- and over-sensitive parenting at opposite ends and sensitive parenting in the middle," he wrote. "There are hints that the mediating physiology may lie along a similar continuum."

Parenting, as behavior and as biology, is not a setting but a scale. Not one way to be, but many. This, of course, is true for fathers, too.

Rilling told me, the way he sees it, all adults have "the same basic core neural circuitry" for caregiving that can be shaped by many variables. "How readily does it get engaged? What's the threshold?" he said. "And then, you know, there are going to be both physiological, bottom-up factors that influence that, like hormones, but also top-down social, cultural influences as well."

Those top-down influences can include society's expectations for fathers, or a man's own expectations for himself. They can include how much and what kind of support he has. There is the stuff of connection within us all, but it takes all shapes. "I say as often as I can," Saxbe told me, "good parents are made, not born."

More research on fathers is coming. A few studies have been published about whether and how the structure of the human paternal brain changes, but with mixed or quite subtle results. As of summer 2021, Saxbe's lab had just started publishing papers from a longitudinal study following at least one hundred couples from around midpregnancy through the first year postpartum, and that work will include functional and structural analysis of the fathers' brains over time. Rilling was beginning recruitment for a longitudinal study following expectant fathers across a similar time period. Both projects are funded by the National Science Foundation, which is notable given that a lot of maternal brain research is funded through the National Institute of Child Health and Human Development at the National Institutes of Health.

Some researchers have told me that, even when they are studying mothers, funders have sent grant applications back to them with the question: What about the offspring? As though maternal development is worth investigating only through the lens of child outcomes, not on the basis of the mothers' own existence. Research on fathers adds another layer. Saxbe told me it is "really siloed." She said she often feels, "if you want to look at adult neuroplasticity, you sort of have to sneak it in." This, despite the fact that understanding what motivates men to care for infants has "a lot of social and political utility."

* * *

THE PARENTAL BRAIN RESEARCH ON any group of parents who are not straight, cisgender people who share DNA with their child is quite thin. What exists is fascinating, but each paper stands like a lone person on a dance floor, waiting for the music to start.

One early, exploratory paper used electroencephalogram, or EEG, to look at what are called event-related potential patterns in fourteen biological mothers and in fourteen mothers who were either adoptive or foster parents. With a net of electrodes attached to the scalp, researchers measured patterns of electrical activity in the cortex that have been linked, through repeated studies, to particular kinds of stimulus processing. The mothers were asked to view images of their own child and other children (familiar and unfamiliar), a familiar adult and an unfamiliar one. Both groups responded to their own children's faces, as compared with others', in a way thought to indicate "greater attention allocation." Importantly, this finding did not significantly vary by biological relatedness.

Within a larger group of foster mothers, oxytocin production and brain activity were linked in interesting ways. The study—conducted by Johanna Bick, then at the Yale Child Study Center, Damion Grasso of the University of Connecticut, and colleagues at the University of

Delaware—evaluated thirty-two women's oxytocin production (measured in this case through a series of urinary samples) when cuddling with their children, within the first two months of child placement and again three months later. At the same time points, the researchers used EEG to measure the mothers' neural activity in response to a series of images of children, including their own and others.

At the first period of testing, higher cuddling-related oxytocin production was correlated with greater amplitude in a measurement linked to "motivated attention" when the foster mothers viewed any infant—not only their own. That changed three months later, when higher oxytocin was correlated with greater amplitude in response to a mother's *own* infant. The results suggest a biological process of bonding in which oxytocin plays a role, or perhaps a "mediating physiology" that places foster parents along a parenting continuum. To put it more simply, the neurobiology of foster parents seems to be changed by parenting, too. Of course, the caveat—it's just one study.

We've already touched on research that found similarities in amygdala activation between primary caregiving fathers and primary caregiving mothers. In fact, those findings came from a study, by Ruth Feldman, Eyal Abraham, and colleagues in Israel, that compared straight and gay couples, in terms of their brain responses, oxytocin, and parenting behavior.

The participants included forty-one heterosexual biological parents (men and women, where the women were primary caregivers) and forty-eight gay fathers who had a baby through surrogacy (half of the fathers were biologically related to their child, and all were considered primary caregivers to their children). Researchers visited parents in their homes, to collect salivary samples for oxytocin assessment and to videotape parent-child interactions "in the natural habitat." Parents' brains were later scanned using fMRI as they viewed those taped interactions, as well as recordings of just themselves and of unfamiliar parents and children.

This paper was key to establishing the idea of a global parental caregiving network. Across all parents viewing the taped interactions with their children, the researchers found mostly consistent engagement of brain regions linked to vigilance, salience, motivation, social understanding, and mentalizing. The researchers wrote that their findings underscore the idea that human parenting may have evolved from "an evolutionarily ancient alloparenting substrate that exists in all adult members of the species" that is activated as needed. "Such an alloparental caregiving system, observed throughout the animal kingdom, may have contributed to the extreme variability and flexibility of paternal care observed through the evolution of our species," they wrote.

There were some important differences between the groups. Mothers showed greater activation of the amygdala than secondary-caregiving fathers did. Those fathers showed greater activation of the superior temporal sulcus than the mothers did. But primary-caregiving fathers had high activation of both of those regions. And there were no significant differences in brain region activation among the gay fathers, biological or adoptive.

Looking across all fathers, those who spent more time directly caring for their children showed a greater increase in functional connectivity between the amygdala and superior temporal sulcus when viewing tapes of themselves with their children. The researchers note that their findings underscore "the central role of actual caregiving behavior" in the development of the parental brain. In other words, experience matters.

Lesbians also have received little attention in the research literature, as of 2021. One study evaluated testosterone levels across the prenatal period in twenty-five expectant couples and found—similar to what's been found in fathers—that in both partners, lower prenatal testosterone predicted better reported commitment, higher relationship quality, and more time spent engaged in baby care three months out. But, contrary to what they expected, the researchers did not find a significant change in prenatal testosterone in the nongestational mothers, compared with "small but reliable" declines in the researchers' own sample of expectant fathers. If a drop in testosterone in expectant fathers is a kind of neurobiological signal of their commitment to care, why wasn't it present in these new parents who were women? One explanation might be that they were already deeply committed.

For gay couples, having a baby can require additional layers of planning and financial investment. The women in the sample were mostly in their thirties, had good incomes, and had been looking forward, together,

to becoming parents. Robin Edelstein, an author on the paper and director of the Personality, Relationships, and Hormones Lab at the University
of Michigan, told me that some of the questions on the standardized scale
the researchers used to assess relationship quality and commitment felt
out of place here: How invested are you in this relationship? Do you see
alternatives to your partner? "When I first saw the numbers, I thought,
is this a mistake?" Edelstein said. "They're all just doing great. So there's
not a lot of variability." A study with a larger sample might have different
results, she said, or better yet one that follows women over a much longer
period, even before they have met their partners.

I asked several researchers to what degree nongestational parents
make up their own category, with findings about biological fathers
applying similarly to all others, and I got mixed responses. Some said
it's possible that a biological connection between parent and child matters in how strong a stimulus that baby is. But I have to think that the
difference, if it exists, is marginal, perhaps one more factor determining a parent's place on the continuum, along with hormones, readiness,
experience, and social support.

The thing is, we don't actually know what studies that look at the
effect of "ownness" on the parental brain are really measuring. Is it a
quality of shared genetic material? The work on foster and adoptive
parents suggests not. Perhaps it is, instead, a state of capture, of being a
spellbound adult whose attention and sense of self have been expertly
infiltrated by a tiny, powerful baby.

Soon after Roberts became a Boot Camp for New Dads coach, he
found himself asking his pregnant friends and coworkers about their
partners: "Is he talking to your belly? If you want, I can sit down with
them. We gotta talk about baby poop. We gotta talk about gatekeeping."

A few years ago, Maine Boys to Men added a new segment to its
program for expectant fathers. After boot camp, coaches lead the group
in conversations about characteristics that define a good mother or a
good father. They create two lists. Then they cross out the titles for each
list and talk about the nature of good parents, or as Maine Boys to Men
executive director Heidi Randall put it, how we are "humanly inclined
to care for our children." The expectant fathers are asked to reflect on
their own parents and on themselves.

Roberts described his own first experience with boot camp as a "golden ticket," an invitation to shape his own fatherhood, to make his own path. This exercise is like that, too, he said, an invitation to choose. "Just don't operate on autopilot," he said. "That's your ticket."

* * *

SOMETIMES THE RESEARCH ON THE parental brain feels deeply old-fashioned. Outdated. Stuck. In paper after paper, mothers and babies exist as a unit in space. Mothers are deemed primary, fathers secondary. Families exist as a child and two adults, one from each of two "strikingly non-overlapping bimodal" genders. This is not the world I see around me.

One clear summer night in 2019, I sat in a canoe on Kezar Lake in western Maine with Logan Nichols-Chestnut, a multidisciplinary visual artist and maker of graphic memoirs. We were both staying at Hewnoaks, an artists' residency made up of a string of cabins built over the first half of the twentieth century into a hill at the lake's edge. We each had left two children at home with our spouses, for some much-desired quiet and time to focus. In this moment, I was happy to just be there, under a sky full of stars and brushed by the Milky Way, framed on two sides by the blue-black of mountain silhouettes. Over and over, we watched streaks of light chase meteors across the atmosphere.

I was at Hewnoaks to work on my book about motherhood, about how different the story of motherhood felt from the truth of it, and how the science of the maternal brain could have helped me to feel better prepared. Nichols-Chestnut was at work on a book about his experience as a trans man and a father, and about his own father, who died before he could meet his grandchildren. I thought then that our work was related but separate, tracking two paths across the same plane.

We stayed in sporadic touch in the years that followed, sending dispatches about pandemic parenting and our books. It would be almost two years before I realized just how our stories converged, after I had returned in 2021 to Hewnoaks for another week and got a note in my inbox from Nichols-Chestnut. He sent me the first two chapters of his book, *The Reciprocal*, which he planned to shop to publishers soon. The chapters were a beautiful rendering of the making of his own queer family—including the decision to have his wife carry their children and to use a friend as a sperm donor, a man their sons call Papi—and of how parents shape the parents their own children become, sometimes in surprising ways. I had asked about the title. Like a reciprocal number, he told me. The number by which you multiply another number to get 1. The inverse that results in a whole. The dissimilar made similar. A binary folded in on itself: masculine/ feminine, parent/child, love/grief.

When we talked by phone later, Nichols-Chestnut told me that his mother was largely absent in his childhood—present physically but not otherwise. His father was not overtly sentimental but consistently caring; he worked a lot but went out of his way to make time for Nichols-Chestnut. He showed his love by teaching. How to do laundry, how to make an omelet, how to iron. Also, how to fix a car, how to build a fence. "It wasn't like, you need to learn how to do this because you're a girl," Nichols-Chestnut said. "You need to learn this because you need to take care of yourself." His father was practical but also patient and attentive.

Nichols-Chestnut and his wife married before he transitioned, but his father didn't come to the wedding, and Nichols-Chestnut didn't come out to him as transgender before he died. Still, he paints such a thoughtful portrait of his father and explores his own experience of gender in such a moving way that by the time I got to the page that includes side-by-side panels of his father demonstrating how to make chicken and dumplings and Nichols-Chestnut cooking the same dish for his sons, my eyes welled up with something like pride. For both of them. "My dad really did show me that this type of caregiving—it can be anyone," he said.

The biology of parenting is strikingly overlapping. I'm not trying to say that mothers and fathers are synonymous, their experiences entirely the same. They typically do have different biological paths of development, and they experience the world as defined by wildly different and incredibly powerful social norms according to their gender. It's just that those differences don't spring from male and female brains made in different molds. Yet the structures and mechanisms in place to explore the parental brain—the funding sources, the questions upon which studies are built, the chosen metrics of measurement—still often assume that they do.

In a recent essay in the *New York Times* marking ten years since his first testosterone injection, Thomas Page McBee wrote that every person everywhere is constantly negotiating "with the political and cultural forces attempting to shape us into simple, translatable packages." He challenged readers to do more of what transgender people are good at because they have to be—to question things that are held out as norms of biology, including around parenting. "What might it mean for all parents if 'mother' and 'father' were not such distinct categories in child-rearing? Who benefits from their continuing separation?"

These questions barely entered my mind when I, as a cisgender woman married to a man, was birthing our biological children in a medical system designed exactly for families like ours. But they are very much on my mind now, and not only because I want to be a better ally to people who continue to be harmed by those institutions. It's also because I now more clearly see the ways those categorical separations are problematic for my own family, too—ultimately, I believe, for all families.

They have not felt beneficial when my husband, who is as much a primary caregiver to our children as I am, is left out of playgroups or online parenting support groups labeled explicitly for mothers, and therefore excluded from really critical sources of information about juggling work and a newborn, finding affordable childcare, navigating special education in our local school system, or finding a car seat that can be installed without pulling out your own hair. They didn't feel beneficial when my former boss denied my request for a four-day flextime schedule, asking why I couldn't just plan to work from home, with a toddler and a newborn, on that fifth day. "When was the last time you spent a day alone with a toddler?" I asked him. He couldn't say.

The pervasive tropes around "mama" culture and "daddy day care" that assume one to be the singular nurturer and default parent and the other to be an as-needed stand-in, are not beneficial. And birthing parents rarely benefit when the biological processes associated with motherhood, including vaginal childbirth and breastfeeding, are so hallowed and essentialized that, when those processes are not possible, they begin parenthood feeling like a failure.

Saxbe told me that a professor she had in graduate school used to say often that anything as important to the survival of a species as parenting will be overlaid by redundant systems. There is no single moment or process that opens the one and only door to the parent-child bond. Parents who miss out on skin-to-skin contact in the moments after birth, for example, have other opportunities to begin that connection. And, likewise, there is no single form that a loving parent must take. Saxbe pointed to her lab's research on prolactin in fathers and the idea that a hormonal system tied to milk production in females may be co-opted in males to facilitate bonding through proximity—a redundancy aimed perhaps at making sure every baby has an alert parent at hand, or every toddler has an attentive adult nearby once their baby sister arrives.

We need much more research on parents of all kinds. Big longitudinal studies that pull in measures of whole family dynamics, that look beyond the maternal-infant dyad in the immediate postpartum period. And smaller studies with more precise categorizations that consider the diversity of family life in the modern world.

We need this. And yet, we know enough.

We know enough to say that every person possesses the capacity to develop a parental caregiving network. We know enough to say that babies change the adults who care for them. We know enough to say that it is love and attention that ultimately shapes and creates the adapted parental brain, not exclusively a person's gender, sex, or method of procreation. Sure, a million questions remain, and we know enough to act.

We can recognize, in birthing places, doctor's offices, prenatal education, and postpartum support groups that parents take all forms. The support pregnant women and new mothers find at this stage in life through other pregnant women and new mothers is important, validating, and often the primary source of necessary physical and mental health information. But if nearly the entire infrastructure of mainstream online and in-person support groups is exclusive to birthing, cisgender women, then not only are we telling other birthing parents that they are on their own but we're sending a message to fathers and partners that this stuff just isn't really for you. This major, brain-changing event is not your major, brain-changing event.

We can recognize and reconsider the hypergendered language we use to talk about parenthood. There is a backlash on social media, among conservative pundits, and within pockets of women's rights activists and birth workers against use of the phrase "birthing people," as if it erases women and mothers or takes something away from them. As a writer, I believe in using specific language when referring to individuals, and precise, inclusive language when referring to groups of people. As a mother, I recognize the power in my birth experience and the strength I gain in my capacity to care for my children. Recognizing those very same things in other people who carry or parent children, no matter their sex or gender, takes nothing away from me. It only affirms what I know to be true.

Perhaps the most important step we can take in helping all parents adapt to caregiving is to implement robust paid family leave programs that support all parents of newborns and adopted children wherever these programs don't already exist, especially in the United States— which is far behind other similar-income countries on this front. As important are incentives that promote uptake of these programs by fathers and other nongestational parents, for whom we know that time spent actually caring for a baby is so vital.

Saxbe is optimistic about the changes underway when it comes to gender norms and parenting. Just look, she said, at the Mandalorian. The starring character of the *Star Wars* series by the same name—with his impenetrable beskar helmet and a demeanor inspired by Clint Eastwood and the samurai characters of Japanese filmmaker Akira Kurosawa—cares for a tiny, powerful alien who checks every box on the cuteness scale: proportionally large eyes, small chin, round cheeks. Plus, those ears. "You have this really manly, armored warrior guy," Saxbe said, "but he's taking care of baby Yoda."

Often men feel intimidated by parenting because it doesn't come naturally to them. But it doesn't come naturally—whatever that means—to anyone. Or rather, it does, but through practice. "Parenting is a skill," Saxbe said. "That's a hopeful message because it suggests that you can train it. You can develop it. It's about your motivation."

If we were to really acknowledge that parenting is not automatic, that instead the parental brain develops through experience, Saxbe said, that could change things, including perhaps the political appetite for paternity leave benefits. "It doesn't have to feel like this thing that you're either biologically born to do or not," she said.

The neuroscience is proving just how true that statement is. And society is shifting, too. Slowly. But it is changing, Saxbe said: "It's a matter of time."

CHAPTER 7

Start Where You Are

When Alyssa McCloskey's first son was born, she was in awe. She was sixteen years old and newly married, and she had just been through more than twenty hours of excruciating "back labor." But then little Tyler arrived and he loved her, she could tell. And she loved him back.

She hadn't planned on getting pregnant as a teenager, she said, but she had tried to prepare herself. She read all the books she could get her hands on. In those first months as a mom, she said, she worried about whether she was doing things right. The responsibility, the feeling that everything she did would be watched and repeated by her son, weighed on her some. But being Tyler's mom was a joy. "It was a pretty magical experience," she said. "I loved everything about it."

A lot of things felt different when McCloskey became pregnant again about eleven years later. This time, her pregnancy was planned and hoped for. But it also was a struggle. Separation of her pelvic bones made it excruciating, even with physical therapy. "I couldn't wait to go into labor," she told me. The pregnancy went past her due date and McCloskey had an appointment for an induction when her water broke. Contractions, however, didn't come, at least not consistently. So McCloskey was given the induction drug Pitocin, and then labor came fast and hard. Too hard. "It felt like my body was going against me instead of working with me," McCloskey said. "I couldn't even breathe, because it was just so intense."

Then her son was born. McCloskey said she had been so eager to feel that overwhelming love again, but when she held Simon for the first time, it was missing. "I felt almost like he wasn't my baby," she said. "It was such an odd feeling, because it was something I had wanted for probably about two years prior to that. . . . I was pretty disappointed in myself."

That feeling of disconnection diminished some as the weeks went by—nursing helped—but it didn't go away. She didn't know how to bond with Simon. He was just a baby. And she was full of guilt. She wondered, "Does he even want me to be his mom?" McCloskey said she worried that Tyler was feeling pushed out of his relationship with her. And, for months, she said, she struggled to leave an abusive relationship with Simon's father, their separation complicated by the fact that he wanted time with the baby and she was nursing, and by her belief that so much of this—the abuse and the struggle to bond—was her fault.

Before Simon was born, McCloskey said, she thought postpartum depression was when a mother had an overwhelming urge to hurt her child, and that was not her experience at all. She started reading more about it online. From her early days with Tyler, she knew what it felt like to have a rewarding connection with her baby. Maybe that feeling was missing with Simon because of a difference in her brain and her hormones this time around, she thought, because of the stress she was under.

For McCloskey, this realization was hopeful. Hopeful and hard.

Recognizing the fallacy of maternal instinct comes with some hard truths. A friend told me they had expected their child to arrive with a kind of upgrade for themselves as a parent, a download of skills and information necessary for the job. Adult 2.0. But it never came. The parental brain grows out of the brain a person already has, one shaped by their genes and their complicated family history, by how they were cared for as a child, and by the coping mechanisms they've developed along the way. By the stress and trauma they have experienced over a lifetime and during pregnancy and the postpartum period. And by the healing and the support they've known, too.

There is no separate parenting brain network—no dedicated, on-demand, prepackaged instinct—that comes online as needed. We start where we are.

Here, we'll look at the many ways the hard stuff of life can affect the brain through the transitions of parenthood. Chronic stress and trauma are powerful influences that shape the neural circuitry for motivation, emotion regulation, and social cognition on which parenting depends. And likewise the upheaval inherent in pregnancy and the postpartum period influences the stress responses we've developed over a lifetime in important and sometimes surprising ways. Researchers have begun using what they've learned to figure out how to better support parents of young children and how to treat those who struggle most, often by taking advantage of the very factor that makes them vulnerable: the brain's own heightened flexibility.

* * *

BEFORE MY SONS WERE BORN, I thought postpartum depression was like the flu. Either you had it or you didn't. I was naive, of course. It's not as if depression in the general population can be diagnosed by a blood draw or a cotton swab to the cheek. Why would it work that way for new parents? Also, I was misled.

Postpartum depression typically is presented to pregnant people as a list of symptoms to watch for and a recommendation that they seek help if, after their two-week allowance for more transient "baby blues" is up, they're still feeling "hopeless or empty." This feels contained. Neat. As if certain people will tick the boxes on the symptom list and others will feel more or less hopeful and full. Steady. Stable.

The more I learned about the parental brain and talked with parents—listened, really—the more I realized that our experiences fall across a broad spectrum, with little distress at one end and debilitating distress at the other. Between them is a range of unease and adaptation. There is no clean cutoff, no precise point along that continuum at which distress tips into disorder. Few people who become parents get through it without any psychological struggle. Perhaps that's why the way we talk about postpartum mood disorders becomes so distilled in the first place. Because we don't entirely know what to say.

"The transition to becoming a parent is one of the most profound things anyone will ever do—hands down," Samantha Meltzer-Brody, director of the University of North Carolina Center for Women's Mood

Disorders, told me. Meltzer-Brody is best known these days for her research on brexanolone, a drug marketed by Sage Therapeutics as Zulresso that in 2019 became the first to receive US Food and Drug Administration approval for the treatment of postpartum depression. But she wears many hats as a researcher and clinician.

It was Meltzer-Brody who called postpartum depression a "garbage-bag term," not unlike the category of breast cancer, which isn't one but many kinds of cancers that present with different symptoms, different prognoses, different treatment options, and different genetic, hormonal, or environmental causes. Similarly, postpartum depression has long been an inadequate catchall for the myriad ways parents can experience psychiatric disorders after having a baby. So people experiencing paralyzing anxiety or obsessiveness might find nothing in the baby books that explains their experience. Those having flashbacks to a traumatic birth experience might never learn that childbirth-related post-traumatic stress disorder is a real and treatable thing.

Many clinicians and researchers now recognize a broader category of perinatal mood and anxiety disorders, or perinatal psychiatric disorders, generally thought to affect about one in five birthing parents (see endnote for more about the challenge of calculating prevalence). The umbrella terms better reflect the breadth of experiences, which also can include eating disorders or rare but serious psychosis. The subcategories overlap, and that can complicate diagnosis and treatment. Trauma shapes depression. Anxiety and depression are often, but not always, co-occurring. The same goes for obsessive-compulsive disorder.

Even those who present with symptoms more readily recognizable as depression may be experiencing different biological mechanisms causing those symptoms. Often postpartum depression occurs when people lack the supports they need to manage the adjustment to new parenthood, including financial resources and supportive partners, family, or friends. Or when they have a prior history of mental illness. Or when they are experiencing chronic or acute stress that undermines their capacity to cope with the stresses inherent in pregnancy, childbirth, and caring for a baby. Other times, and often in the most severe cases, Meltzer-Brody said, postpartum depression seems to hit "out of the blue" in a way that feels "incredibly biologic."

The *Diagnostic and Statistical Manual of Mental Disorders*, sometimes referred to as the bible of psychiatry, does not recognize postpartum mood disorders explicitly. It considers perinatal depression to be a subtype of major depressive disorder that begins during pregnancy or in the four weeks afterward. Many birthing parents are screened for postpartum depression only at their standard six-week checkup—if they ever are. Yet it's widely accepted, including by the World Health Organization and the US Centers for Disease Control and Prevention, that postpartum depression can occur any time in the first year postpartum. One recent study followed hundreds of women who received prenatal care at a·Michigan hospital and found that, among the 325 who screened negative for depression and post-traumatic stress disorder at six weeks, 8 percent switched their status and screened positive for one of those conditions by three months postpartum. Many birthing parents struggle for weeks before they ever get a chance to talk to their doctors. And many others struggle, without help, afterward. Scientists have begun trying to link the timing of depression's onset to particular neurobiological triggers.

For some, symptoms begin in pregnancy, but pregnant people are not routinely screened for risk factors. And while postpartum depression generally shares the same symptoms of major depressive disorder in other contexts—including loss of interest or pleasure, withdrawal, or hopelessness—it also can look different from how depression often is described, especially when accompanied by symptoms of anxiety or obsessiveness that may seem opposite from a loss of interest. As in the general population, postpartum bipolar disorder is common and underdiagnosed, partly because the typical screening tools look for depressive symptoms but not manic ones.

What is somewhat clearer is the toll that depression can take on parents and babies. A baby needs an attentive parent, to keep them safe and clean and fed but also to engage with them in ways that are important for brain development. Depression can interfere with those things, though it doesn't always. Depression during pregnancy, particularly more severe depression, is associated with an increased risk of premature delivery. Postpartum depression has been linked to behavioral challenges and lower cognitive development in children, though often the effect sizes in these studies are small—meaning the association with poor child outcomes may be weak—or the findings are dependent on whether the depression persists over time or on what other kinds of support that parent and baby have in their lives.

This point is important because people with postpartum depression can feel like their struggle has unquestioningly undermined their baby's future. As if the presence of their distress, in the face of an overwhelming life transition, has soured the milk, or turned the child. But babies are resilient. We know they are good at hooking the hearts of adults, and not only the people who birthed them. Plus, new parents' brains possess an incredible capacity for change and adjustment. In this sense, the presence of perinatal mental illness is *not* deterministic. What may be more deterministic is the absence of other caring adults in a family's life, a scarcity of the time and resources that all new families require, or a lack of access to effective treatment.

Postpartum depression can have serious and potentially lifelong health consequences for parents themselves. Suicide is a leading cause of pregnancy-associated death, alongside homicide (most often at the hands of a partner), and thoughts of suicide or self-harm during the postpartum period are surprisingly common, with one analysis finding between 5 percent and 14 percent of mothers reporting ever having thoughts of harming themselves. Depressive symptoms make such thoughts more likely.

As Darby Saxbe and her colleagues described, the transition to parenthood is a "critical window" into a person's long-term health, including—in big and important ways—their mental health. About 40 percent of people who experience postpartum depression have never had a depressive episode before, but they may have another. Postpartum depression, especially if left untreated, increases a person's risk of recurrent depression and bipolar disorder later in life.

None of the science discussed in this book will provide *the* key to solving postpartum mental health so that more families can get a better start. If such a thing existed, it might sit in the pockets of government officials and policy makers who make choices about whether and how to support vulnerable families and address inequality in their communities. A few years ago, a group of researchers from California looked at data from across the globe tracking the prevalence of postpartum depression. They analyzed 291 studies from fifty-six countries, includ-ing data from nearly three hundred thousand women. They found the global prevalence rate of postpartum depression to be about 18 percent, but that varied considerably from country to country—38 percent in Chile versus 3 percent in Singapore, for example. Some of that vari-ability likely had to do with differences in awareness, cultural framing of the disorder, and quality of research from country to country. But the countries with the highest rates of postpartum depression also had higher rates of economic and health disparities across society. Child-bearing people who are stable and supported have a better chance of making it through the tumult of new parenthood without a crisis.

There's a lot that researchers can do—and have been doing—to figure out what exactly causes postpartum depression and how best to prevent it and treat it, in ways that don't depend quite as much on the whims of politicians or on solving the most intractable societal problems.

* * *

A LOT OF MELTZER-BRODY'S RESEARCH is aimed at dissecting the nature of postpartum depression, picking threads from the diagnostic tangle and following them back to their source. She is part of an international consortium of researchers who pooled their detailed clinical data on thousands of people from across nineteen health care institutions and used it to look for subtypes of postpartum depression based on partic-ular characteristics, such as when a person's symptoms appeared, how severe the symptoms were, and whether they also experienced anxiety or suicidal ideation. In 2016, that group launched an app where women who experience postpartum depression can submit their own informa-tion to a research database. Some participants are then asked to provide DNA samples in spit tubes shipped to their homes. Three years after the launch, with help from creative agency Wongdoody, the project was rebranded as Mom Genes Fight PPD, with an upgraded app design, a social media campaign, an influencer event in Los Angeles, and a video ad that manages to be both catchy and devastating. "It has totally super-charged the whole project," Meltzer-Brody said.

As of fall 2021, the consortium had collected genetic data from about twenty thousand women and was getting ready to publish the results of its first round of genome-wide analysis. The goal is to create a database of samples from one hundred thousand people—hopefully enough to provide meaningful insight into the genetic risk factors for different subtypes of postpartum depression, which could lead to improved screening or better treatment.

"Twenty-five years ago, you had breast cancer and everyone got the same treatment," Meltzer-Brody said. "Now we treat you based on your genetic signature of the cancer. And there's wildly different outcomes, in the most positive way, based on that specificity. And in postpartum depression, we're still sort of like, everyone's getting the same thing, regardless of what the underlying subtypes are."

One day, such precision psychiatry might be available to postpartum people, too. But there's an important distinction here, Meltzer-Brody said. Breast cancer is typically site-specific. A tumor can be biopsied and analyzed. "We can't do that in people's brains," she said. "Therein lies the problem."

One thing researchers have been doing is using brain imaging to try to get a sense of what postpartum depression looks like in the brain. Imaging studies could be an important tool for understanding the mechanisms by which the disorder impacts parenting and which to target for treatment. But so far, they are quite limited.

If postpartum depression is many different subtypes, it's going to require large sample sizes—like the one Mom Genes is trying for—to really understand it. Imaging studies to date mostly have looked at the brains of one or two dozen people with postpartum depression at a time. They almost never follow people with postpartum depression over time, in longitudinal studies. And so far, the results are quite mixed, in part because the criteria for inclusion—months postpartum or symptomology—vary from study to study. So do the stimuli used to evaluate neural activity, which may be pictures or cries recorded from a mother's own baby, or stimuli that are meant to be positive or negative but have no personal relevance to the person in the scanner.

Researchers recognize that imaging studies can only do so much. The goal is to look for results that hold true across studies and "above and beyond" differences in a given study group, said Aya Dudin, a doctoral researcher in neuroscience at McMaster University. One such finding relates to the amygdala.

In people with serious depressive symptoms in the postpartum period, the amygdala's response to negative stimuli, such as distress cries from a baby, is generally thought to be blunted. That effect may be dose-dependent, with a more muted response the more severe a person's depressive symptoms are. That's opposite from the hyperreactive effect seen in major depressive disorder in the general population.

Dudin is coauthor on a pair of fascinating studies that highlight the challenges of distilling imaging results into simple narratives. This work compared women who were depressed and not depressed, with and without children. When the researchers asked women without children to view images of smiling infants—positive baby-related stimuli—the amygdala response did not differ by depression status. Among the mothers, however, those with depression showed a *stronger* amygdala response to the smiling pictures of unfamiliar infants than the mothers without depression did. The researchers also asked the mothers to view their own babies, and again the amygdala in depressed mothers reacted strongly. But the researchers noticed something interesting. In nondepressed mothers, the amygdala reacted much more strongly to their own baby than to other babies. In depressed mothers, the difference in reaction between "own" and "other" was smaller.

The researchers called this a "blunted unique amygdala responsiveness to own infant." It's as if the radar for baby cues was turned up in depressed mothers and not well tuned. And some researchers have suggested this might reflect a characteristic of postpartum depression—an amygdala that responds too much or too little, depending on the context, but that misses the range in the middle that perhaps best maintains that balance between parental motivation and vigilance.

Other studies have tried to pinpoint depression-related differences in more reward-related brain regions, in the circuitry essential for emotion regulation and executive functioning, in white matter connections, and in the distribution of neurotransmitter receptors. Because a person *can* be anxious or depressed and still be a responsive parent, researchers have tried to suss out which connections in the brain support caregiving in the presence of those symptoms. It all makes for a nuanced and often frustrating picture, like so many squiggly lines on a Magic Eye poster that you just can't make out.

It may be that postpartum depression in someone who has a history of depressive episodes looks different in the brain than it does in someone whose first-ever episode is during the postpartum period, Dudin said. But most imaging studies necessarily sort people into yes/no categories that can't detect that nuance. "It's a binary system," she said, "and we know that all mental health and mental illnesses are heterogeneous just by nature."

A basic principle of the brain, and one important for understanding mental illness in general, is that it works by dynamic tension. This is certainly true in parenting. Tending to a baby requires a push and a pull. Parents must pay attention but not overly obsess. React but also regulate. Nurture but be vigilant. Researchers sometimes frame this as "reciprocal inhibition" between circuits of brain activity that seem to lead to opposing ends. Pup-directed aggression versus pup grooming. Parental defense versus parental care.

The balance of these things seems often (but not always) to be related to stress: how much of it a person experiences, when and for how long, and what capacity they have for absorbing more. There's a growing acknowledgment that, to understand the parental brain, we need to know more about how stress affects it, from pregnancy to the postpartum period.

* * *

THINK ABOUT STRESS IN THE body and you probably think about cortisol. It has been dubbed the body's "stress hormone," and so we tend to think that less is always best. If you've been following along here, you know what I'm about to say: that's not quite right.

Cortisol is produced when a stressful situation triggers a system that includes the hypothalamus, the pituitary gland that sits just below the hypothalamus, and the adrenal glands perched atop the kidneys. This is the HPA axis. It is the body's control center for responding to stress, and it is also molded over time by exposure to acute and chronic stressors. Cortisol produced by the adrenal glands increases blood glucose levels and makes sure the body has the energy it needs to respond to a challenge or to maintain a high alert. But, like the HPA axis generally, it is involved in many more processes in the body related to adapting to a changing environment, in conditions we might consider very stressful or very ordinary.

Cortisol levels are generally cyclical, higher in the morning and declining toward the evening. They also vary minute by minute, in response to the stimuli we encounter as we move through the day. This kind of multilevel variation is an important facet of cortisol. Cortisol is a change agent, involved in memory, immune response, and quite literally getting out of bed in the morning. It also seems to play a fundamental role in the processes of neuroplasticity and learning. In people with chronic stress or major depressive disorder, the daily cortisol rhythm may flatten or show extreme spikes and a slow recovery to lower levels. One researcher told me cortisol is the "currency" of stress. Like a glut of cash in the economy, dysregulation of cortisol affects neural systems in complex ways.

Psychiatric disorders related to chronic stress are thought to cause atrophy in the hippocampus in humans. Because the hippocampus is part of a feedback loop regulating HPA activity, stress can create a cascading effect, with impairment of the hippocampus leading to further dysregulation of the brain's stress response. Antidepressant medications may work partly by reversing volume reductions in that brain region. Meanwhile, the effect of stress on the amygdala—that salience detector—is just the opposite. In humans and in other animals, stress and stress-related disorders have been correlated with both greater volume and increased activity in the amygdala, which could be linked to increases in fear and anxiety.

A lot of what we understand about stress and the brain can be traced back to the work of neuroscientist Bruce McEwen, a giant in his field who died in 2020. McEwen and his colleagues were the first to show that the rat hippocampus had receptors for corticosterone, which is the primary glucocorticoid in rodents and considered more or less an analog to cortisol in humans. That meant the stress hormone circulating in the body made its way into the brain. The researchers went on to detail how corticosterone shapes neuroplasticity in that brain region and elsewhere. Over his career, McEwen explained how dysregulation of the body's stress response can produce "wear and tear" on otherwise adaptive processes, to disastrous effects. He expanded on the idea of allostasis and popularized the notion of "allostatic load," or the price the body pays when it reacts to stress too much or too little, or fails to correct once an acute stressor has passed. Central to McEwen's thinking was the fact that cortisol is not the body's "bad guy" but rather a critical mediator of its capacity to respond and predict.

This is an important point for making sense of cortisol's role in the context of new parenthood. Cortisol production increases exponentially during pregnancy and remains high in the very early postpartum period. Less, it turns out, is not always best. Plasma cortisol in the third trimester is as much as three times higher than it is before pregnancy—a level that would be considered clearly pathological in other contexts but is entirely normal in pregnancy.

Cortisol is thought to aid in a fetus's maturation by making more glucose available during development, and it is important in labor, delivery, and milk secretion. It is passed to a developing fetus, but the placenta can block harmful levels from reaching the fetus by converting cortisol to an inactive form. Amazingly, pregnant people also have protection from what would otherwise be damaging health effects from super-high cortisol. That's partly because increased estrogen drives an increase in a protein in the blood called corticosteroid-binding globulin that—as the names suggests—binds with cortisol and reduces the amount that's "free" and available to cells. And a person's cortisol reactivity—the spike when faced with a stressor—repeatedly has been found to be blunted during pregnancy.

Cortisol generally declines—probably quite precipitously—to more typical levels by about three months postpartum. But in those first days, it remains high, particularly for first-time birthing parents, and researchers have suggested that it plays a role in driving them to pay attention and respond to their babies in those early hours and days when they may have no prior experience to draw on. Higher cortisol levels have been linked to brand-new mothers' attentiveness toward their babies, as measured by affectionate touch such as kissing and patting, sympathetic responses to infant cries, and attraction toward other cues. The cortisol research in fathers is quite spotty, but one study found that, compared with experienced fathers, new fathers showed stronger cortisol reactivity in response to infant cry sounds.

In rats, corticosterone seems to help shape early caregiving experiences into a "maternal memory" that rat mothers can call on later, after they've been separated from their pups. We can't say whether elevated cortisol aids the creation or retention of early postpartum memories in humans, or how it shapes learning to parent. But it may. Those first days with a baby are jam-packed with newness. New parenthood is immersion learning at its most intense.

The benefit of higher cortisol seems to fall off, however, for mothers at least. By a few months postpartum, higher maternal cortisol may be either inconsequential or possibly a detriment to caregiving. Mothers with higher daily cortisol levels at between two and six months postpartum performed worse on measures of executive functioning and demonstrated less parental sensitivity during play sessions in one study, though the evidence on this point has been mixed.

Importantly, the HPA function of birthing parents and babies becomes "attuned," their cortisol levels and rhythms following similar patterns. This effect is strongest, or at least most consistent, in breastfeeding parents and babies, though milk may be just one means of establishing this link (see: redundant systems). Some amount of HPA attunement may be heritable or established in utero. And some could be the result of parent-child interactions in the first months of life, in how each responds to the other's distress.

But the narrative of how cortisol and HPA function during pregnancy and the postpartum period is a messy one. There's too much variation from study to study, in what each group of researchers is measuring and when, to get a clear picture of a hormone that does not fit into a linear story line anyway, but instead fluctuates across different time scales, over the course of a day, in any given moment of stress, and in the context of other hormones. This is true for so much of the story of how hormones influence parental caregiving, but especially so with cortisol. "We think we maybe know," said Jodi Pawluski, the psychotherapist and neuroscientist, "but no one can pinpoint it really well."

I started to see cortisol like the particularly frazzled member of a stage crew at a community theater. Harried yet effective at making all the necessary adjustments—replacing a missing prop just before the curtain, fixing a broken set piece on the fly—to keep the bodies onstage performing and connecting with their audience even, and most especially, when a crisis comes up. Cortisol is a central part of the crew. But it is not the only one.

Neurotransmitters generally fall into two categories: excitatory or inhibitory. These are sort of like uppers or downers for the synapses, ramping up activity or slowing it down. Gamma-aminobutyric acid, referred to as GABA, can do both but is considered the primary inhibitory neurotransmitter in the nervous system of vertebrates. Certain GABA receptors in the hypothalamus are thought to play an essential role in regulating activity of the HPA axis, in preventing it from getting overexcited. Think of GABA signaling as the stage crew's voice of reason.

Pregnancy seems to make this GABA activity more potent and better at blunting that stress reactivity in the hypothalamus. That effect is driven, at least in part, by an increase in allopregnanolone, a neurosteroid produced mostly by metabolism of progesterone, which of course rises dramatically in pregnancy, too. Jamie Maguire, a neuroscientist and director of the Maguire Lab at Tufts Graduate School of Biomedical Sciences, told me that this increase in allopregnanolone is so significant that, on its own, it would have serious sedative effects. Except there's a counteraction. Maguire and colleague Istvan Mody documented that, in pregnant mice, the number of certain GABA receptors drops significantly during pregnancy, like a check against too much inhibition.

Researchers think these nuanced changes in GABA control may help balance the scales of a pregnant person's stress response, at a time when sky-high steroid hormone levels, including progesterone and cortisol, are important for the progression of gestation, but when neither a sky-high nor a bottomed-out stress response would be beneficial.

It's a tricky balance. Acute stress itself can throw this regulation of the HPA axis out of whack. And chronic stress has been linked to deficits in GABA-driven inhibition. Then the end of pregnancy basically throws those stress scales up in the air. Progesterone and allopregnanolone levels plummet around birth. The number of GABA receptors rebounds. Meanwhile, other hormones, including cortisol, are in flux and not necessarily all tracking the same timeline or intensity.

Progesterone and estradiol drop so precipitously at childbirth that researchers have suggested that the body experiences a withdrawal state to which some people are especially sensitive, and that sensitivity could be a cause of postpartum depression. Other research has pointed to the ratio of estradiol to progesterone during and after gestation as important, with a higher ratio linked to depression. Plus, it's thought that chronic stress could interfere with changes in the oxytocin system and disrupt adaptations that reinforce the rewards of caring for a baby. And based on animal literature, researchers think that birthing parents may experience changes in the central immune system that could affect mood. There is, in short, a lot going on and, frankly, many opportunities for it to go wrong.

Cortisol has been a major focus for Alison Fleming, who along with colleagues, first identified the link between cortisol levels and maternal responsiveness in 1987. She and others have more recently described the "bimodal effect of cortisol." The hormone is an important part of priming a new parent to be alert and attentive, but there is a just-so element to it, what Dudin described to me as a "Goldilocks effect"— not too much or too little. Fleming recently coauthored a review paper titled, "Mothering Revisited: A Role for Cortisol?"—a reflection of the fact that cortisol and the HPA axis still mostly have been treated like an emergency-response system in the parental brain and are not typically incorporated into models of the neurobiological changes that lead to adaptive parenting. But perhaps they should be.

* * *

McCLOSKEY WENT LOOKING FOR THERAPY, for herself and for her sons, and eventually she was referred to Mom Power, a "strengths-based" program created at the University of Michigan for mothers facing adversity that partly targets those who may have had postpartum depression and never received care. By the time she started the program, McCloskey had left her ex for good, had put up firmer boundaries—personal and legal—around his presence in her life and his son's, and had found a new home for her family in Ypsilanti, Michigan.

McCloskey was skeptical of Mom Power. She had read a lot of parenting books and wasn't sure what more Mom Power could teach her. But she was still struggling to connect with Simon. She was more checked out than she wanted to be.

So every Monday afternoon for ten weeks through summer 2021, she logged on to the video platform where the group had gathered since the pandemic started. During one of the first sessions, the group leader asked the mothers to watch a video montage of mothers and babies interacting, as the song "Wind beneath My Wings" played in the background, and imagine that they were singing the song to their babies: "Did you ever know that you're my hero / And everything I would like to be?" OK, sweet, McCloskey thought. Then the participants were asked to watch it again and this time imagine their babies were singing the song to them. McCloskey broke down sobbing.

"You don't always think of yourself that way as a mother," she told me. "You are hard on yourself. You don't know if you're doing a good job, and the facts are that your kids—obviously they rely on you. And they think that you're the greatest thing, because . . . you're all that they have."

It was a cathartic moment for her, and an empowering one, more so because of what came next. Mostly, practice.

The group wrote scripts for how they hoped to respond to their children in stressful moments. They checked in with each other from week to week to describe what had gone well and brainstorm about what to do differently. Importantly, she said, she learned about pausing before reacting. When Simon was struggling, she started thinking, "let me help him," instead of shutting down. She started explaining to her son when she felt her own frustration growing, instead of letting her emotions build. "I never even considered doing that before," she said. It wasn't just the ideas that helped but the plans they made: "Here's the equation. Here's the answer. Now you can go implement it."

Just about every person expecting a child has hopes for what kind of parent they will be. They've dreamed about the connection they will feel to their newborn. Or they have imagined their relationship with a future toddler or ten-year-old. Maybe they've researched child development and parenting theory and plotted out their own. This can be an important part of the transition to parenthood, thinking our way into the role. The thing is, those plans are put in motion not by innate instinct but by complex neural processes—conscious and subconscious behaviors—that occur in a brain that may already be shaped by neuro-psychiatric disorders and differences.

Human parenting often is treated like a psychosocial phenome-non. But how we connect, how we worry, how we bond—those things are shaped by the structure and function of our brains. This is some-thing that the animal research has acknowledged for a long time. How a mother rat licks and grooms her pups affects their DNA methyla-tion, which influences how genes are expressed, and alters offspring HPA function in ways that can last into adulthood. Higher licking and grooming leads to lower stress responsivity in the offspring, and vice versa. Because those patterns also alter gene expression in the medial preoptic area, which we know plays a central role in initiating maternal behavior, those licking and grooming tendencies may be repeated in the next generation.

In humans, too, parenting has a physiological basis. Factors from a parent's life, and not only whether they have a postpartum mood dis-order, can affect how intensely their reward or motivation network responds to a baby's cry, for example, or how they experience that shift in neural activity from hypervigilance to a more regulated state. A large body of evidence has linked chronic or extreme stress in infancy and childhood to an increased risk for mental health disorders over the life span, and specifically to alterations in the connection between the amyg-dala and the prefrontal cortex, essential for emotion regulation.

In the last decade or so, researchers have tried sorting out some of these factors by connecting early life experience and later parent-ing in humans, whose life trajectories are quite a bit more complicated than laboratory rodents'. They've found that mothers who experienced trauma or abuse as children may have differences in brain regions related to processing infant cues, empathy, or regulating their emotions. One study compared twenty-four mothers who experienced sexual or physical abuse as children and twenty-eight who had not. Those who had not been abused were more sensitive in their interactions during a fifteen-minute free play period and while helping their child with a puz-zle. They also had higher gray matter volume in a brain area involved in "emotional empathy," or perceiving and experiencing what the child feels, while those who had experienced abuse had higher volume in areas of the brain involved in "cognitive empathy," or mentalizing the needs of the child. The researchers suggested the latter group may lean on mentalizing hubs to compensate for deficits elsewhere.

Poverty can have a profound influence on child brain development. That may be true in parental development as well. Pilyoung Kim, who was a coauthor on some of the earliest parental brain imaging studies, now directs the University of Denver Family and Child Neuroscience Laboratory. Much of her recent work has focused on trying to close the socioeconomic gaps in parental brain research.

Kim's lab scanned the brains of fifty-three first-time mothers who were within about ten months postpartum and had low or middle incomes. The researchers assessed the mothers' exposure to stressful circumstances through interviews and home visits, including their levels of food insecurity, housing quality, and exposure to community violence, as well as a measure of whether their income met their household needs. More stress exposure was associated—no surprise—with more anxiety symptoms among the new mothers. When the mothers were asked to listen to the sound of an infant crying, more stress correlated with reduced activity in the insula, which is a key salience region, and in cortical areas important for processing emotional information and for regulating one's own emotions. Dampened activity in certain of those brain regions also was linked with lower maternal sensitivity when the researchers observed the mothers playing with their children.

There are lots of other factors than can shape people's physiological capacity for managing stress, including their exposure to systemic racism, their immigration status, or their identity as queer or transgender parents in a world that still makes little room for them. This capacity is also influenced by their exposure to a wide variety of protective factors, at the individual level and at the community level, that are particular to their circumstances. The field of parental brain research, which is overwhelmingly White, has barely accounted for these things, though Kim in particular has called for an increased focus on how cultural differences interact with exposure to stress.

It's important to note that, for now at least, studies looking at differences in the parental brain and linking them to metrics of caregiving include very small sample sizes that measure a limited number of demographic factors and use narrow metrics of behavior. They are a snapshot, a blurry one at that, and one that reflects an average effect. They are not absolute truths about human nature or any specific individual's experience. What they do tell us is that parenthood is not a static thing, a tiny gold baby bottle added on to the charm bracelet of the brain. Understanding that at a deeper level can change things.

There is no certain story line in the data yet about just how addiction affects the parenting brain, but the findings to date fit a general theory that Helena Rutherford of Yale's Before and After Baby Lab and her colleagues put forward a few years ago, which suggests that addiction disrupts the brain's reward and stress circuitry. Infant-related reward responses may be turned down and stress responses turned up. Then there's the fact that stress drives cravings and parenting stress seems to be especially potent.

Rutherford has led a lot of the imaging work related to addiction and the parental brain. She often presents her research to clinicians specializing in addiction, who have told her that the neuroscience has changed the conversation they have with patients who are parents. "It gives them a very concrete mechanism to talk to them, to say . . . 'This is one reason that you might be struggling, because the areas of the brain implicated in addiction are also those that are important for parenting,'" Rutherford said.

And it's not just talk. Rutherford hopes that the research will lead to more targeted support for parents with addiction—training, for example, in emotion regulation or mindfulness, techniques to reorient the stress circuitry and help parents more consciously focus on engagement with their babies as a rewarding experience.

Parenting programs offered in treatment for mothers with problematic substance use can vary quite widely in their methods and rarely use evidence-based approaches, according to recent systematic reviews of those programs. Often they are focused on teaching information about child development or "parenting skills," such as limit-setting and changing child behavior through time-outs or rewards rather than through harsher discipline strategies. But these programs have lower success rates in people with limited resources. Plus, it may be hard for parents to set limits and cope with the escalation that may cause in a toddler's behavior, at least at first, without control of their own emotions. They may have few opportunities to meaningfully practice those skills if they are separated from their children while in treatment or through the child welfare system.

Skills-based parenting programs often fail to acknowledge the particular neurobiology or life history of parents with addiction, said Amanda Lowell, an associate research scientist at the Yale Child Study Center. She is involved in training and efficacy research in a program at Yale called Mothering from the Inside Out, based on the work of psychologist Nancy Suchman. It's more of a therapeutic approach than a specific curriculum. The program's entire focus is mentalization and cultivating the curiosity it takes to know another person's state of mind.

How it typically works is, in one-on-one treatment, a therapist models that process by being curious about the mother's mind, and together they reflect on her child's. "The idea is that parenting can feel more rewarding if we enhance the parent-child relationship, and then caregiving should improve," Lowell said. "When it feels more rewarding, and when the stress of parenting is lower, that kind of turns the substance use piece on its head." In studies so far, participants show improved reflective functioning, or a capacity to make sense of one's own mental state and emotions and those of another person, and that corresponds with more sensitive caregiving, with the effects lasting through a year postpartum.

Providing better care for parents with addiction is important for lots of reasons. About one in eight children in the United States live with an adult who has a substance use disorder. Notably, that statistic is based on data from between 2009 and 2014, which means it does not capture the continued and dramatic growth of the nation's opioid use epidemic in the years since. (There is the separate but related fact that a huge number of women are prescribed opioids to cope with the pain of recovering from vaginal delivery and C-section, and about 2 percent of those go on to develop a "new persistent use" of the highly addictive drugs.)

The stakes are high, but so is the potential for change. All that habit upheaval, all those shifting neural connections—researchers think they present an opportunity. Drug use falls dramatically in pregnancy and the early postpartum period, and generally climbs again in the later postpartum period. It may be that the neurobiology driving parental motivation basically interrupts drug-related motivation, making new or expectant parents more likely to commit to treatment. The question for researchers is how to reinforce that shift, to make it stick. "This is a unique time in a mother's life, where the neuroplasticity is really ripe for intervention," Lowell said.

Mentalization also is an important part of Mom Power, the program in which McCloskey participated. Mom Power started at a primary care clinic for adolescents and young adults in Ypsilanti and now runs at mental health centers and clinics in eight states serving mothers of any age who have depression, a history of trauma, or other factors that could affect their start in parenting. The goal is "to really scoop them up," said Maria Muzik, medical director of the University of Michigan Perinatal Psychiatry Clinic and one of the creators of Mom Power. That means helping mothers feel supported and nurtured in relationships with group leaders and with their peers, while also filling tangible needs for things like financial literacy and self-care skills. Woven throughout is a focus on understanding and interpreting a parent's own emotional responses and the ways children communicate their emotions through behavior.

Studies have found that Mom Power similarly increases reflective functioning and reduces parenting stress. It may also change neural activity. Mom Power organizers worked with maternal brain researchers James Swain and Shaun Ho to measure the brain activity of a small group of mothers before and after the program and compare those scans to those of mothers who did not participate but instead had information mailed to them at home. In response to their babies' cries, those who had gone through Mom Power showed a greater increase in specific activity and connectivity in brain regions related to reading emotional cues and to mentalization.

Muzik said she was pleased but not surprised by the brain imaging results. Mom Power gives parents a safe place to be with their kids, to talk and reflect on their experiences, and to practice how to do things differently. The result, she hopes, is "an altering experience in your whole body."

* * *

NOT EVERYONE WHO IS STRESSED during pregnancy develops postpartum depression. Not every child who is neglected goes on to struggle as a parent themselves. No particular sequence of life events is strictly definitive of how a person develops as a caregiver.

Some researchers have investigated this some-not-all reality by looking at how a person's genes shape the link between their childhood and their parenthood. For example, if a mother experienced abuse or neglect as a child herself, she is less likely to maintain breastfeeding when she becomes a mother and more likely to develop postpartum depression. But, researchers found, the chance of those outcomes increases if she also has a particular variation in a gene that codes for the oxytocin peptide. Stressful life events, like a death in the family or a serious illness, are associated with the development of postpartum depression. But when women who had experienced those things also had a specific variation in a serotonin transporter gene, their risk for depression in the late postpartum period was higher.

Every parent enters into the role with their own mix of genetic factors, life experience, and current stressors. Muzik aptly described it as background music for the brain. "It can be loud. It can be quiet. It can be very disturbing or it can be a nice, soft music," she said. "We cannot undo this music. We cannot get rid of it. It shapes us. It's who we are, but we can quiet it down, and we can put new tunes over it."

On the one hand, this is a reassuring thought. None of it is purely deterministic, and the work we do to change the music matters. But I admit, I also find it hard to face. In this mixing board that is my brain, some tracks are predetermined. However much effort I put into parenting, there are facets that I can't entirely change. Certain sounds remain.

Sometimes this idea is paralyzing. I get stuck in a loop, thinking about the mothers who came before me, who shaped the genes that shaped my brain that shapes my mothering that shapes my children's brains.

My grandmother was an army nurse. She went to France during World War II, met my grandfather, married him in a bombed-out church, and began having children almost as soon as the war was over. As a girl, I knew her as someone with soft cheeks and a rough edge, quick to tell a joke and curse the Yankees, deeply invested in helping the neediest people in her community, and ever with a cigarette between her fingers, a drink in her hand, and her beloved, mangy miniature poodle by her side. Now, I think about the fact that, in very short order, she came to understand the ravages of war, returned home to a brand-new city to live among a family—my grandfather's—whom she had never met before, and had a baby. Then another, my mother. Her own mother died soon after.

I live just a few miles from the first apartment my grandparents shared, at the edge of Portland's Back Cove, a tidal basin that hosts the most brilliant sunrises and the bleakest winter grayscapes. I imagine her, holding a newborn, watching from her apartment window as the egrets moved, slow and stilted, among the grasses, and I wonder, how did she feel?

I don't have to wonder how my own mother felt at the end of her first pregnancy. It is still so raw for her, so hard to face, that we had never talked about it at length until I was writing this book.

She was eight months along and leading a Girl Scouts troop meeting more than seven thousand miles from home, in Okinawa, Japan, where my father was stationed in the US Air Force, when she thought she was going into labor. At the hospital on base, they told her it wasn't labor and sent her home. But the baby wasn't moving. Eventually—two weeks later—a doctor at the hospital confirmed there was no heartbeat. Ending the pregnancy, he told her, was against his faith. He sent her home. To be swallowed up by despair and anger and the weight of things beyond her control. "I waited another three weeks," she said, "and I went nuts." Finally, she and my father returned to the hospital and saw a different doctor, who agreed to induce.

My mom's story is full of rage. Justified and unremitting. At the doctor who prolonged her suffering. At the nurse who came into her hospital room insistent on checking the baby's heartbeat and who couldn't understand when my mother said there was none. At the priest who refused a baptism. Afterward, the wife of the base commander told people to give my parents space. So friends stayed away. My grandmother arrived from across the ocean, and one day Mom went with her to the commissary, where they ran into a close friend whose due date had been just a few days apart from my mother's. "She stood in front of the baby," Mom told me.

Soon after, my parents received a humanitarian reassignment back to the United States. "I didn't talk about it," she said. "I exercised like crazy to get back in shape, and you just kind of forget—try to forget."

"You don't forget," I said.

"True."

My sister was born about two years later. Being pregnant again was excruciating, Mom said. Having a baby was healing. And hard. My mother was dedicated to tending to our physical needs when we were young—my sister, my brother, and me—to keeping a home. And she was anxious. *Is* anxious. "The worry never goes away," she said. "No matter how old you guys get. The worry for your child never goes away. It just ages somehow."

I feel that worry for my own children. And sometimes it seems like a chain extended through time, grown link by link. This lineage feels heavy and undeniable. Yet when I read the research on how maternal care may be passed from generation to generation, that chain feels heavier still, and that feeling, like a finger on the scale, is one I do not trust.

Studies about the intergenerational transmission of maternal care typically compare just two points on a life span full of complexity. They look at a tiny part of a person's genetic makeup or discrete aspects of parenting behavior, but not in the context of a whole relationship. A whole family. They may measure affect and touch in short frames of time. But not the feeling of climbing into flannel sheets as a kid. Not the smell of your grandmother's kitchen. Not your mother's handwriting. Not their laughter, which does not come easily but is sharp and bright.

The findings themselves are mixed and messy, containing conflicting— even opposite—results or ones that change depending on which demographic variables are added to the analysis. "There is so much noise, and we are trying to find patterns in the noise," Viara Mileva-Seitz told Abigail Tucker, author of *Mom Genes: Inside the New Science of Our Ancient Maternal Instinct*. Mileva-Seitz was lead author on several gene-environment interaction papers and a doctoral researcher in Alison Fleming's lab in Mississauga, though she told Tucker that she left the field and now raises sheep with her family and works as a photographer. Scientists studying maternal genetics "are at the base of this humongous mountain," Mileva-Seitz said. "We are not sure how to climb it. Everybody is just picking at it in various ways."

Sometimes these studies are based on measures that, to me—not a scientist, just a person who thinks—seem dubious. Take, for example, one that correlated a mother's "unresolved" childhood trauma to her disengagement from her own child's distress, where the state of her trauma was assessed by measuring slips in grammar during a structured interview about her childhood memories and attachment relationships, and the amount of her disengagement was measured by fMRI. The leaps required to get from childhood adversity to an adult's "linguistic breakdowns" to meaningful neural patterns seem a bit too much.

This might be what Sarah Richardson, science historian and director of the Harvard GenderSci Lab, calls "cryptic causality." The long jump from a narrow finding to a broad conclusion, across an expanse of time. An effect whose edges seem to grow fuzzy or even disappear when you look at it in a real-life context.

In her book *The Maternal Imprint: The Contested Science of Maternal-Fetal Effects*, Richardson argued that much of what is held up as fact—specifically about how pregnant people shape their child's long-term health through in utero effects—is based on studies with small effect sizes that are expanded into "complex chains of causality" and used to create "biosocial narratives charged with urgency by the specter of fetal harm." That includes some of the foundational work on high cortisol during pregnancy and more recent studies that have linked an expectant mother's diet to her daughters' cancer risk (and her granddaughters' and her great-granddaughters'), based on quite nuanced research in rats. Those findings are publicized under headlines like the one deploring "The Nutritional Sins of the Mother," and, Richardson wrote, they leave many childbearing women feeling like "inadequate vessels" with real, measurable consequences for their own mental health and that of their families.

It's not that pregnancy doesn't matter for child outcomes. It's that the intrauterine environment is not *the* determinative, immutable factor shaping long-term health. Richardson wrote that the field of developmental origins of health and disease is full of unreplicated findings that are propped up by "social assumptions about where agency and responsibility lie for offspring outcomes"—the mother.

A different but related research literature looks at how exposure to adverse childhood experiences, or ACEs—things like emotional, physical, or sexual abuse; substance use; mental illness; poverty; or community violence—affects a person's long-term health. These effects are cumulative and widespread. They have been validated by large studies that include tens of thousands of people with robust effects showing that the more trauma a person experiences as a child, the higher their risk of later heart disease, stroke, death by suicide, or depression, among other things.

Dr. Nadine Burke Harris has long been a leading voice on ACEs and in 2019 became the first-ever California surgeon general. In 2020, under her leadership, the state launched a first-in-the-nation program to pay providers in its Medicaid program—including prenatal care providers—to screen patients for ACEs in order to address the conditions for which they may have a greater risk.

How you are cared for as a child really and truly does matter for your health and, almost certainly, for the health of your offspring. We tend to look for linear narratives—made link by link—but a huge array of factors determines how any given child's life unfolds. They include fathers and kin. Family dynamics and community ones. Individuals and institutions. The problem of childhood trauma shaping adult health is a public health issue, Burke Harris told me when I interviewed her in 2018. "It's too big for all of us," she said. "If it's too big for all of us, it means we all take a little bite."

There is a certain subgenre of parenting content on social media that celebrates the neurobiological connection between baby and parent—mother, mostly—with posts that encourage women to nurture their babies, to respond to their cues, to nurse them to sleep, to reject notions of baby training, and to embrace the labor of supporting healthy infant brain development to promote their long-term health. Every time I see them, I feel a little bit glad that the story of the responsive parental brain and its connection to a baby's development is reaching a bigger audience. *And* I feel a deep pang of concern for the parents who worry that they are doing it wrong. That they have damaged their infant by sleep training when they were desperate for sleep themselves, or simply want a more predictable schedule. That they can't be a responsive parent because their child is in day care, because their baby cries all evening, every evening, and they don't know how to help, or because they struggle with postpartum depression. That they have worried too much, fraying the line that connects them to their baby or, worse, charging that connection with harm.

Fleming's lifelong work has focused on the physiological and behavioral links between mothers and babies. How each shapes the other. And yet, she told me, she understands quite clearly that these links are part of a much bigger picture, in which—apart from the extremes of abuse and neglect, and sometimes even then—parents have only so much influence over the trajectory of their children's lives. "There isn't a single linear line from one point early in life to when you become a mother," she said. "Lots of things happen along the way. And, if you think you're screwing up with your kid—well, you know, I mean, stop it. But on the other hand, they have a lot of life to live."

Parents matter. And so do many other things.

"You knew I was going to say that, right?" Fleming said, laughing. A year and a half earlier, we had almost the exact same exchange. "I did know you were going to say that," I told her, "but maybe I needed to hear it again."

* * *

THERE IS A LOT THAT we can do to make pregnancy and new parenthood go better for everyone—parents and babies. There is a wide gap, especially in the United States, between what we know serves birthing parents best and the care they are getting today.

In 2016, the US Preventive Services Task Force recommended that all pregnant and postpartum women be screened for depression. The task force is made up of doctors who review the evidence for preventive screenings and procedures and give them a grade based on safety and efficacy. Most insurers in the United States, including private insurers and Medicaid programs in most states, are required under the Affordable Care Act to cover those services given top grades with no out-of-pocket costs to their customers. This recommendation rightfully was seen as a huge win for maternal mental health. But screening to identify people who are already in crisis is hardly enough.

In 2019, the same task force made another recommendation. Clinicians should refer pregnant or postpartum women to counseling if they are *at risk* for perinatal depression—before symptoms occur—and those services should be covered as preventive care, the group said. The endorsement was based on a review of twenty studies. It means that many pregnant and postpartum people who have risk factors such as a history of depression, elevated anxiety, complicated pregnancy, or a history of particularly stressful life events can—at least in theory—receive preventive care in the form of counseling at no additional cost to them. (I repeat, at no extra cost to them!)

Except doctors have no widely used, standardized screening tool to identify risk for perinatal mood disorders. The task force acknowledged this and issued some basic parameters for screening. As of fall 2021, the American College of Obstetricians and Gynecologists, the primary professional organization for the field, had not issued guidance on how to implement the task force's recommendation. Then there's the fact that the United States has widespread shortages of mental health providers, especially those who accept payment from Medicaid, which covers more than 40 percent of births in the United States. All this prompted one ob-gyn I spoke with to call this an "unmanned mandate."

We know that the pandemic has been an incredible stressor for parents during childbirth and afterward. It will be years before the toll it has taken on new parents is fully accounted for. I think of the single mother I interviewed who left the time-warped reality of the NICU and arrived in the time-warped reality of a city in its first days of a lockdown, so many of the supports from family and friends she had planned on now suddenly unavailable to her. Of all those who found themselves cluster-feeding a newborn and homeschooling older children, the days on an endless loop. Or those who couldn't fall asleep even after the baby was fed because they worried about their family's financial security and their physical safety.

But the pandemic has brought about at least one shift in health care that could help, by expanding access to telemedicine and normalizing remote delivery of care. "Convincing depressed postpartum women to show up to the hospital with their newborns has always been a struggle, a struggle that is even greater for low-income women who may lack childcare or access to transportation," Mary Kimmel of the University of North Carolina Center for Women's Mood Disorders, and Lauren Osborne and Pamela Surkan, both of Johns Hopkins University, wrote in a commentary published in February 2021. They called on insurers to recognize telemedicine as a tool for reaching those hard-to-serve patients and to pay providers more to deliver it.

Better treatments, of course, would make a difference, too. For all the well-warranted excitement around Zulresso, the first drug approved in the United States for treatment of postpartum depression, it remains inaccessible to most people. The development of Zulresso was based on the changes in GABA signaling that occur through pregnancy and the postpartum period. It is a proprietary form of allopregnanolone that must be delivered by injection over a three-day hospital stay. Like high levels of naturally occurring allopregnanolone, the drug has a sedative effect and can cause dizziness and fainting.

In women with moderate to severe depression, Zulresso was found to be fast-acting, with more significant results in those with more severe depression. It does not work for everyone, said Samantha Meltzer-Brody, whose research on the drug is funded by Sage Therapeutics. The reality of many postpartum depressions requires many paths to prevention and treatment. But for those in whom it does work, she said, it can cause a "robust state change." Importantly, that change lasts long after the drug is administered.

Researchers are trying to figure out just why Zulresso's effects last. Jamie Maguire and colleagues found that allopregnanolone and its synthetic analogs alter the oscillations of brain activity in a specific part of the amygdala shown many times over to be important for both parental behavior and the expression of fear and anxiety. They suggested that this might shift the synchronization of the amygdala and the prefrontal cortex into a healthier network state. "We think that it resets, and it kind of is stable there until there's another shift," Maguire told me. Whether or when a person experiences another episode, another change in network state, likely varies according to each person's circumstances, genes, and stress.

Maguire's work challenges the notion that postpartum depression is a kind of brokenness. Or an absence. A missing maternal instinct. "You can shift from the unhealthy state to the more healthy state," she said. "It's just that we need to restore that balance."

Yet only a handful of facilities in metropolitan areas across the United States offer Zulresso. Its rollout was stymied first by concern over the price tag—about $34,000, not counting the inpatient stay—and insurers' reluctance to cover the cost. Plus, for many new parents, a three-day hospital stay without their baby is a big barrier. The pandemic didn't help.

Zulresso is Sage Therapeutics' first drug on the market. Most of Sage's sales staff was among the 340 or so people laid off in spring 2020. The company cited few people seeking treatment during the pandemic and too few physicians willing to prescribe it. As of late 2021, Sage told stockholders that it planned to focus sales efforts on only those locations already offering the drug.

Sage has another drug under development, also targeting GABA signaling, but this one could be taken orally, at home, and used for depression outside the postpartum context as well. The drug had a rocky start in clinical trials, but postpartum results published in June 2021 were promising, with significant improvements in depression scores compared with placebo at three days of treatment and bigger gains forty-five days out.

Still, the antidepressant medications known as selective serotonin reuptake inhibitors, or SSRIs, remain the primary pharmaceutical intervention for postpartum depression, prescribed to up to 10 percent of pregnant and postpartum women in the United States, Canada, and elsewhere. SSRIs are thought to work by keeping more serotonin in synapses, by preventing the uptake or absorption of the neurotransmitter into the nerve cell, resulting in better mood and more receptivity to psychotherapy. But precisely how they work in the general population is still a bit unclear. How their function may change during the perinatal period is a big question mark—though there is good evidence that it does.

That's because the central serotonin system changes across pregnancy and the postpartum period. It's thought that it upregulates during pregnancy, resulting in more serotonin cycling in the body and the brain—at least according to studies involving mothers' blood and cerebrospinal fluid samples. Rodent studies have found significant serotonin-related changes in cell activity, metabolism, and receptor expression in a brain region known as the dorsal raphe, which is a major supplier of serotonin to the forebrain.

But scientists still know very little about how serotonin, in rodents and humans, behaves typically across pregnancy and the postpartum period or how exactly it influences parental behaviors, and they know even less in the context of postpartum mood disorders. One recent study, led by Pawluski, looked at how sertraline, marketed as Zoloft, interacts with the typical plasticity in the rat hippocampus in late pregnancy; it contains this line, which seems emblematic of the literature on serotonin generally: "This work has generated more questions than answers."

What researchers know is that serotonin interacts with hormonal and neural systems that change in complex ways during pregnancy and the postpartum period. Serotonin influences dopamine activity, for example. And all the reproductive hormones that are dramatically in flux—estrogen, progesterone, oxytocin, prolactin, and glucocorticoids—are known to influence serotonin activity. "It's all linked," Pawluski said. But how?

Remarkably few studies have evaluated the efficacy of SSRIs in the postpartum context, perhaps because of the challenges of recruiting people, perhaps because of the assumption that the drugs work well enough given their track record in other contexts. In February 2021, the respected Cochrane Library published a systematic review that concluded there "may be a benefit" to taking SSRIs for postpartum depression, compared to a placebo, but the certainty of the evidence was "low or very low." The studies available for that group's analysis were small in size and in number, and they had high rates of attrition.

"So we are actually giving a medication that could or could not be helpful," Pawluski told me. "Maybe it's a placebo effect, who knows. Even if it's placebo, that's important if you're feeling better. That's how I feel. But ultimately the idea is to correct or normalize a system that's not working well." And, she said, researchers can't say for sure if that's what SSRIs taken in the postpartum period are doing.

These drugs have been an important tool for treating perinatal depression, and doctors generally advise pregnant and postpartum people who are taking them to keep doing so if the drugs help. I don't want to minimize their value in that. But it's also clear that we need better medications or at least more information about the ones we have. Meeting either goal will depend on learning more about how depression works in the postpartum brain specifically.

Given the state of the research, that could take a while. Meanwhile, knowing what a dramatic neurobiological transformation new parenthood is and how much that change is influenced by stress should be enough to invest in proven supports for birthing parents. That includes more maternal care providers, midwives, and doulas, particularly in the hundreds of rural counties in the United States that are considered "maternity care deserts," with *no* hospital-based obstetrical care and little access to providers. Also needed are more home visits and greater access to telehealth services, more well-designed support groups, and a universal paid family leave policy. There is good evidence that such changes could reduce postpartum mood disorders.

We don't need a precise understanding of the mechanisms by which the HPA axis shapes the brain in pregnancy and the postpartum period before we can push for a "normalization of what the body is actually going through," Molly Dickens, a stress physiologist whose work focuses on motherhood, told me. Normalize it, as in normalize the need for more support. Pregnancy "pushes the body right to the edge." If a person struggles in the process, "that's normal." Getting through it without at least some symptoms of a mood disorder, Dickens said—"that's the fucking miracle."

In her book *Ordinary Insanity: Fear and the Silent Crisis of Motherhood in America*, Sarah Menkedick wrote that new motherhood involves mourning. She mourned the loss of her old self and the loss of the mother she thought she would be. Yet there is so little space for grief in the postpartum period, so little recognition that one stage of life is left behind and a new stage begun. One that is largely unknowable until you're in it.

In the United States, so much of the ritual that would have helped make sense of this life change—among communities of women and between generations of birthing parents—has been stripped away or lost to human migration across town or across an ocean, subordinate to that "toxic individualism" in family form that Mia Birdsong writes about. "Postpartum depression," Menkedick argued, "might be the only ritual American mothers have to express their grief."

I balked at this line when I first read it. Postpartum depression is biological, I thought. It occurs in populations across the globe with widely divergent cultural expectations and practices around birth and the postpartum period. But rituals are manifest recognition, a conscious accounting of things. Perhaps it's true that, for some parents, depression is the accounting, the outcome in the absence of acknowledgment of what their body and their brain are going through.

I wonder whether giving expectant parents and the people around them a better understanding of how this new life stage could feel might help them to make new rituals, or return to old ones. At least it might make those losses less surprising and offer people a clearer sense of what they may gain. This would require naming the various factors that can influence that trajectory, including the experience of childbirth itself.

* * *

SOMETHING AMAZING HAPPENED A FEW years ago on the pathbreaking parenting podcast *The Longest Shortest Time*, hosted by Hillary Frank. In 2014, Frank had interviewed famed midwife Ina May Gaskin, whose 2003 book *Ina May's Guide to Childbirth* is part of the prenatal canon. The book's message is that women's bodies know how to deliver a child and typically can do so "naturally" as long as fear doesn't get in the way. Without fear, Gaskin wrote, birth can be quite a pleasurable experience.

This was a revolutionary idea for many birthing parents at a time when elective and unplanned C-sections were on the rise. It also drove the notion that "natural" birth was the right way to deliver and the birthing parent held the key—her preparation, her mindset—to making it happen.

Frank told Gaskin that she read the guidebook while pregnant, and it made her feel strong, where before she was scared. It helped her believe that she could manage childbirth without drugs or procedures. But then the day came, and Frank ended up with a series of interventions, including Pitocin, an epidural, and an episiotomy, which needed to be repaired a week later. "In the end, I felt like I had failed," she told Gaskin. "I thought I could do it. I believed I could do it, and I couldn't. Doing it naturally felt like something to achieve. And looking back at those books, I've got to admit, I felt upset. I felt angry. Ina May doesn't have anything to tell me about what happens when you can't do it."

Gaskin responded that her goal is to help people avoid unnecessary medical procedures, but telling women that everyone can go through childbirth without pain—"that's a big lie." Frank stopped her: "I was under this impression—and maybe it was the wrong impression—that you believed that all women could have, if not a pain-free labor, then at least a relaxed labor."

No, Gaskin replied. "I probably need to write some more stuff if I've left you with that impression."

And then she did.

Five years later, in 2019, Gaskin released an updated version of her guidebook, based on her conversation with Frank and the nearly four hundred comments collected after the podcast aired. She incorporated more about C-sections and other interventions—both on avoiding them and coping with them—and more about the uncertainty of birth and the range of ways it can go. She also explicitly rejected the use of the phrase "the golden hour" to refer to the time immediately after birth, often described as a critical window for attachment, that many families miss out on when birthing parents are recovering from C-sections or if babies need NICU care. "It makes it sound as if bad things will automatically happen if temporary separation places you and your baby in different places for a time," Gaskin wrote. "This is simply not true."

I love this conversation for so many reasons. For the strength and warmth the two women show for one another. For their openness. For the fact that Frank said things that so many women felt, and that Gaskin listened.

I also love it because it acknowledged childbirth for what it is: An experience that the human body is capable of performing and that can be made easier by steadiness in the face of fear or by giving birthing people the right supports at the right time. *And* one that is incredibly intense, that almost uniformly pushes a person to the brink of what they can do physically and psychologically and sometimes to the very edge of life, that is shaped by forces that reach well beyond the particular biology of the birthing person on the day of delivery.

For all the many other things it can be, childbirth also is an inherently traumatic experience. As much as 6 percent of mothers develop childbirth-related post-traumatic stress disorder, characterized by invasive negative or disturbing thoughts, avoidance of triggers, and hyperreactivity. *Six percent*. Many more, around 17 percent, report some PTSD symptoms in the days and weeks following birth.

Like everything else, there is no clear formula for how or when childbirth-related PTSD develops. Sharon Dekel, assistant professor of psychology at Harvard Medical School and director of the Dekel Laboratory at Massachusetts General Hospital, worked with colleagues to assess the birth and postpartum experiences of 685 women and found that the course of delivery matters. Having an unplanned C-section increases the risk of PTSD threefold. Medical inductions, complicated births, and sleep deprivation prior to birth are risk factors, too. So is experiencing a dissociative state—the feeling of being outside one's body or disconnected from what's happening—during birth, though there's evidence that dissociation can be protective against later depressive symptoms for some.

Among the study group, women who had a history of sexual assault—as many as one in five women in America—had a significantly higher rate of complications, premature deliveries, and unplanned C-sections, and they experienced more acute stress during delivery. A birthing parent's age, education level, prior mental illness, and, perhaps to a lesser degree, previous pregnancy stressors such as miscarriage, stillbirth, or prematurity, can influence outcomes, too.

Childbirth-related PTSD often occurs alongside postpartum depression. Dekel's work found that the risk for the double diagnosis increased twofold in the case of preterm deliveries. PTSD is not always recognized as co-occuring with depression, but parents may require particular kinds of treatment for processing that trauma.

Dekel's goal is to tease out the factors that can cause childbirth trauma, in order to develop better prediction and screening for those

most at risk. That includes both objective measures of trauma and subjective ones, and their interactions. If a birthing parent hemorrhages
and there is a real risk to her life, that is clearly an objective stressor.
But Dekel also asks women about their internal experience of the birth
and the immediate aftermath. Did they feel afraid? Did they feel a loss
of control? Did they feel angry? A person's emotional response to childbirth may be the most important predictor of all, Dekel said: "What is
traumatic for one person may be different than what is traumatic for
another person."

Yet very little attention has been paid to screening birthing parents
for traumatic experiences, and the complexities of how trauma can
weave itself into the experience of new parenthood—into how birthing
parents feel about their bodies, their babies, their sense of themselves in
this new role—are dramatically underappreciated.

Dekel has interviewed hundreds of women in her lab; many of them
had the means to seek professional help, yet they often have told her
that they had never talked with anyone about their traumatic childbirth
experience. "They felt shame," Dekel said. "They felt guilty. They didn't
want to overtraumatize their friends who are also pregnant. . . . Many
times they weren't really sure what was happening to them, because
they're not necessarily depressed."

Dekel told me she often explains it to her students this way: If a person gets in a car accident and suffers post-traumatic stress as a result,
they may not be able to drive for a long time or ride in a car. They may
not even be able to cross the street, because any reminder of cars could
be a trigger. "For the mother who has traumatic childbirth and who has
PTSD as a result," Dekel said, "the baby is the trigger."

But the baby can't be avoided. "That makes the pathology worse, the
recovery possibly delayed," she said. "Then you think about the expectations of society and how you are supposed to bond with your child.
It's a very difficult place to be."

Lots of brain imaging studies have looked at the functional and
structural brain changes that underlie PTSD, often in the context of
combat trauma and particularly focusing on activity in the amygdala, the hippocampus, and the prefrontal cortex and on reductions
in global brain volume. No studies have looked at childbirth-related

PTSD. At the time of writing, Dekel was recruiting participants for what could be the first. She and her colleagues also were in the process of documenting another important outcome of distress in childbirth: growth.

Dekel began her career studying the potential for psychological growth in the context of war, captivity, and disasters, including in people who were at the World Trade Center when the towers were attacked on September 11, 2001. Intensely stressful events can "shake your world assumptions," Dekel said, altering how a person thinks about themselves and their own strengths, about their relationships with others, and about how they make meaning in their lives. In fact, it may be that distress is a requirement for psychological growth, the very impetus for it.

It fits, then, that a majority of women report psychological growth following childbirth. In a sample of 428 women, Dekel and colleagues found that, by some measures, women who had objectively stressful childbirth experiences, such as an unplanned C-section, reported the highest levels of growth around their appreciation for life. The message isn't that trauma equals growth, Dekel said. Symptoms of PTSD were negatively correlated with growth outcomes. Rather, stressful circumstances *can* lead to growth, particularly when the right supports are in place.

Very soon after the pandemic began, Dekel's lab began recruiting for a new cohort of mothers, including those who delivered within the first wave of COVID-19 in the United States, when things felt especially precarious and labor and delivery policies were in flux. Not surprisingly, mothers who tested positive or were suspected of having COVID while pregnant or during delivery experienced high levels of acute stress, with half showing clinically significant symptoms of PTSD, about double the rate of women who delivered in the same time frame but who were COVID-negative. Across the study group, Black and Latinx women were almost three times more likely to have a clinically significant traumatic stress response to childbirth in the early months of the pandemic.

But Dekel told me that in the broader sample of pandemic mothers they've collected, as well as in the earlier study, a pattern has emerged. In parents for whom the stress of childbirth does not tip into PTSD, distress can instead build a sense of strength in themselves. "This might lead to better bonding with your child because your sense of competence possibly has been strengthened through the birth experience, even if it's traumatic and possibly especially if it's traumatic," Dekel said. Bonding then leads to more competence and more certainty. It's a feedback loop, Dekel added, and it's possible that the direction of that loop is opposite, with the bond coming first and the sense of strength following. Either way, the two seem to be linked, driving a change in outlook and a sense that "your level of existence is higher than what it was before you were a mom."

It strikes me how much of this depends on framing. On the stories people carry with them into childbirth and whether they have the support they need to process what happens to them as it unfolds. On *how* they are cared for during childbirth, and not only which tests and treatments are delivered. Consider that one in six women in the United States report being mistreated—shouted at, ignored, scolded, violated, or forced to accept treatment they didn't want—during pregnancy and childbirth. Women of lower socioeconomic status and women of color across income levels report even higher rates.

In May 2021, Congresswoman Cori Bush of Missouri told a House committee of how she was twice denied critical care during pregnancy. In one case she was instructed by a doctor to go home and let her pregnancy abort; only after her sister threw a chair down the hallway did the medical staff provide Bush with the care that saved the pregnancy that would lead to the birth of her daughter, now an adult. "This is what desperation looks like—that chair flying down the hallway," Bush said. "This is what being your own advocate looks like. Every day Black women are subjected to harsh and racist treatment during pregnancy and childbirth. Every day Black women die because the system denies our humanity. It denies us patient care." It is trauma upon trauma.

Just as cortisol is not the "bad guy," the stress of pregnancy and childbirth is not necessarily damaging. Or at least it doesn't have to be. Bruce McEwen wrote that a stressful experience may be labeled good, tolerable, or toxic depending on how much support and control a person feels in coping with it.

One of the more unusual birth experiences I've heard to date came from Cristina Lois. Lois's story struck me because of the number of objectively traumatic events involved and Lois's perspective on them. "My initial plan was to have the most natural birth experience," Lois told me, "and it went completely opposite of what I wanted."

Dekel introduced me to Lois, who also happens to work at Massachusetts General Hospital as a physicist in medical imaging research primarily studying Alzheimer's disease. For a long time, Lois said, she wasn't sure she wanted to have children. That changed in 2013, as soon as she saw her positive pregnancy test.

She was ecstatic, and her pregnancy went quite well. But at thirty-seven weeks, doctors told her they wanted to induce. She was thirty-six years old at the time, which made her doctors more cautious, and an ultrasound indicated that the baby wasn't growing as expected. But Lois, who is from Spain, knew the United States has higher induction rates than many other countries and she didn't want an induction. She delayed, over doctors' objections, for two more weeks and then was induced. "It didn't go very well," Lois said. Her labor started. And then stopped. Eventually, she went in for a C-section.

Soon, her son was out and he was healthy. But, Lois said, she could see "faces of concern and people moving around and people talking to each other, and at some point they were taking pictures." Her baby was on her chest but she couldn't focus on him. Eventually someone from the medical team told her they had found a mass on her ovary that could be cancer. Did she want to have the ovary removed or to be stitched up to await more tests?

Lois was very familiar with the research on ovarian cancer. She knew how deadly it can be. Her baby had just been born and suddenly, she thought, "I might be on my way out."

"Take it out," she told them. The preparations started, and then the doctors realized they were wrong. It was a large fibroid—benign— wrapped around the ovary. They could remove it easily.

Within a few days, remarkably, Lois and her family were home. She focused on recovering and feeding her son, Roque, while her husband took care of her and cooked and cleaned. About ten days postpartum, she started having pain in her chest. She called her doctor and was soon rushed to the hospital by ambulance. She had a pulmonary embolism. "It was like, 'What else?'" she said. She was discharged a few days later with a long course of blood thinners and home visits from a nurse.

The thing that strikes me about Lois is that, as we talked about the nature of childbirth and trauma, it isn't these events that she came back to again and again. She said she gets upset sometimes thinking about the decision to induce and then to do a C-section, but mostly she said her providers were doing the best they could. Instead, she emphasizes just how hard everything that came after was, all the much more typical experiences of new parenthood. The sleep deprivation. The feeling of being overwhelmed, of wishing for more hands to help. The challenge, later, of going back to work before she was fully ready. The looming thought that parenthood is forever. "It's a huge change," she said.

Those first weeks as a parent, she said, "I don't think it's a happy time for anyone."

The truth is, I don't know anyone who made it through to parenthood and beyond those postpartum months without at least some significant distress. Distress—right alongside joy and wonder—from years of miscarriages or months of debilitating sickness in pregnancy. From the roller coaster of adoption or surrogacy, or from complications in childbirth. From worry over a newborn with medical needs. From depression or anxiety or cracked nipples or guilt. From all the ways that having a new baby can bring up old trauma or create new trauma, in a person or in a family.

We act as if parenthood is this thing that a person just comes upon in the path of their life, this glittering gemstone that's been sitting there in its place all along. When really, this brilliant gem has been forged through heat and pressure and time. And it is us. By ignoring this reality, we let so many parents down. We fail over and over to give them the support they need. And we also fail to hold a place for them, to see in them all that this transition can mean, all they stand to gain in making it.

Lois said she is a different person today than she was before Roque. She loves her career, but she has more perspective on it. She and her husband divorced, a difficult start to parenthood having added strain to their marriage. Now, she said, she is less prone to panic when something unexpected happens, more prone to plan. More prone to joy, too. She and Roque ride bikes together. They build volcanoes with baking soda and vinegar. They turn on music and dance. Children find happiness in little things, Lois said, and "that's kind of contagious."

CHAPTER 8

The One in the Mirror

"Tell me again—what is your book about?" the mother of my son's pre-school classmate asked. We had met up for a picnic on the beach on one of those perfect spring evenings when it feels like summer but the throngs of tourists visiting Maine have not yet arrived, which meant we were able to spread out on a picnic table just near the playground. Our children mostly entertained themselves, and we could actually talk to one another. She and I had become friendly during drop-offs and pickups but, as those friendships so often go, we hadn't really gotten to know one another yet.

"It's about how becoming a parent changes the brain," I said.

"You mean, how our children fry our brain cells?" she said, with a belly laugh—this mother of three kind, smart daughters who had recently opened her own store selling artfully curated home goods that had become one of my favorite places to find treasures for friends. Who had cultivated a community of makers around her. Who had begun selling her own geometric prints that could brighten a room and also convey meaning for the moment.

"Well, no, actually," I said. "Not exactly."

This is almost invariably the reaction I get when the topic of my work comes up, including from some of the brightest, most capable women I know. I see it coming. Their eyes get wide with recognition. "Oh," one will say, "you're going to explain to me why I can never find anything when we're rushing out the door in the morning?" They assume I am writing about the phenomenon of "mommy brain," because this is what they know about parenting, that their own brain feels like Swiss cheese and the whole world seems to recognize their impairment.

"You watch people get pregnant and know they'll be emotionally and intellectually absent for 20 years," writer Lucy Ellmann said in a 2019 interview about her novel *Ducks, Newburyport*, even as her work was described in the same interview as "furiously feminist." "Thought, knowledge, adult conversation and vital political action are all put on hold while this needless perpetuation of the species is prioritised."

In July 2021, a *New York Times* headline declared "'Mommy Brain' Is Real," and a few months later the *Washington Post* seemed to retort, "Is There Really Such a Thing as 'Mommy Brain'?" Yes, there is. And we'll get to that. But how the parental brain affects the broader context of our lives is so much more than the poor word recall or missed appointments we characterize it by. My friend's response was a knee-jerk one. It's not entirely untrue. But neither is it the whole story.

We already know that having a baby makes parents vigilant and attentive—protective—when it matters most. We know that it pulls them close to their child, to tend to their needs and to shape their baby's developing social brain. The "mommy brain" narrative is so problematic because it makes it seem as if a mother pours herself into caregiving to the detriment of everything else, as if our skills for parenting are strengthened at an overall cost. But there is no dedicated parenting circuitry separate from the rest of our brain. The parental brain, with these new skills and capacity to care, is the same one we use to navigate the rest of our lives. So it follows that we carry those strengths into other domains.

The problem is, there just isn't a lot of science looking at the brain in the bigger context of a parent's life. Not much at all. So here, we stretch. This chapter will look almost exclusively at gestational parents, because the research considering how the neurobiological transition to fatherhood affects a man's life generally, apart from his direct interactions with his child, reflects society's views on how fatherhood affects a man's life generally—which is to say, it is barely considered. And, once again, other nongestational parents are mostly absent from this part of the science to date. But many of the premises explored here apply across all parents who funnel attention and energy into the transformative work of parenting.

This chapter examines the findings to date and then looks just beyond, to see what meaning we can make of it, for mothers and others. I've tried to be clear about where the science ends and where my own "wishful thinking"—call it an educated guess—begins.

* * *

AS MANY AS FOUR OUT of five expectant mothers report increased forgetfulness during pregnancy. But five out of five birthing parents have been told that their cognitive function will be diminished by having a baby. So, how do we make sense of what's real and what may be the long-term effects of those nineteenth-century claims that children stunt their mothers intellectually by stealing their "vital power"?

In 1986, researchers surveyed fifty-one women, mostly medical professionals and administrators, and found that twenty-one of them reported transient symptoms of what the authors labeled "benign encephalopathy of pregnancy," including forgetfulness, confusion, and trouble reading. Since then, a handful of studies have tried to quantify cognitive decline in pregnancy and the postpartum period, with mixed results.

It's possible that pregnant people aren't always reliable reporters of their own cognitive symptoms, as evidenced by one study in which researchers administered tests of attention, memory, language, and executive functioning to pregnant and nonpregnant participants and found no differences between the groups, even while the expectant mothers reported having more complaints about their brain in the week prior. And some studies that find declines might be influenced by confirmation bias, or the willingness of the authors to see an impairment where they already believed one to exist. But when researchers analyze the data across studies in such a way as to try to account for that potential bias, they find that deficits in particular kinds of memory remain.

A 2012 analysis of the research up to that point found mostly small effects, including a small working memory deficit in pregnancy and a slightly larger one in the postpartum period. Delayed recall—the ability to recall a list of items after, in this case, ten minutes have passed—was moderately impaired in pregnancy and slightly less so in the postpartum period. And there were small effects on prospective memory functions, like remembering an upcoming doctor appointment. The researchers, Marla Anderson and Mel Rutherford of McMaster University, found a deficit in processing speed, which was worse during pregnancy than in the postpartum period, and suggested that it matched the pattern in women's reported experiences. This may be what's behind the broader picture of memory and pregnancy, they wrote: not so much a decline in cognitive ability but the need for slightly more time to do the same task, to recall a word or find the keys, with a trend toward improvement after childbirth.

A more recent analysis that focused on pregnancy found similar memory impairments plus small deficits in measures of executive functioning, such as problem-solving and cognitive flexibility—processes that involve the frontal cortex for relatively more complex tasks. The emphasis here is on "small." The authors, from the Baby Brain Research Project at Deakin University in Australia, wrote that while the average deficits are big enough that pregnant people and those close to them may notice, they aren't likely to lead to poor job performance or significantly impair their ability to complete important tasks.

Average, of course, means that some birthing parents will not experience any impairments and others will feel greater effects. Depressive symptoms could amplify working memory problems for pregnant people. Interestingly, one study found fetal sex may play a role. In a study of thirty-nine mothers, those who had daughters performed worse during pregnancy and across the postpartum period than mothers who had sons, specifically on complex tasks that presented a challenge to working memory. The reason for the difference is unclear, though researchers point generally to the complex ways that a fetus and the "maternal periphery" interact, in a "bidirectional relationship." The memory differences between the mothers of daughters and a nonpregnant control group, however, did not reach statistical significance.

In humans at least, memory deficits may compound with multiple pregnancies. A study that tested memory performance in 254 pregnant women throughout their pregnancy and again between twelve and fourteen weeks postpartum found that, beginning in about the second half of pregnancy, those who had prior births scored worse on memory tasks, and the biggest deficits were seen in women who had three or more children.

This finding might be entirely unsurprising to anyone who has struggled to get comfortable with a growing belly at night and then woken at the crack of dawn with a toddler, or who has managed the very different sleep schedules of an infant and her siblings. But the researchers quizzed the mothers about their sleep and tried, as best as possible, to control for differences in quality or quantity. The effect remained.

Notably, while some studies on cognitive function include data on fathers, I have seen none focused on measuring average forgetfulness in new fathers, who also can be depressed and sleep deprived.

Liisa Galea, a neuroscientist at the University of British Columbia and editor in chief of the journal *Frontiers in Neuroendocrinology*, regularly forgot where her car was parked when she was pregnant with her second child, a daughter, and the experience fueled her interest in studying pregnancy and cognition. She said it's important to talk about this effect so that pregnant people can feel their own, real experience acknowledged. "We don't want to talk about it, because perhaps we are worried it's going to affect women's career choices or show a diminishment of their mental capacity," she said. In reality, these effects are typically "minor blips" in memory function. But by ignoring them, she said, we could be missing a bigger picture of cognitive function and parenthood, one that might include changes for the better.

Researchers have some pretty good working theories about how these memory troubles occur. Some research has linked cognitive performance to changes in the default mode network, but the hippocampus, an important center for mapping out and retaining the details of our very social lives to be stored and retrieved as memory, has received the most attention. The hippocampus also is an important center of new neuron production. In pregnancy and across the postpartum period, the architecture and activity of the hippocampus change.

Remember that structural study by Elseline Hoekzema's group, which mostly found that the brain decreases in volume across pregnancy? Her group found that the hippocampus shrinks, too, but then rebounds some in the two years after childbirth. She and her colleagues hypothesized that these changes contribute to the patterns of subtle memory deficits that pregnant people experience, including a rebound of memory by about two years postpartum (though participants in their own study did not show significant differences in memory performance before and after pregnancy). The volume change might be the result of changes in neurogenesis, they said, with a decline in the creation of new neurons across pregnancy and a rebound in the postpartum period.

Rats also experience a drop in working memory as their due dates approach, and scientists understand at least a bit more about what's happening there. For a study published in 2000, Galea and her colleagues placed pregnant rats into a circular pool of water with a platform submerged just below the surface. During a series of tests, the pregnant rats were really good at learning the quickest path to the place where they could rest—at least, at first. In the first trimester they took less time and covered less distance to the platform than nonpregnant rats. But as pregnancy progressed, they took longer and swam farther before finding the platform. Their spatial memory performance declined, the authors wrote. When the researchers later measured the brains of the pregnant females, they also found a trend toward smaller hippocampal volume.

In the more than two decades since that paper was published, researchers have documented multifaceted changes in the hippocampus of the pregnant rat, including a reduction in new cell production, particularly in late pregnancy, and decreased dendritic spine complexity. First-time rat mothers have impaired memory and a decrease in new neurons in the hippocampus into the early postpartum period, too. But their memory function improves again around the time of weaning, and, remarkably, it's better on certain measures than virgin rats' memory. (Studies of California mice, in whom fathers are closely involved in pup-rearing, have found similar changes in hippocampal plasticity in mothers and fathers.)

Here's the thing about mother rats: motherhood is *beneficial* for their brains over the long haul, even "neuroprotective." Rats who have one or more litters see less age-related decline in neurogenesis in middle age and follow what researchers have said could be an "altered aging trajectory," based on a variety of factors. While caring for offspring and afterward, they seem to be protected from the detrimental effects of stress on learning. In later life and long after having pups, mother rats perform better than nonmothers in maze tasks testing their spatial memory and cognitive flexibility, and those who had more litters performed faster than those who had just one, suggesting that benefits "may accrue" through multiple pregnancies. In the same study, older mother rats were found to have fewer deposits of amyloid precursor protein, the breakdown of which contributes to the plaques associated with Alzheimer's disease in humans.

Evidence for a long-term neuroprotective effect of human parenthood is thin but intriguing. As detailed in chapter 5, a person's reproductive experience and genes interact to influence brain health later in life, but much more work is needed to sort out exactly how. Meanwhile, those studies using large databanks to look at brain age have provided some first indications of possible aging-related benefits to parenthood, but that work is just beginning.

What about the expanse of life between the immediate postpartum period and a person's eighth decade? There's basically no research into how reproductive history affects cognitive function through the years—or decades—of managing household schedules and meal planning and the rituals of childhood and adolescence. Through balancing work and life. We know that rats who have had litters are more efficient at foraging and better at hunting crickets than nonmother rats, but we're stuck with an abbreviated story about human mothers that says they are compromised.

One study comparing executive function in teen mothers, adult mothers, and peer groups without children found interesting effects of motherhood and age. Teen mothers performed worse than their peers in measures of working memory, a finding the authors say could be related to the stress of teen pregnancy. But they performed significantly better in attentional capacity, about in line with the adults, which makes sense, given what we know about the development of the maternal brain and the importance of attention in caregiving behavior. It also suggests that with some aspects of cognition, depending on the context, motherhood is additive.

Several researchers told me that the science so far mostly doesn't get at cognitive function in ways that are really meaningful in the context of parenthood. It uses tools that are standardized for testing across the

general population. What's missing is relevance. How do you quantify
a person's performance relative to the pace and intensity of learning a
baby's needs and how to meet them? By what statistical method do you
account for the way that caring for a child adds to the cognitive load a
person managed before they became a parent? How do you measure
human parental memory, the consolidation and adjustment of those
memories in the face of a growing child, or the capacity to retrieve and
make use of them when parenting multiple children?

Researchers have just begun to parse out some of these questions,
using memory tests that include parenting-specific stimuli and a more
nuanced analysis of the brain in the context of pregnancy. Their limited
findings so far are encouraging, pointing in one case to "general cognitive enhancement effects." Forgetfulness and lapses in attention may be
real. But the singular focus, to fit a story line about female impairment,
feels a bit like deriding a great artist who is engrossed in her work for
leaving dishes in the sink.

* * *

WE CAN'T TALK ABOUT COGNITIVE performance in new parenthood
without talking about sleep. But first—my youngest was up between
2 a.m. and 4 a.m. last night and his brother woke for the day about two
hours later—let me get another cup of coffee.

Sleep loss is a nearly universal experience among new parents.
Almost everyone I have interviewed in the process of writing this book
talked about how hard it is to go months upon months without real,
consistent sleep, hard in ways far beyond what they had imagined
before having children. The ways other people joked about sleep when
they were pregnant somehow didn't help. "Congrats on the baby! You'll
never sleep again!" Ha. Ha.

Emily Vincent, the pediatric nurse from Cincinnati, told me that
she felt traumatized by the sleep deprivation she experienced when her
oldest, Will, was a baby. He nursed to be fed and nursed to be soothed,
and she felt pressure—self-imposed but also societal—to keep nursing
and to avoid or limit bottles and pacifiers while doing so, because that's
the advice she received during parenting classes at her hospital.

The night she brought her daughter home two years later, she said,

"I cried like a baby." She told her husband, "'I can't do this again. I can't wake up every hour.' . . . And my husband just held me and said, 'You can and I'm here and I love you and it's going to be fine.'" That night, baby Margot woke just twice, and this time around sleep came a little easier for Vincent. Margot slept more and Vincent also started therapy, antidepressants, and exercise to help cope with the anxieties that sometimes kept her up even when the baby didn't.

With a little distance, Vincent said, she feels mad about her first postpartum experience. For a long time, after her twelve weeks of maternity leave ended, she woke every two hours at night. The sleep loss was painful and disorienting. She talked about being at work, dressed and ready for her day, but having little memory of how she got there, something she jokes about now but that was not at all funny at the time. "I wish that somebody would have told me," she said, "that breastfeeding is great . . . but if you're not sleeping for X amount of time, it's time to switch to a bottle."

For all the books and blogs and sleep consultants offering advice on what a baby needs to go to sleep and stay asleep, that conversation often ignores what a parent needs to function. Or it offers unhelpful bromides about sleeping when the baby sleeps or allowing a partner to trade off nightly feedings, the latter of which depends on having a helpful partner and a baby who takes a bottle, and runs counter to what many parents are told about best practices in breastfeeding.

Vincent was very familiar with the "ABCs of safe sleep," the standard medical advice for putting babies to sleep alone, on their backs, and in a crib, to avoid suffocation and other risks. But, she said, medical professionals push that standard without offering clear guidance on *how* to get a baby who wants to be held to sleep in a crib. That leads many desperate parents to co-sleep anyway, if they weren't already choosing that route to start with, or to try one of an array of baby sleep devices on what was, until very recently, a mostly unregulated market.

We know from the broader body of sleep research that sleep deprivation doesn't just cause sleepiness. It's bad for your health. Long-term sleep loss, characterized by less than seven hours a night, increases a person's risk for cardiovascular disease, depression, diabetes, anxiety, and more. When it comes to the brain, sleep loss has profound effects that are very relevant here. "Without sleep, our cognitive and emotional abilities become markedly disrupted," a group of sleep researchers at the University of California, Berkeley, wrote in a paper for the journal *Nature Reviews Neuroscience*. The problem isn't just the absence of sleep, they said, but also the extended time awake.

Genetic variations can make people more or less sensitive to the effects of sleep deprivation, but generally chronic lack of sleep undermines or at least alters a bunch of cognitive processes that are essential to parental behavior. Sleep deprivation is known to hamper memory-encoding activity in the hippocampus. It's linked to decreased activity in prefrontal regions important in sustained attention. It reduces connectivity in the default mode network and impairs the brain's ability to, essentially, switch off that network during activities that require on-task attention.

Of particular note, acute sleep deprivation alters dopamine signaling and activity in the reward circuitry. The result, the authors wrote, seems to be a hypersensitized reward system, with amplified responses to pleasurable things—like desirable food—but also an "over-generalized" response, or an impaired ability to differentiate between rewarding and unrewarding things. Researchers have tested this in relation to a sleep-deprived person's ability to accurately gauge changes in monetary value during gambling tasks or to rate desirable or undesirable foods when hungry. At the same time, sleep deprivation increases amygdala activity and disrupts connections essential to the work of interoception and to accurately reading other people's emotions and one's own. I read this and thought about studies of people with postpartum depression that have found hyperactivity in the amygdala and a blunted ability to differentiate their own baby's rewarding cues from others'.

Both the amount of time a mother reports sleeping and her "sleep satisfaction" fall steeply across pregnancy and the first three months postpartum, according to a study that included thousands of German parents interviewed annually over six years. Fathers also experienced a dip in sleep and sleep satisfaction, though it was less dramatic. For both parents, things improve slowly from that three-month low, but none of the measures recovered to prepregnancy levels within the six-year study period.

Yet we know almost nothing about how sleep interacts with the changing neurobiology of the parental brain. Some, but not all, parental brain imaging studies try to control for sleep deprivation by quizzing participants about sleep quality. None that I know of looks at its influence on the brain directly, even while huge questions hang over the parental brain literature. For example, to what degree is sleep loss shaping the observed changes in the parental brain, alongside (and in concert with) hormones and caregiving experience? And what, if any, protective effects might occur within the parental brain to mitigate the otherwise deleterious effects of sleep deprivation?

The nature of parenthood—parents' inability or unwillingness to be part of studies that include sleep manipulation, for example—surely is an obstacle to more detailed analysis. Another is the particularities of sleep in the postpartum period. It's complicated.

"Newborn sleep deprivation is the worst kind you can possibly get," Stanford University neuroscientist Robert Sapolsky told journalist Katherine Ellison for her 2005 book *The Mommy Brain: How Motherhood Makes Us Smarter*. There is the sleep loss, and then there is the unpredictability. The body adjusts its nighttime cortisol levels, he said, in preparation for the challenge of getting up for a feeding or to settle a restless baby. "If you go to sleep anticipating you could be woken up any second during the night, you're always physiologically preparing for the stressor of waking up," Sapolsky said.

Lots of studies have linked sleep loss with postpartum depression, though not always in a simple less-sleep-equals-more-depression way. In one study, researchers at the University of North Carolina at Chapel Hill and the Center for Sleep and Cognition at Beth Israel Deaconess Medical Center in Boston measured depressive symptoms and sleep in twenty-five first-time mothers for weeklong periods in the third trimester of pregnancy and across the first few months postpartum. The women wore wrist actigraphy monitors that track movement, similar to an Oura Ring or other consumer health-tracking devices. They also completed sleep logs and surveys about their quality of sleep.

The study was relatively small, but it followed the same women over time and it was comprehensive, looking at subjective and objective measures of sleep. It measured total sleep but also other factors, including how fragmented or efficient a mother's sleep was, with efficiency being a measurement of how much she actually was asleep while in bed. Total sleep duration was *not* correlated with depressive symptoms, the researchers found. In fact their study and others have found that the total hours of sleep mothers actually get may not be so far off from the seven to eight that are recommended. The problem is, it's fragmented and inefficient, with those qualities, plus a mother's own rating of her sleep disturbance, linked to mood.

Sleep interventions could be an important tool for preventing depressive symptoms, including "sleep education or prescribed naps," the researchers wrote. Others have suggested a key to better sleep postpartum might be in establishing healthier sleep patterns during pregnancy, especially an earlier bedtime, and that prenatal education and public health messaging should emphasize this point.

Christine Parsons, a psychologist and associate professor at Aarhus University in Denmark, has been a coauthor on influential papers looking at how the brain processes infant cues and how those neural responses change with caregiving experience. She told me she recently started investigating sleep and the parental brain, recognizing the dearth of studies that cover the two. She's curious, for example, about how the parental brain processes infant cries during sleep and whether there are differences between men and women, or perhaps primary and secondary caregivers.

"You combine a new stimulus that is incredibly important and takes on, for many, many new parents, just a whole new meaning . . . and then you're not sleeping," she said. "You've got this coming together of two factors that I think probably compound each other as well."

There is no way around the fact that babies wake to feed through the night, especially in those first months. For the vast majority of parents, sleep disruption is an unavoidable part of the experience. But there are things that can help. First off—you know it—paid leave. It's hard to take those prescribed naps while working. It's hard to rest if you're also worried about how to pay the bills while on leave without pay. Clearer messaging for expectant parents about just how their sleep patterns will change and what that will mean for their brains and their bodies could help, too, so that they can anticipate those changes and put a plan in place for real support.

Vincent told me that, despite all the prenatal preparation she did, reading books and attending parenting classes and talking with her doctor, despite the snide or funny warnings other parents gave her in passing, there was never a point where she was offered time or space to "step out of the happy, excited land and really prepare and focus" on what new motherhood could mean for her, as a person with a body and a brain that will go through massive adjustments, beyond pregnancy. It could have made a difference, she said.

* * *

LET'S SAY WE ACCEPT AS fact that some memory function and attentional focus can be lost—albeit temporarily—as an "expense" during the early transition to parenthood. We already know there's some return on that investment. The circuitry for social processing, a person's capacity for reading social and emotional cues from other people and responding to them in a meaningful way, seems to be strengthened in parenthood. It's possible that those changes—gains, even—apply in other relationships, too, particularly other close bonds. Like those with our partners.

About a decade ago, Shir Atzil and colleagues scanned the brains of fifteen mothers and fifteen fathers—couples—as they observed videos of their own infant and another infant. Within couples, they found, brain areas associated with mentalizing, empathy, and motor responses were activated similarly between mothers and fathers as they viewed their own babies. The study was small and exploratory, but these correlations suggest that "parents may share in real time their intuitive understanding of the infant's state and signals," the authors wrote.

A separate study, led by researchers at Bar-Ilan University in Israel, scanned forty-two couples, about half of them same-sex couples and all of them first-time parents, and then followed the families over six years to examine the neural and hormonal underpinnings of co-parenting and family dynamics. The findings were nuanced, but among them, the authors noted that parents who showed greater connectivity between motivation-related areas of the striatum and the ventromedial prefrontal cortex, an area linked to empathy and emotion regulation, also demonstrated more collaborative co-parenting over time. Prior research has associated that particular link in brain regions with cooperation and behavior flexibility, among other things that serve the kind of altruism that family life requires.

Neuroscientists recognize that this method of looking at the brains of two people when they do something separately, even if they engage in the same task, like watching a video of their child, is quite limited. There is too much distance there. Human relationships don't exist as moments of observation but rather as continual, evolving interactions in which individuals read and influence the mental states of others and are influenced by them in return. Some have suggested that people engage in mutual mind reading, where their brains act together in a "we-mode."

The capacity for that kind of connection between two people is not unique to parenting. It may be a fundamental characteristic of human sociality. But it's likely that for many parents with partners, working together to care for a baby is the most intense and complex collaboration they've ever engaged in, one characterized by heavy demands, high stakes, and big potential gains. It would only make sense that, just as a parent's capacity for reading and responding to their baby is strengthened, their capacity for reading and responding to their partner is, too.

Two-person neuroscience, looking at brain activity in multiple people interacting with one another in real time, is logistically and statistically challenging. The technology available to do it is still quite limiting. There isn't much of it yet, but it is certainly where the field of social neuroscience is headed.

In one recent study, an international group of researchers measured the neural responses of twenty-four mother-father couples with young children using functional near-infrared spectroscopy, or fNIRS, which involves light emitters and sensors placed across the skull to measure blood flow at the very surface of the brain. Activity in the participants' prefrontal cortex was measured as they listened to laughter and crying, from infants and adults, and to static. When the couples were tested as they listened to the sounds while in the same room as one another, at the same time, hubs of attentional regulation and cognitive control seemed to sync up more than when they were tested separately. That effect did not occur when control pairs, who were not real-life couples, were tested together.

The couples matched brain signals more strongly when listening to neutral or positive sounds than when listening to cry sounds, which the authors suggested may be adaptive. Both parents reacting with stress to a baby's crying could be detrimental for everybody, they write. The results, they said, reflect the potential for parents' brains to work in concert with one another "to coordinate joint impending behaviors"—a skill that has clear benefits in raising a child but is useful, too, in the bigger picture of building a life together.

There is another study that Atzil coauthored about how mothers relate to other adults, and this one I think about all the time, as I watch parents greet their kids at school pickup or at the playground or while sitting with my sister on her back porch as our kids run around us and splash in a kiddie pool.

Atzil and neuroscientists Talma Hendler of Tel Aviv University and Ruth Feldman of the Interdisciplinary Center in Herzliya scanned the brains of mothers as they viewed different interactions between other infant-mother pairs. In some of the videos, the mothers engaged easily and affectionately with their babies. In others they were disengaged, anxious, or uncoordinated in their responses. When the mothers viewed the videos of the "synchronous" interactions, their brains responded more strongly in regions related to reward and mentalization, and in those involved in simulation, or the embodiment of someone else's actions in one's own mind. The researchers suggested that the mothers detected social synchrony in other mothers by reflecting it in themselves. In other words, a mother saw a healthy mother-child interaction, and her brain responded by simulating that interaction as if it were her own.

This made sense to me. I have clung to my friendships with other mothers these past few years. They offer joy and solidarity as we navigate this shifting terrain of kids and marriage, particularly through a time of harrowing politics and a global pandemic. And they help me sort myself out, in tangible ways—with advice on car seats or navigating the rules of play dates in the time of coronavirus—and in perhaps less tangible ways.

New parenthood is so much change at once that sometimes the experience can feel like wearing someone else's clothes, this uniform of responsibility that doesn't fit quite right. But then I watch one of my brilliant friends walk down the street hand in hand with her daughter, or I hear another give her son clear, firm directions about what he is or is not allowed to do, or I listen to them talk about their worries or their loneliness or their parenting wins, or we trade messages on a snow day or a pandemic day, cooped up, at wit's end—"my kids are monsters," one will say—and in all this it's like my brain grabs a freeze-frame from the scenes as they roll by and tags them: "Mother." I see myself in them, and it all fits a bit better.

The results from that paper, Atzil told me, aren't just about mother-to-mother interactions. The process of taking care of a child, of being responsible for regulating another person's allostasis, provides parents with a new internal model that they can use to interpret the social world around them, one that now incorporates all the experience they've had in paying attention to another person's needs and figuring out how to meet them.

Some parental brain experts have been so bold as to suggest that this new internal model could be a force for social change. The pull of an infant—the features that make up her *Kindchenschema* but also her laughter and babbles and smell—acts on adults in fast ways and in slow ones. It elicits quick attention from caregivers and it slowly builds their expertise in empathy and compassion, wrote a group of researchers that includes Marc Bornstein, then a senior investigator at the National Institute of Child Health and Human Development, and University of Oxford researchers Morten Kringelbach and Alan Stein. They frame this as the power of "cuteness," where "cute" describes all those positive features that make babies a sensory force.

Cuteness, Kringelbach and colleagues propose, can prompt people to expand their moral circle, or "the boundary drawn around entities deemed worthy of moral consideration." They offer, as an example, the global response to images of three-year-old Syrian refugee Alan Kurdi, whose body washed ashore in Turkey after the boat he and his family took to try to reach Greece capsized.

People looked at the image of that boy, his tiny face pressed into the sand, and they read the words of his father, Abdullah Kurdi, as he explained how he had tried many paths to get his family to safety in Canada where his relatives were waiting for them with jobs and a place to stay, and how, when nothing else worked, he put his family in a smuggler's raft, and they and others tumbled into the sea, and he tried to keep his sons afloat, holding one up and then the other. And then Alan was gone, along with his mother and his older brother. "What was precious is gone," Abdullah Kurdi told the *New York Times*.

"Rocketing across the world," the boy's story captured the attention, at least for a while, of politicians and the public like nothing else had before, not even the scale of more than eleven million people displaced at that point, the *Times* reported. Maybe that's in part because so many people saw those images and responded with a simulation of their own child. The same brain regions that are active when they press their hand against their own child's soft, round cheek. The familiar flicker of parental anxiety. So much joy, so close to despair.

"Like a Trojan horse," Kringelbach and his colleagues wrote, "cuteness opens doors that might otherwise remain shut."

There is remarkably little research on whether caregiving itself, and that response of reflecting it in others, possesses the power to open doors. In fact, we often hear how parenthood can make people more insular. This is the notion of parental aggression in action, an adaptive mechanism to protect against outside threats. One series of studies found that priming people to think about babies or caregiving before presenting them with pictures or information about members of an "out-group" increased their bias against that group, but only when the group also had been primed to be perceived as threatening. Very little research—almost none—has looked at how caregivers respond to one another, which is especially remarkable when you consider just how big a role parent-to-parent relationships play in adult life.

It's notable that the large majority of parental brain studies to date start with questions examining the root causes of pathology. Elsewhere there has been considerable investment in brain imaging research that asks questions deemed valuable for the sake of illuminating human nature and not only for solving a problem—in the fields of sports psychology, for example, or in studying the neural circuitry that motivates monetary investments or to more fully describe the nature of leadership. Yet exploring the development of parenting for the sake of understanding this fundamental experience somehow is a harder sell, even when it focuses on the parent-child relationship. "Even just the social neuroscience literature—it's all about empathy for peers," Darby Saxbe, the developmental psychologist, told me. "Don't we have to start with, kind of, where all that stuff evolves from, which is looking at the most fundamental first social relationships that anybody has?"

In 2016, the journal *Hormones and Behavior* ran a special issue on parental care in honor of Jay Rosenblatt. In it, Feldman wrote that Darwin's theory of evolution held at its center the idea that human nature is "primarily ruthless," driving perpetual competition for survival. But, she said, Rosenblatt and colleagues, who focused on the biological underpinnings of caregiving and connection, demonstrated that "social collaboration, interactive synchrony, and the capacity for reciprocity are no less 'biological' and 'primary' than the brutal acquisition of resources." While her research and others' has told us much more about how those biological mechanisms work, particularly between parents and babies, there's so much more to learn.

We've seen that, for humans, child-rearing has always been a cooperative act, and it seems that the parental brain incorporates a function—simulation—for recognizing in others the capacity for this kind of work. What does that mean for how parents relate to one another, at a neural level and in their lives at large? Perhaps parenthood is a factor for doubling down on commitments to social in-groups, but could it also break those barriers down, by making caregiving an in-group of its own?

It certainly seems that way, if you look at how effective community and political organizing around the status of motherhood is. Donna Norton is executive vice president of MomsRising, an advocacy organization focused on universal paid leave, immigration, gun safety, criminal justice reform, and other issues affecting family security. Part of what mobilizes parents to volunteer, Norton said, is a desire to protect their children—and not only their own. "Being a mother makes you often feel connected to your community because you just need your community more," she said. "You need to reach out to other people. It's impossible to just raise your kids alone. It takes a village."

Maybe one function of the parental brain is to recognize those villagers when we find them.

* * *

THERE ARE NO STUDIES I can point to that say explicitly that parent-hood makes a person smarter, but I believe it can. For all the nuanced findings this book has explored, there is this simple fact: parenthood requires a person to be immersed in exactly the kind of enriched environment—lots of sensory input, complex social demands—that is known in neuroscience to enhance cognitive functioning, and not only in the postpartum period but for years or even decades afterward.

I can't cite any data that proves for sure that parenthood makes a person more efficient, but I'm pretty sure that it does. Just ask them. But also, consider that shopping list. Before a person becomes a parent, they are responsible for managing their own basic needs. Afterward, they have their own and their child's to manage. Same hours in the day. Same brain.

I don't know of any research that has found having a child makes a person bolder, braver, or more resilient per se. But how else could so many parents live with a brain that makes them acutely aware of potential threats to the thing they hold most dear and, at the same time, closely attuned to the social and emotional needs of that small creature? This path requires boldness.

I can't point here to any studies that say that parenthood makes a person more creative than they were before. Without a doubt, it can. "There's a kind of evolutionary division of labor between children and adults," psychologist Alison Gopnik wrote in *The Philosophical Baby: What Children's Minds Tell Us about Truth, Love, and the Meaning of Life*. "Children are the R&D department of the human species—the blue-sky guys, the brainstormers. Adults are production and market-ing. They make the discoveries, we implement them. They think up a million new ideas, mostly useless, and we take the three or four good ones and make them real." I would argue that simply living adjacent to and growing alongside those "blue-sky" thinkers offers parents some-thing else, too: awe.

For something to elicit awe, according to psychologists who study this feeling as something measurable, it must be vast, to remind us of our smallness. Either literally, like space or the ocean stretched out across the horizon line. Or figuratively, like a spiritual awakening, or perhaps watching an infant slow-blink to sleep and recognizing the fleeting moment in the great expanse of time. It must also prompt a person to alter their mental representation of the world in some way. Being a parent, it seems to me, provides an almost infinite number of opportunities in which both conditions for awe may be met. If we look. And awe is thought to be a potent creative force, that vastness making room for new ideas or connections between old ones.

But sure, let's focus on forgetfulness.

In 2017, Molly Dickens, the stress physiologist and writer, was working for Bloomlife, a start-up focused on maternal health, when she interviewed six-time US track and field outdoor champion Alysia Montaño about how Olympians prepare for labor and about competing as a pregnant professional athlete. Montaño talked about facing questions around whether her running was safe for her baby. "The part that enraged me," she told Dickens, "was when I started to recognize that people have this diminished view of pregnant women—the view that women lack the intellectual capacity to just know her body, to understand it, to respect that it's giving a life, yet still be able to function and move."

She told Dickens about how her sponsor had withheld money when she had failed to place at the 2014 national championship, when she raced while thirty-four weeks pregnant. Two years later, Montaño would tell the full story, this time for the *New York Times*.

It was ASICS that threatened not to pay and then dropped her. Montaño had a similar experience with Nike. Kara Goucher, a long-distance runner and also an Olympian, reported similar treatment from Nike and from the United States Olympic Committee and USA Track & Field—lost pay, lost time with her son, lost health insurance, and disrespect from the same company that marketed its products to women with a big message: "Dream Crazy."

"The sports industry allows for men to have a full career," Montaño said in a video op-ed for the *New York Times*, "and when a woman decides to have a baby, it pushes women out at their prime."

Montaño and Goucher broke confidentiality clauses to tell their stories. Less than two weeks later, inspired by them, sprinter Allyson Felix published her own op-ed in the *Times* about how Nike had offered her less money after she had a baby and refused to guarantee that she wouldn't be punished if she didn't perform at the top of her game in the months around pregnancy. Felix, who would soon after become the most decorated US track and field athlete ever, asked, "If I can't secure maternity protections, who can?"

Their actions spurred a movement, pressure from Congress, and changes in Nike's policy. They're not done.

In 2020, just as the pandemic hit and Montaño gave birth to her third child, she and Dickens launched a nonprofit called &Mother. As in, champion and mother. Athlete and mother. Scientist and mother.

Dickens was a postdoctoral researcher at the University of California, Berkeley, in 2013, studying stress, reproductive hormones, and fertility, when she became pregnant with her first child. She wanted to take four months of leave, but the National Institutes of Health fellowship that funded her postdoc position offered eight weeks. So she decided to try to pause her fellowship and go without pay to give herself the remainder of the time. Her husband's income and insurance policy made the choice possible. When Dickens informed the human resources office of her plans, she said she was told, "No one has ever asked for this."

One week after her daughter was born, Dickens was offered an interview for a tenure-track position on the other side of the country. She asked to interview after she was back from leave but was told the position couldn't wait. A few weeks later, she flew across the country with her newborn and her husband and participated in a two-day interview, with breaks every two hours to pump milk. She felt like she had done well. She didn't get the job. The same year, the journal *Nature* published an entire special issue asking, "Where are the women?" in science. It explored gender bias and the need for more women in leadership roles and on scientific advisory boards, but it devoted little space to parenthood.

"There's no acknowledgment that sustaining a woman through this part in her career will boost how many women can stay in science," Dickens said. A career in science can be a career forever, she said, and the failure to accommodate people through the relatively short period when their family demands may be most intense is shortsighted. "How many women who would be—I'm sorry, like, studying women's health, studying pregnancy, studying maternal health, how many women that would have been studying that drop off at this point?"

Her comment is particular to science but the problem exists across industries, including the news industry where I've spent most of my career. The barriers to balancing a job in media with motherhood are lower than they once were but still quite severe—a fact that not only hampers the careers of journalists and equity in the newsroom but severely undermines the social discourse that journalists play a key role in shaping. In the same vein, how much richer might the landscape of professional sports, and our collective image of what women can do with their bodies over the whole course of their adult life, be if more room was made for mothers?

Now &Mother is working publicly and behind the scenes to make sure athletes get contracts that include parental protections. They're trying to establish standards within sports that make motherhood feasible, for things like protected time off and lactation support during travel and competitions. They are working to make contract language public so that athletes know what to ask for and how. The goal is to make a way forward in this industry that might serve as a model anywhere—everywhere—that has discounted the value of what people bring to the table *after* they become parents.

Beyond the implicit value of athletes being able to keep their careers after motherhood, when they know their bodies can do it, the Tokyo Olympics demonstrated quite clearly what the value of mothers in sports can be, to fans and to sponsors. Mothers in competition was a major story line of the games, powerful and joy-filled but hard won. Felix, who is now sponsored by Athleta and sits on the board of &Mother, brought home a bronze in the 400-meter race and gold from an electric 4×400-meter relay.

Making paths like hers easier for other athletes requires subverting old ideas about what women are allowed to do once they become mothers, about what they're capable of doing, Dickens said. The work of &Mother is interesting to me in part because it seems to take this broader struggle about who a person is after pregnancy and make it really visible. There's a perception about what the body of a pregnant or postpartum person can do, and there's a perception about what the brain of a pregnant or postpartum person can do. In neither case do they match reality.

"That's exactly it," Dickens said. "How do we reset that?"

CHAPTER 9

Between Us

T. Berry Brazelton answered his cell phone when I called in early 2016. The famous pediatrician whose decades-old writing had helped me reframe my own postpartum experience was about to turn ninety-eight, and I was on the cusp of my first anniversary of motherhood. Hartley would turn one a few days later. Brazelton didn't know me, but a mutual acquaintance had connected us, and he agreed to meet me for lunch.

A few weeks later, we met at the Colonial Inn in historic Concord, Massachusetts, which sits about halfway between the North Bridge, where minutemen fought British troops on the first day of the American Revolution, and the Orchard House, where Louisa May Alcott wrote her classic *Little Women* ("I am angry nearly every day of my life, Jo," Alcott's Marmee tells the headstrong second-oldest of her four daughters, "but I have learned not to show it; and I still hope to learn not to feel it, though it may take me another forty years to do so"). My husband dropped me at the door and went off in search of the library to pass the time with Hartley.

Brazelton had traveled to Concord with a caregiver from his home on Cape Cod to attend a funeral that afternoon of a former colleague from Boston Children's Hospital. Over the din of a busy dining room, I told him my story, explaining what his words had meant to me during some particularly dark days and how they spurred my interest in the neurobiology of new parenthood. Listening back on the recording from our conversation, I can hear myself sigh as if in relief when he started talking, slow and certain.

All doctors should talk with new mothers about depression, he said. Some depression in the postpartum period is nearly universal, maybe even essential. Productive. "You're frightened and you don't feel adequate and you're working very hard to pull yourself together, to start facing this child that you've fallen desperately in love with for the first time in your life," he said. "You realize what a major responsibility that is and what a turning point in your life it is. . . . I see getting disorganized and thrown into a frenzy like that as a major opportunity to reorganize yourself and pull yourself back together and become the person—the new person that you want to be."

This had been his philosophy, more or less, since he began practicing in Cambridge in 1951, at a time when, according to the obituary that would run in the New York Times two years later, "the conventional wisdom about babies and child rearing was unsparingly authoritarian." Infants were seen as unfeeling and best kept to a rigid schedule. Brazelton took a very different, often unorthodox approach. He recognized that babies could communicate with adults, from day one, through their behavior.

Using that framework, he played a key role in repopularizing breast-feeding. He advocated for parental leave and promoted the importance of having parents present when their children had to be hospitalized. Through his practice, his writing in magazines and books, and a long-running Lifetime channel TV show, What Every Baby Knows, Brazelton prioritized empowering parents by teaching them to understand their babies' language.

When he started in the field of pediatrics, he told me, "everything that went wrong with the child was blamed on the parents. And the parent was already feeling inadequate and guilty, so it re-enhanced the feeling of failure. It seemed to me that was the opposite of what we ought to be doing. We ought to be building up a mother's self-esteem, so she can pass that on to her child."

Brazelton said he was encouraged when the US Preventive Services Task Force issued a recommendation just a few months before our meeting for all pregnant and postpartum women to be screened for depression, and he hoped a movement among pediatricians to be more involved in maternal mental health would grow. By that point, I felt sure he would agree with me: Shouldn't we also be better preparing people for the brain changes they'll experience, before their baby is born?

"I don't think that most mothers are ready for that kind of information," Brazelton said. "It would scare a lot of people. I don't think they'd want to think their brains are going to change. They'd be frightened about which way it was going to go." If mothers raised the topic with him, he said, he would be glad to talk about it. Otherwise, it might add too much to their fears.

I fumbled my words, dismayed. The conversation until then had been so reassuring, if a touch paternalistic. But here suddenly was the very heavy idea that women can't handle information about their own bodies, their own brains. "Isn't that a very, in a sense, old-fashioned idea?" I asked, self-conscious even as I said it about posing such a question to someone of Brazelton's experience and stature. After all, I said, it used to be that women weren't told much about childbirth, out of concern about whether they could handle the anticipation of such a formidable physical experience. That's changed, to a large degree. Isn't the brain something to talk about more openly, too?

Brazelton took the question differently than I meant it and talked about the challenges of working mothers who lack social support. Our lunch ended soon after. People were gathering at the church.

It's hard to overstate how progressive Brazelton was for his day, how much he pushed against the culture in medicine. He listened to mothers at a time when other doctors mostly dictated to them. His impulse was to "let people tell you what they need," and that's the approach he would take with the neuroscience, too.

I knew what he was saying. I had withheld what I knew from my own friends when they were pregnant, afraid to scare them and nervous about what revealing my own struggles would say about me and my motherhood. But the idea that this was an acceptable decision—the *right* one—left me deflated.

How was I or any expectant parent, deluged with adorable onesies and congratulations, supposed to actually know what information we needed about our own development, when new parenthood was never described to us as the dramatic neurobiological change that it is? When popular pregnancy apps use headless diagrams to track weekly changes to a pregnant person's body and ignore the brain altogether but for a mention of forgetfulness? ("Not to worry, though," one such app reassures in the third trimester, "your brain will plump back up a few months after delivery.")

Baby books don't hesitate to tell a pregnant person what to expect when it comes to childbirth or feeding methods, about what to eat and how much, about what to buy for baby gear, or about how to feel (lucky, joyful, blessed). But this fundamental thing, how the brain changes— this we should keep between us, among those who have experienced it firsthand. At least until the next person we know has a baby and finds themselves running the postpartum gauntlet. Then, *maybe*, we let them in on the secret?

No.

In the time since I met Brazelton, years spent researching the parental brain and talking to people who have made this big life transition, many of whom felt as blindsided as I did, I have moved beyond feeling just a little let down that this parenting icon didn't like my idea. Now, I'm pissed. Not so much at Brazelton himself (a little bit at Brazelton) but at the whole collective of people and institutions that has made mothers think that pregnancy and new parenthood is a bodily challenge and a logistical challenge but one that they can more or less step into. As is. With their maternal instinct ready and intact. I feel angry that all other parents have been treated as peripheral or invisible or exempt. This is a charade. And everyone knows it but the people who most need to know it.

I am under no illusion that this science will be *the* thing that finally unravels the patriarchal norms that undermine mothers and other new parents. After all, generations have told us—continue to tell us—that we've got the story wrong. But I am certain that it can help, like one more seam ripper at the task.

I want expectant parents to know the story of this science so that they can be better prepared as they enter this new stage of life. There is no more important motivation for me in writing this book. But there are bigger reasons, too, for this science to be a prominent part of the public discourse, reasons that stretch across society and over time.

Because this science could reshape how we think about a person's physical and mental health over the whole course of their adult life. Because it compels us to reimagine how we measure and support the bonds that matter most in a child's life. Because, for all the vulnerability this science reveals about the parental brain, there is strength in it. And what would happen if we truly embraced that?

* * *

THE NEUROSCIENCE OF THE PARENTAL brain is young. You might say it's a four-year-old full of interesting, as-yet-unanswerable whys and hows and whats. Let's consider a few, starting with one that seems obvious but for which we have no good answer.

How might the changing brain affect childbirth? Orli Dahan, who studies the philosophy of science at Tel-Hai College in Israel, recently pointed out that the neuroscience of the parental brain focuses on how these changes prepare a person for parenthood but skips over labor and delivery almost entirely. Scientists don't know the precise brain mechanisms involved in coordinating or sustaining labor, or how exactly those mechanisms are affected by environmental factors or medical interventions. Dahan suggests that humans may have evolved the capacity for an altered state of consciousness during birth that includes changes in focused attention, time distortion, and pain reduction, and that some of the brain changes researchers have documented could serve that function. It's possible, she wrote, that the brain "is an active and crucial actor during birth and that birth, itself, is a process that requires brain neuroplasticity."

What about the gut-brain connection? A fair amount of attention has been paid in recent years to the ways delivery and feeding methods can affect a growing infant's microbiome. And there's an increasing understanding of the connection between the brain and the community of bacteria that live in a person's bowels, particularly through immune- and stress-related systems, including the HPA axis. Microbiome differences have been correlated with anxiety and major depressive disorder, for example. But what happens in a person's gut during pregnancy and the postpartum period?

Studies have found that the microbiome changes across pregnancy in ways that, by the third trimester, are thought to support energy storage in fat tissue and to fuel the development of the fetus. There are indications that disruptions in the birthing parent's microbiome could play a role in their perinatal mental health or specifically in the tenuous balance of their stress response and the fluctuation of hormones at childbirth. But researchers haven't put together the pieces yet to figure out how or, truly, whether they do.

And what exactly are all those fetal cells doing in a gestational parent's body? In chapter 4, we touched on the fact that fetal cells take up residence and can remain in a birthing parent's body long after the umbilical cord has been cut. The science describing the phenomenon of fetal microchimerism is, in a word, bonkers. The name refers to a chimera, a mythological monster made up of parts of multiple creatures appearing as one, as in a female lion with the head of a goat protruding from its back and a snake for a tail, in the Greek tradition. As in, you are no longer alone in a body of your own genetic makeup. In reality, you probably never were.

This is an exchange, sometimes referred to as "cell trafficking," though it is uneven. Babies carry cells from the parents who birth them—and even from older siblings or perhaps grandmothers—through their own infancy and on into adulthood. But gestational parents are the recipient of more cells than they distribute. The intact fetal cells with which a birthing parent is "seeded" during pregnancy are unlikely to be "accidental souvenirs of pregnancy" but could have a distinct evolutionary point, according to a 2017 summary of the literature published in *Nature Reviews Immunology*. That point may be to alter the parent's immune tolerance, lowering the chances of the body rejecting the growing fetus and increasing a birthing parent's rate of success over time, from pregnancy to pregnancy.

Fetal cells are found in small amounts in the blood of all pregnant people—100 percent—and are increased by common pregnancy problems, such as preeclampsia and miscarriage. But the cells are thought to proliferate and colonize tissues throughout the body after childbirth to varying degrees. One group of researchers from Arizona State University suggested that these pluripotent outside cells might be a kind of biological envoy, working to direct bodily resources toward an infant's needs, sometimes at a cost to birthing parents. They have been found in breast tissue, including mammary glands, and animal research suggests they play a role in promoting milk supply. They've been found in cesarean scar tissue and are thought to migrate to sites of injury to help in wound healing and perhaps even to slow the effects of aging.

In mice, researchers have found that fetal cells become neurons and integrate into mouse mothers' brain circuitry. In one study, the brains of fifty-nine human mothers who had carried sons were autopsied, and researchers found evidence of microchimerism, measured as the presence of male DNA, in about two-thirds. This proxy for microchimerism was found across multiple brain regions, and the study provided some of the strongest evidence to date that it persists. The oldest woman in whom male DNA was detected was ninety-four years old.

There are lots of questions left to answer, and so many of them center on the fact that pregnancy and childbirth do not make up a discrete and separate health event, distinct from a birthing parent's life course, though that's often how we treat it. We are somewhat conscious of the fact that a person's prepregnancy health can influence their health during pregnancy. It's also true that their health during pregnancy and the postpartum period can shape the trajectory of their health over the rest of their life. One's organs—brain included—don't simply fit back in place, in their original shape and size and function. If new parenthood is a stage of development, with lifelong effects on a person's physical and mental health, then it should be a well-considered factor in the design of health care, research, and the development of new treatments.

This has not been the case.

Instead, as neuroscientist Liisa Galea and colleagues at her lab at the University of British Columbia wrote in a 2018 opinion piece, reproductive experience is "a critical determinant of female physiology that has been grossly overlooked."

The problem is tightly woven with the ongoing neglect of biological sex in research generally. In 1977, the US Food and Drug Administration prohibited mothers and potential mothers—any woman of childbearing age—from inclusion in most clinical trials. Males were generally treated as the default, representative of all. The decision followed high-profile ethical breaches and the tragedies of babies harmed by prenatal exposure to the nausea antidote thalidomide or to diethylstilbestrol (DES). And many researchers preferred this anyway, so that they wouldn't have to account for women's hormonal "variability."

Women pushed back, calling the blanket ban a threat to their health, and a 1985 federal task force concurred. Soon after, the FDA and the National Institutes of Health recommended women's inclusion in clinical trials. But little changed. In 1993, Congress mandated that all clinical trials funded by NIH include women unless researchers could give a good reason not to.

But the law didn't require researchers to report on what they may have learned from those women. In the two decades after it took effect, only about 17 percent of studies on treatment options for coronary artery disease—the number one killer of women in the United States, and a disease that often presents differently in women than in men—included sex-specific outcomes, and that figure did not improve over time. Numerous other studies have chronicled underrepresentation in recent years. In 2016, the NIH began giving favor in its funding decisions to preclinical trials that use male and female animals, and the agency has put in place various programs to support researchers in doing so. Other major funding agencies around the globe have taken similar steps to push for the integration of sex and gender variables in research.

There are indications that the trend is improving today, though unevenly. In a recent analysis, Galea and colleagues evaluated thousands of papers published in the fields of neuroscience and psychiatry in 2009 and 2019 and found significant improvement in the use of male and female subjects over time. But, while 68 percent of studies included two sexes at the later time point, only 19 percent followed what the researchers called "optimal design" for actually identifying any sex differences. (These results were published as a preprint in November 2021 and not yet peer reviewed as of writing this.) There are real consequences to this, including bad science.

When the Society for Women's Health Research looked at nearly 150 mouse studies, published between 2013 and 2018 and evaluating potential Alzheimer's treatments, the group found that only one-third included male and female mice and far fewer analyzed their data by sex. The authors noted that a large majority of the mouse studies reported at least partly successful results, but those did not translate into successful clinical trials in humans, "which begs the question, why not?" One reason, they wrote, may be that the disease develops and progresses differently in females, and women make up nearly two-thirds of all diagnoses in the United States.

Of course, if women are neglected in science, it follows that pregnant people have been studied even less. Until January 2019, they were officially listed under federal policy as "vulnerable to coercion or undue influence," a classification that made enrolling pregnant women in research studies a bureaucratic feat. The FDA has issued specific guidance for the inclusion of pregnant people in clinical trials, but meanwhile people continue to face decisions every day about how to treat allergies or chronic hypertension or mental illness while pregnant, with little information to guide them. Few new drugs are evaluated specifically for safety and effectiveness during pregnancy before they go to market. "The default assumption has long been—and, to a large extent, still is—that it's essential to protect pregnant women from research, rather than ensure they benefit from its rapid progress," journalist Carolyn Y. Johnson wrote in the *Washington Post* in 2019.

Pregnant people become postpartum people who become people with a reproductive history. Around 83 percent of women in the United States have birthed a child by the time they are forty years old. Yet we know remarkably little about how that major life stage affects their long-term health.

Those fetal cells within a birthing parent's body are doing *something*. Fetal microchimerism has been implicated in autoimmune disorders, including thyroid disorders and lupus, for which people who have had pregnancies are at higher risk, and possibly in the exacerbation of symptoms of multiple sclerosis. When I read that fetal cells "have been proven to invade maternal skin," with their presence linked to "unexplained inflammatory skin disorders," I thought, maybe that explains the persistent dyshidrotic eczema I've had since becoming a mother and for which I've seen multiple doctors without resolution—an invasion. Fetal cells have been found in higher numbers in the presence of other types of diseases, too, within tumors or diseased organs, in the case of hepatitis C, for example. What the cells are doing there exactly—propelling the disease or repairing the damage—"is still an unresolved issue," according to a 2021 review led by Diana Bianchi, a medical geneticist and director of the Eunice Kennedy Shriver National Institute of Child Health and Human Development.

Studies looking at human health and disease "need to include complete pregnancy histories, including elective terminations and miscarriages," Bianchi and colleagues wrote. The biological connection between a birthing parent and a child truly is lifelong, even "at the most basic, granular, cellular level."

Hormone levels change more dramatically during pregnancy and the early postpartum period than at any other point during most people's lives and, while they level off after childbirth, they don't return to pre-pregnancy levels, maybe ever. Numerous studies in rodents and humans have found persistent changes in hormone levels and the expression of hormone receptors, with estrogen and prolactin levels reduced in mothers, compared to nonmothers. Those hormonal changes, along with other neurobiological and immunological ones, are surely driving some of the documented differences in the prevalence or severity of diseases according to reproductive history, but in most cases—as with Alzheimer's disease or the association between the number of pregnancies or pregnancy complications a person experiences and their risk for cardiovascular disease or stroke—researchers don't know how.

There's a lot that remains unstudied, a lot of questions still unanswered. And there are brand-new questions that will never be answered unless they are first acknowledged. For example, could it be that pregnancy fundamentally changes how the brain processes fear? It's a fairly well-studied phenomenon—though not one that's widely known in clinical care—that changes in estradiol and progesterone alter the effectiveness of exposure therapy, which is often used in treatment of anxiety disorders and involves exposing a person to the things they are fearful of but without a negative outcome. The thinking is that exposure allows people to create new "safety memories" attached to a stimulus, to essentially override fear memories. Studies of rats and humans have found that, in individuals with low estradiol and progesterone, during the follicular phase at the start of the menstrual cycle or at any point while taking contraceptive pills, this override, or the fear extinction process, is impaired.

A while back, psychologist Bronwyn Graham and her colleagues at the University of New South Wales became curious about how the long-term changes in hormone levels associated with reproduction might alter fear extinction. What they found was surprising. In both rats and humans, lower hormones after pregnancy didn't simply result in incremental changes to the cycling effects on fear extinction. They erased those effects. Mothers' capacity to extinguish their fear through exposure therapy no longer varied according to their hormone levels. Why? Graham's lab began trying to answer that question—a question that led to more questions.

Rats with reproductive experience seem to be using completely different parts of their brains to extinguish fear, Graham's lab found. Most notably, they do not engage their amygdala, that brain region often referred to as the "fear center." This finding has not yet been published or peer reviewed as of writing this. Graham said it was so unexpected that her group spent a year testing it and testing it again. They found that when mother rats were conditioned to a fear (in this case, the fear that a specific noise would be followed by a shock to their feet) and then had their amygdala deactivated, they subsequently were able to extinguish their fear just fine (through exposure to the sound with no shock).

Most of the findings by Graham's lab have, so far, been focused on what the brains of mother rats are *not* doing, which is an important step in the science but not the ultimate goal. They aren't using their amygdala to eliminate their fear. Nor are they using a specific type of receptor, called the N-methyl-D-aspartate or NMDA receptor, involved in synaptic plasticity and important for fear extinction in nonmother rats. "The issue is, we haven't figured out what they *are* doing," Graham told me. But, she said, "we can provide plenty of questions."

That the amygdala is not involved in fear extinction for rat mothers "is such a surprising finding," Graham said. "But one thing that I say to my lab all the time is, if we hadn't studied this system so comprehensively in males for so long, would this be surprising? Or would it just— maybe it's just that we have accepted as dogma that this is the way the brain works, but it actually only works that way under a very specific set of circumstances that for social and historical reasons have become the status quo of what we actually research."

Young children extinguish fear differently than adults do, and the neural process is different still in adolescents, Graham said. Why couldn't the process be different following pregnancy, which marks the start of yet another developmental phase?

I am eager to see where Graham's research leads. The notion that pregnancy changed the way my own brain processes fear or overcomes it *feels* correct. More importantly, figuring out how exactly fear extinction works in people who have had babies could lead to more effective treatment for those struggling with anxiety disorders. For this reason and for all the other questions pending—plus all those that haven't yet been asked—it's important that pregnancy and new parenthood be recognized and talked about as the profound and largely still-unexplored transformation it is. Otherwise, who knows how much we will miss?

* * *

WHEN I BEGAN WRITING THIS chapter, the United States was poised to pass a bill that would have dramatically increased access to affordable quality early childhood education and that would have brought the United States at least closer to being in line with the nations of the world in offering paid leave to new parents. Then the Build Back Better provisions for paid leave were cut dramatically and the whole bill was hung up in the Senate, largely because of opposition from West Virginia democratic senator Joe Manchin. The fact that quality education for the youngest children and especially paid leave are so far out of reach for so many families is a particularly American kind of shame.

Only five other countries—none of them high-income nations— have no national paid leave policy, and all but a handful of countries offer mothers twelve weeks or more. Most of Europe, as well as Canada, Chile, India, Iran, Russia, Venezuela, and others offer at least twenty-four weeks or more, and some nearly twice that much. Among eighty-three countries that offer paid paternity leave as of 2021, the average was sixteen weeks, according to Claire Cain Miller's reporting at the *New York Times*.

Why does the United States still lack such a policy, more than a century after mothers here formally began lobbying for one?

It can't be that economists simply have failed to show how paid leave benefits workers, employers, or the broader economy. Apart from all those functional programs operating around the globe, the evidence from state-based programs here in the United States indicates that, even among the peculiarities of this capitalist society, paid leave checks each of those boxes. It has the potential to bolster household financial security, to increase labor force participation, and to lower employee turnover–related costs for employers, or at least not result in broad negative effects on business.

The barrier to getting paid leave in the United States is not that public health experts have failed to adequately demonstrate the health benefits for babies and birthing parents. In fact, the health effects are dramatic and no longer a matter of debate.

Paid leave has been linked to reductions in the proportion of babies born preterm or at a low birth weight, with the largest effects for the children of Black women and unmarried women, a result that may be related to lower job- and income-related stress during pregnancy. Birthing parents who have access to paid leave are more likely to keep breastfeeding and to maintain a regular schedule of doctor appointments for their child, and focused time with a newborn is thought to set up the start of family life in ways that have long-term benefits for child health and development, particularly for children in lower-income families. In the measure that matters most, several studies have found that longer paid leave policies are associated with significant decreases in infant mortality rates.

For mothers, the health benefits are multifaceted and long-lasting. For starters, people simply need time to recover from childbirth, which often involves major surgery and sometimes involves life-threatening complications. Women who take paid leave of any length have a considerably lower risk of needing to be hospitalized for any reason in the year after birth, and each added week of leave (paid or unpaid) makes them less likely to report a state of "poor physical well-being" during the first year postpartum. The higher breastfeeding rates, and longer periods of it, associated with paid leave can benefit a person's long-term health by lowering their risk for diabetes, high blood pressure, and breast or ovarian cancer. Twelve weeks or more of paid leave has been found, over and over, to lower rates of postpartum depression, and longer leaves may have a small effect of protecting against depression even at age fifty and beyond.

As awareness has grown around the massive disparity in outcomes for Black birthing people and babies, a lot of attention has been paid to making changes within obstetric care, addressing the effects of systemic racism among doctors and within health care institutions, making sure that expectant parents' concerns about their own health are heard and addressed during pregnancy and birth, and filling the gaps in health insurance coverage. Overhauling the model of obstetric care is critical, but the problem is bigger than that.

In the United States, pregnant people are treated as important only during the standardized appointments that they are supposed to attend during pregnancy and immediately after, Joia Crear-Perry, an ob-gyn and president of the National Birth Equity Collaborative, told me. "We don't make room for their existence outside of that," she said. "We don't support them. We have people trying to get to a doctor's appointment in the middle of a workday. We've given them no paid leave, tell them not to bring their other kids, tell them not to eat in the office. We make it the opposite of what people need to actually thrive."

What people actually need may be fewer but more targeted prenatal visits to the ob-gyn and better integrated care, where their doctor can help them to connect with other providers or services to deal with factors affecting their pregnancy, such as homelessness or job stress or childcare for other children, she said. What people actually need may be postpartum care delivered at home and by a broader set of providers, including midwives. What people most certainly need is paid parental leave. That message has become an important part of Crear-Perry's work.

"Unpaid leave policies were written to support an outdated idea of a family—one in which the father supports everyone. But that's not how most families look today," she wrote in a 2021 commentary for Bloomberg Opinion. "Failure to recognize this undermines maternal health, especially in Black and brown communities, and is one of the reasons the U.S. is the most dangerous rich country in which to give birth."

We know all this. And yet—this inaction has nothing to do with the value of paid leave to children and families and everything do with what values our leaders hold. As Danielle Kurtzleben of NPR wrote in 2015, about opposition to family leave and also mandated sick leave, "You could write an entire book about the complicated forces at work here, but a mix of a few big factors has helped set this scene: The aftermath of World War II, business lobbying, a diminished American labor movement, and the American love of individualism and bootstrap-pulling all have combined to help keep the U.S. alone in not giving its workers paid leave." I'd add to that list the belief in maternal instinct and biology as destiny—women hold the capacity to care for children, their highest and best use—plus the absolute primacy of the maternal-infant bond.

That's what's behind conservative commentators' derision of US Transportation Secretary Pete Buttigieg's decision in 2021 to take paternity leave when he and his husband adopted newborn twins, their comments all a variation on a theme: Dads don't need time with babies! Newborns need their mom! There's no mom in this family, so what's the point? "In terms of bonding with dad, the most important time is a little later in the child's life," podcast host Matt Walsh wrote, among a series of tweets that cited his experience as a father of four who never took paternity leave. "Dads will do much more bonding in toddler years than in early infancy. Infants are focused almost entirely on mommy. It's biological."

That is belief, not biology. Biology tells us that babies connect with more than just their birthing parent. In addition to all the ways that fathers can support their partners—birthing or not—through the transition to parenthood, they also have an important role to play as part of the social world their baby is growing into. From a child's first months, fathers help to shape their brain development in ways that can influence their emotion regulation as toddlers, their confidence, their capacity to connect with peers, and their readiness for school. And, as important, time with a baby changes fathers, too, in ways that can adapt them for their lifelong role as caregiver.

Many feminist scholars have long been "unnecessarily biology-averse," economist Nancy Folbre told me by email. Biology so often has been used to justify inequality. "And," she wrote, "maybe most of us are unconsciously afraid of the very obvious possibility that forces largely beyond our control shape our lives and want to minimize it."

What happens if we look at those forces square on?

In her 2021 book *The Rise and Decline of Patriarchal Systems: An Intersectional Political Economy*, Folbre wrote that "confidence in women's natural or God-given propensities for self-sacrifice enabled the masculine pursuit of economic self-interest." Whether or not it was actually rooted in biology, women long experienced pressure to perform "compulsory altruism" and care for others, leaving men free to succeed in the capitalist economy, until the script for "doing gender" became almost synonymous for "doing care." Much of the anger directed at feminist campaigns comes from the fear that, if women move away from traditional roles, the level of care that's available to others—men, children, the sick, the elderly, employers—will decline. "This is not an entirely unrealistic fear: the renegotiation of gender roles requires a renegotiation of broader norms of obligation for the care of others, provoking resistance from all those hoping to avoid paying a larger share of the costs," Folbre wrote.

There is a risk to highlighting how the neurobiology of parenting—or caregiving in general, perhaps—captures adults, Folbre told me. Not everyone wants to be captured. "Maybe some biological fathers don't want to be around young infants because they know they will become attached—'stuck,'" she said. "Maybe the increase in childlessness among women relates to the perception that becoming a mother entails irreversible commitments that cannot be easily tailored to fit other priorities."

But this is exactly why I think this science is a necessary tool for shifting gender norms. Anyone can feel stuck or claimed or attached in parenthood, in ways that are to some degree beyond their own free will, even when a child is entirely wanted and planned for. That's part of the process of parental brain development. Your self is extended, and you are not entirely your own anymore. But this is not something particular to one gender. The capacity for this kind of transformation shapes deep and committed caregiving, and is a basic characteristic of the species.

This science is a way to contest the notion that care is distinctly female. It is not.

Men already are dramatically more engaged in fatherhood today than in generations past. If enough fathers can then feel that tension between ambition and obligation, between drive and care, if they can experience the costs and the return on investment, and importantly if they know how to name it—out loud—maybe they'll join in on the call for substantive paid parental leave, quality affordable childcare, reasonable workplace standards that allow for a balanced life, and living wages for direct care workers, including childcare providers. Perhaps that shared sense of capture can speed the renegotiation of norms that Folbre describes.

Getting there might require relinquishing old ideas about the nature of infant development and who, exactly, matters in a baby's life.

Let's consider the fact that, while John Bowlby did a huge amount of good in helping people to recognize and meet infants' needs, he also once wrote that the separation of mother and child was a lot like smoking or radiation. "Although the effects of small doses appear negligible, they are cumulative," he wrote. "The safest dose is a zero dose." This was a conclusion he made based on studies in which rhesus monkey mothers, who engage in exclusive maternal care, were separated from their infants for days at a time.

So much research on new parenthood, including a lot of the brain science in this book, is grounded in Bowlby's development, with Mary Ainsworth, of attachment theory. That means it is rooted in the idea that the connection between a mother and her baby is the most important, most fundamental, and also most developmentally loaded relationship there is. It is true that this connection is important, fundamental, and developmentally loaded. It is also true that all the close connections a baby has are important, fundamental, and developmentally loaded. Yet mothers and babies are still most often studied as a unit in space.

Around the time that I was wrangling with my own feelings about attachment theory, I came upon the book *Different Faces of Attachment: Cultural Variations on a Universal Human Need*. Published in 2014 and edited by Hiltrud Otto and Heidi Keller, it compiles essays by scholars of human development and anthropology that argue there is *no* set design by which an infant's attachment develops, nor one single definition of "maternal sensitivity." Instead, they maintain, these things vary widely according to cultural context and, in fact, in most families around the world, the care that leads to attachment is not contained within a mother-infant dyad but rather is socially distributed, with other adults and older children playing critical roles.

Despite decades of people offering evidence that attachment theory is too narrow, that it isolates mothers and babies from their social context, it has remained predominant and largely unchanged. "It's kind of like gravity," said Thomas Weisner, anthropologist, professor emeritus at UCLA, and a contributor to the book. By that he meant it is ubiquitous, it is seen as accepted science, and it shapes how we see the world.

That's partly because attachment theory became an industry. Researchers hired people to teach them how to code their observations in a Strange Situation experiment, created by Ainsworth, which involves observing how a child behaves when their mother leaves them alone in an observation room, when a stranger enters, and when the mother returns, and then grading the child as securely attached or insecurely attached and, in the latter case, avoidant, disorganized, or resistant. Various attachment scales were developed to determine someone's attachment style at different ages, including into adulthood, and Weisner said prominent journals came to see the Strange Situation as a gold standard for research without fully acknowledging its limitations.

The problem isn't necessarily with the tests themselves but with the fact that they became so embedded in our cultural understanding of mothers and babies, to the exclusion of other valid evidence. Weisner said the outcomes from this one tool of measurement, involving a single interaction, became conflated with the thing it was trying to measure, the social trust developing between a baby and the people in her realm.

In reality, the care of human infants has always been distributed. In every community where children are raised, Weisner said, there are people who have become specialized in caring for them, so that the task of soothing babies in distress—of meeting their allostatic needs—is theirs to solve. These people typically include mothers. But they also can be fathers and grandparents, aunts and uncles, and others. Much of

Weisner's early research focused on the role played by older siblings and cousins around the world, who might dote on infants who spend most of their time with mothers but then assume a direct role in caring for children as young as one or two.

Broadly speaking, Weisner said, the more economic pressure there is on a mother and the more value placed on community cooperation, the more likely she is to have a circle of soothers to help. And, rather than deviating from the attachment norm, this process could, in fact, be an important part of a baby learning culturally relevant social trust. Babies "are prepared to be super responsive to the environment, but in ways that will make them fit socially, into the social world that they're in," Weisner said. If that world involves multiple caregivers, "that is the environment that they're going to respond to and feel secure within."

Figuring out how to account for the realities of a social world within attachment theory is a problem for researchers to solve. But it's also a problem for the rest of us to consider, as we work to build networks of care for our own children and sometimes come up against people or institutions that maintain that, very simply, a mother is enough. What if we paid childcare providers as the social educators and specialized soothers they are, rather than treating them like backstops to "deviant" mothers? What would it look like to build a community system of specialized soothers who could support brand-new parents at home?

Cultural context is a major component missing from the parental brain research to date, Linda Mayes, director of the Yale Child Study Center, told me. Mayes said researchers don't know yet which aspects of parental brain structure or function may be shared across the globe or which may be particular to the mostly White study participants in the WEIRD nations where much of the research has taken place. "Are we talking about a universal phenomenon?" Mayes said. "I presume we are, but we really don't know much about that."

If the theory that many of these brain changes are shared across mammalian species is true, then they should be generally universal in humans, and there is some limited evidence that this is the case. In one study, researchers observed the behavior of 684 first-time mothers from eleven countries and found that, at a very foundational level across social groups, mothers "preferentially and systematically" respond to their crying babies by picking them up, holding them, and speaking to them. You could file that in a folder of studies that demonstrate the obvious, except this study also looked at brain scans for a smaller group of mothers in the United States, China, and Italy, and found that baby cries consistently activate regions involved in automatic motor and speech responses before conscious decision-making occurs. In that sense, the researchers wrote, the behavior of human mothers is very much in line with the approach-and-retrieve caregiving behaviors of other mammals.

Even if changes to the parental brain are generally universal, that does not necessarily mean that all parents, across or within cultures, experience those changes in the same way, Mayes told me. It could be that the brain changes involved in directing attention toward a baby's cues in those first weeks make one mother feel intensely hypervigilant, but in a different cultural context—perhaps one with a bigger support network at the ready or in which young adults are more likely to witness family members or friends making the transition to parenthood before they do so themselves—that sense of preoccupation might be less intense, or described as something else altogether. Also unknown is how the neurobiological changes that are adaptive to parenthood might occur differently, or over an alternate timeline, in someone who has had extensive involvement in caring for children before having their own.

"There's much to be worked out in that regard," Mayes said.

Future parental brain science will tell us important and fascinating things about how humans build and adjust their social brains in infancy and over a lifetime, and it will give us new paths to treatment for postpartum mood and anxiety disorders. It will be fascinating, I am certain. And yet, I keep coming back to the idea that we already know what we need to know to do better for new parents.

Crear-Perry, the ob-gyn, has been a vocal advocate for the idea that a person's race is not a risk factor shaping their health outcomes. There is nothing inherent to Blackness that makes a person more biologically predisposed to deliver a child preterm, for example. Rather, racism is the risk factor, the way it wears on the body and the way those effects compound an already inadequate system of support. Crear-Perry told me there is no need for even one more study proving that racism causes biological harm. "The question is, are we going to do what we need to do to mitigate those harms?" Yet, she said, "I have yet to go to a meeting where somebody doesn't say, 'We still need more science.'"

We don't need even one more study to know that new parenthood is a time of monumental change at every level of a person's life, including for their brain. Social policies in the United States and its broken system for health care delivery have utterly failed to account for that fact. The question is, are we going to do what we need to do to help new parents thrive?

* * *

DONALD WINNICOTT PROPOSED HIS THEORY of "primary maternal pre-occupation" in 1956, and about half a century later researchers began to map the neural changes that underpin the particular kind of vigilance he described. A theory with a circuitry to match—"it looks so prescient," psychiatrist and researcher James Swain told me.

In 1989, Sara Ruddick published her theory of "maternal thinking," describing mothering as work that, at its core, requires a person to really see a child's vulnerability and to respond to it. To strategize about how to protect and nurture and train a child, how to build "proper trust," and how to balance one's own obsessiveness with humility, a conscious awareness of the separateness of a child's life from a mother's own. Supporting it all is what Ruddick called "attentive love."

"Attention is akin to the capacity for empathy, the ability to suffer or celebrate with another as if in the other's experience you know and find yourself," she wrote in *Maternal Thinking: Toward a Politics of Peace*. "However, the idea of empathy, as it is popularly understood, underestimates the importance of knowing another *without* finding yourself in her. A mother really looks at her child, tries to see him accurately rather than herself in him."

Ruddick wrote, too, about how it is not only women or gestational mothers who engage in maternal thinking. Rather it is "an activity governed by a *commitment*"—not a choice, but a fact—of body and mind and energy. "Anyone who commits her or himself to responding to children's demands, and makes the work of response a considerable part of her or his life, is a mother," she wrote. Through all the ways that parents can fail their children and then try again, parenting becomes "a hard, uncertain, exhausting and also often exhilarating work of conscience." A process.

When I reread Ruddick's work today, I think, this is prescient. Attention, motivation, emotion regulation, social cognition, theory of mind (the same and the separate)—this is the constellation of the parental brain.

Ruddick's theory is not mentioned or quoted in any of the hundreds of journal articles on the neuroscience of parenting I've compiled in the process of reporting this book. Nor, as far as I can tell, is the work of other feminist scholars—Adrienne Rich, Audre Lorde, bell hooks, among many others—whose work in the 1970s and 1980s and since has tried to excavate the reality of caregiving as a practice from beneath the false narratives of morality and instinct that have buried it. Winnicott's work, on the other hand, appears often. Perhaps that's because Winnicott was a pediatrician and psychoanalyst. Ruddick was a philosopher. And mother.

How do we bridge the divide between basic science and lived experience, between what's been tested and what's tested us, between the feminist thinking that has long offered a way for people to see themselves in motherhood and the neurobiology that seems to support it?

We do it here, on these pages. And also in our lives, every day, in the stories we tell ourselves.

Ayesha Mattu remembers thinking childbirth and the postpartum period would feel like a rite of passage. That idea was shaped by stories about her relatives giving birth in Pakistan, the married women of the family gathered around them offering reassurances: "This is normal. We are here. You are becoming something, something more."

When Mattu delivered her son at a hospital in San Francisco in 2010, things went very differently from what she had expected. She had a difficult labor—eighty-nine hours—followed by a C-section during which her anesthesia wore off. At home with her son, she felt she was constantly breastfeeding though he never seemed to be getting enough milk. Her husband would leave for work in the morning and come home in the evening, and she would be in the same chair she had started the day in, nursing. Mattu said she struggled to recognize herself. She struggled to feel the motherly love she had expected. "I felt like an alien of some kind," she said. "Why had I chosen to do this, when it seemed like a sentence?"

Around nine weeks postpartum, Mattu began to feel the love for her son bloom. Still, it took time for her life as a mother to come more into focus. In those first months and years, Mattu said, she was intensely focused on her child. She felt like her husband—the world maybe—was waiting for her to somehow go back to the person she was before. And she couldn't. Each of them, on different timelines, had to find their way into their new roles as parents. As she did that, her attention expanded.

She realized that the intense love she felt for her son—"this is exactly how every mother feels about their child," she said. "Then, I want to do everything I can to provide that type of safety and security for every child." Mattu said she became motivated to "get really healthy psychologically" through therapy and her own work on her relationships. She became more consciously engaged on issues of climate justice and racial justice. And she very purposefully stepped into the role of "auntie" to the other children in her life. That includes her nieces and nephews, but also her friends and her neighbors.

Mattu and her husband, who are Muslim, have long been part of an intergenerational *halaqa*, a Quran study group, that meets once a month and more frequently by Zoom since the start of the pandemic. They were one of the first couples within the group to have a baby. When her son was a year old, Mattu took him on a trip with the group to a seaside town and because of weather and travel issues, they arrived at almost 3 a.m. When her son woke for the morning just three hours later, a friend took him and told her to go back to sleep. "And I just felt that feeling of being so deeply loved and known and that my baby was safe, and then I could rest," she said. As more babies have arrived in the group, she's tried to provide that security for them, too. Because they need it, and because she needs it. Because her son needs it—to be safe and known.

In the United States, the tendency can be to make motherhood very small, very focused on your own child's success, where everyone else is a competitor. But this part—about being an elder and a nurturer of the next generation—"that's actually what motherhood should activate us into, I think."

Those early days were overwhelming. Mattu thinks she had post-traumatic stress from the delivery, and her physical recovery was complicated. She wishes she had been better prepared for what those first weeks would be like, and she tries in her role as an auntie to help others prepare. "I felt completely changed, and I had no narrative for that." Now, with some distance, she said, she can recognize what that "breaking open" also was: a beginning.

Reproductive psychologist Aurélie Athan thinks we might all be at a beginning. Athan's work in recent years has focused on the idea of *matrescence*, a word she helped to repopularize that was coined by anthropologist Dana Raphael in the 1970s to describe the transition to motherhood—as significant as adolescence. Mothers and others are becoming more aware that new parenthood is a metanoia, she told me, a change of the mind as well as a change of the brain.

It's not so much that parenthood offers the path to enlightenment. Rather, enlightenment can come from many places, and parenthood is one. This point seems almost obvious, when you think about it. New parenthood is an intensely physical and emotional experience that involves an acceleration of development and inclines a person toward prosocial behavior, toward empathy and reliance on others. Yet, Athan said, "that story [of transformation] has been missing in the transition to parenthood, because it's so ubiquitous. Everybody mostly does it."

The more people who recognize and embrace parenthood as transformative, the greater the potential for "a larger shift to consciousness," Athan said, one that demands the replacement of systems that harm people and the climate in favor of life-supporting social structures and technologies that prioritize collaboration and mutual assistance.

This is the kind of statement that I am prone to be skeptical of. Except—parenthood does change how we think and how we relate to one another. What I think Athan is suggesting is not so much a sudden political awakening as a slower, potent shift in the framework of human society so that caregiving isn't something that happens at the margins but rather is the goal—a goal that might be achievable only through recognition of the biological nature of human sociality, what it takes to support the processes that build it, and the fundamental role that the changing parental brain plays in shaping connection across society.

We have learned so much since Antoinette Brown Blackwell called for women to embrace science as a tool to answer the beating questions at the center of their lives. Motherhood is not a ready-made mode created in the image of the Madonna. It is a developmental stage like any other, one that requires major neural reorganization and the slow acquisition of new skills. This adaptive state, born from attention and a capacity to extend oneself to understand and meet another person's needs, is not unique to birthing mothers but something all humans can grow into—a fact that has been true through all of human history and that remains true today.

Athan spends a lot of time these days with health educators of teens and young adults, training them in how to teach reproductive identity development. This is not the "there's an egg, there's a sperm, and use a condom" conversation, Athan said. She tells educators, before they talk about contraceptives, to ask students, what kind of family did you come from? What kind of family do you want? Do you want to have children at all, and what would that look like? How would you like to have them? The goal, she said, is to consciously frame parenthood as a potential major event for their future selves.

"What do you want to do with it?" Athan asks.

* * *

ONE FALL AFTERNOON A FEW years ago, I followed Hartley around the basement level of the Portland Museum of Art, searching for distractions. My husband sat inside a theater there watching a children's musical. Our youngest was in his lap, giggling and waving his whole body at the performers. For Hartley, the show was too much. Instead, we visited the bathroom and the café. We read and reread the signs posted outside an interactive exhibit under construction. We tried all the chairs in the lobby. We rode the elevator. That's where I met Jochebed.

The marble statue of the mother of Moses, circa 1873, sits tucked into an alcove next to the bank of elevators. In one arm, she holds her infant son, who reaches for her covered breast, oblivious to his own fate. Her other hand grips the edge of her seat, her upper body pitched forward over her baby. Her gaze is not on him but extended out to the world, or to some space beyond herself.

Her expression, not only on her face but in her whole body, is not the biblical view of motherhood I was accustomed to seeing, of calm resolve and unquestioning devotion. In her, I saw emotion so intense it seemed almost paralyzing—desperation and determination, doubt and fortitude. The utter urgency of her child's needs, like a thousand threads, pulls at her own expanding consciousness even as she sees the world, with all its beauty and its dangers, anew. The tension of that state, stretched in opposing directions, is exhausting.

I didn't yet know the story of Jochebed, told glancingly in the Bible's Book of Exodus. I didn't realize that this baby was Moses, born under an edict from the king of Egypt that every boy birthed by an Israelite should be thrown into the river. This sculpture was created by Franklin B. Simmons, a nineteenth-century artist celebrated for his portrayals of American Civil War heroes and statesmen. His statue of Ulysses S. Grant, sword in hand, stands on a pedestal in the center of a grand rotunda on the museum's main floor. Simmons, who was born in Maine but lived and worked for much of his life in Rome, also made work representative of religious ideals. Maternal sacrifice, for one.

Perhaps Simmons's Jochebed is searching her mind for a plan to save the baby whose life, at three months, she can no longer hide. Or perhaps the artist intended this to be the moment at which she begins to rise from her seat to place the infant in a basket made of papyrus and pitch and send him down the Nile in a last-ditch effort—one she couldn't have been certain would succeed—to save his life. The statue, which casts a likely brown-skinned woman in white stone, was celebrated in Simmons's time for its success in contrasting inner turmoil and outward repose, but also for the "exquisite delicacy and loveliness" of Jochebed herself, as one early-twentieth-century art writer put it, for how it captures "the mystic beauty, the very ideal of maternity."

I kept coming back to Jochebed as I learned more about parenting and the brain. I thought about how her brain would have been shaped by her prior pregnancies and by the reality of giving birth under oppression to a son who almost certainly would not live. How would the trauma of that experience have shaped her? Would the biology of pregnancy and parenthood—that attentive love, that capacity to know the minds of others—have equipped her to cope, compelled her to act, to read the world around her and try to find a way? I had never seen in her a delicacy or a godliness. But the paralysis I had seen before was replaced, at least in part, by something else now: power.

Raise it up. Put it on a pedestal. Let it be seen.

NOTES

PREFACE

xiv   **"earned by care"**: Sara Ruddick, *Maternal Thinking: Toward a Politics of Peace* (Boston: Beacon Press, 1995), 42. Here she is describing maternal authority versus fatherhood.

xiv   **life-supporting practice of mothering**: Alexis Pauline Gumbs, China Martens, and Mai'a Williams, eds., *Revolutionary Mothering: Love on the Front Lines*, illustrated ed. (Oakland, CA: PM Press, 2016), 9.

CHAPTER 1: AT THE FLIP OF A SWITCH

1   **Naturally**: "It comes naturally," the mother swan in E. B. White's classic *The Trumpet of the Swan* tells her mate as she starts the labor of nest building. "There's a lot of work to it, but on the whole it is pleasant work."

5   **I found an inkling**: T. Berry Brazelton, *Infants and Mothers: Differences in Development*, rev. ed. (New York: Dell, 1983), 44.

6   **"wholesale remodeling"**: Jodi L. Pawluski, Kelly G. Lambert, and Craig H. Kinsley, "Neuroplasticity in the Maternal Hippocampus: Relation to Cognition and Effects of Repeated Stress," in "Parental Care," ed. Alison S. Fleming, Frederic Lévy, and Joe S. Lonstein, special issue, *Hormones and Behavior* 77 (January 2016): 86–97, https://doi.org/10.1016/j.yhbeh.2015.06.004.

6   **"baby blues"**: Michael W. O'Hara and Katherine L. Wisner, "Perinatal Mental Illness: Definition, Description and Aetiology," in "Perinatal Mental Health: Guidance for the Obstetrician-Gynecologist," ed. Michael W. O'Hara, Katherine L. Wisner, and Gerald F. Joseph Jr., special issue, *Best*

Practice & Research Clinical Obstetrics & Gynaecology 28, no. 1 (January 2014): 3–12, https://doi.org/10.1016/j.bpobgyn.2013.09.002.

6   **the creation of new neural pathways:** Mariana Pereira and Annabel Ferreira, "Neuroanatomical and Neurochemical Basis of Parenting: Dynamic Coordination of Motivational, Affective and Cognitive Processes," in "Parental Care," ed. Alison S. Fleming, Frederic Lévy, and Joe S. Lonstein, special issue, *Hormones and Behavior* 77 (January 2016): 72–85, https://doi.org/10.1016/j.yhbeh.2015.08.005; and Pilyoung Kim, "Human Maternal Brain Plasticity: Adaptation to Parenting," in "Maternal Brain Plasticity: Preclinical and Human Research and Implications for Intervention," special issue, *New Directions for Child and Adolescent Development* 2016, no. 153 (Fall 2016): 47–58, https://doi.org/10.1002/cad.20168.

7   **regions seem to shift in size:** Elseline Hoekzema, Erika Barba-Müller, Cristina Pozzobon, Marisol Picado, Florencio Lucco, David García-García, Juan Carlos Soliva, et al., "Pregnancy Leads to Long-Lasting Changes in Human Brain Structure," *Nature Neuroscience* 20, no. 2 (2017): 287–96, https://doi.org/10.1038/nn.4458; Elseline Hoekzema, Christian K. Tamnes, Puck Berns, Erika Barba-Müller, Cristina Pozzobon, Marisol Picado, Florencio Lucco, et al., "Becoming a Mother Entails Anatomical Changes in the Ventral Striatum of the Human Brain That Facilitate Its Responsiveness to Offspring Cues," *Psychoneuroendocrinology* 112 (February 2020): 104507, https://doi.org/10.1016/j.psyneuen.2019.104507; and Pilyoung Kim, Alexander J. Dufford, and Rebekah C. Tribble, "Cortical Thickness Variation of the Maternal Brain in the First 6 Months Postpartum: Associations with Parental Self-Efficacy," *Brain Structure & Function* 223, no. 7 (September 2018): 3267–77, https://doi.org/10.1007/s00429-018-1688-z.

7   **The imprint of that circuitry:** Alexander J. Dufford, Andrew Erhart, and Pilyoung Kim, "Maternal Brain Resting-State Connectivity in the Postpartum Period," in "Papers from the Parental Brain 2018 Meeting, Toronto, Canada, July 2018," special issue, *Journal of Neuroendocrinology* 31, no. 9 (September 2019): e12737, https://doi.org/10.1111/jne.12737.

7   **those changes last:** Edwina R. Orchard, Phillip G. D. Ward, Sidhant Chopra, Elsdon Storey, Gary F. Egan, and Sharna D. Jamadar, "Neuroprotective Effects of Motherhood on Brain Function in Late Life: A Resting-State fMRI Study," *Cerebral Cortex* 31, no. 2 (February 2021): 1270–83, https://doi.org/10.1093/cercor/bhaa293.

8   **environmental complexity:** Edwina R. Orchard, Phillip G. D. Ward, Francesco Sforazzini, Elsdon Storey, Gary F. Egan, and Sharna D. Jamadar, "Relationship between Parenthood and Cortical Thickness in Late Adulthood," *PLoS ONE* 15, no. 7 (July 28, 2020): e0236031, https://doi.org/10.1371/journal.pone.0236031.

9   **not only from their babies:** Shir Atzil, Talma Hendler, Orna Zagoory-Sharon, Yonatan Winetraub, and Ruth Feldman, "Synchrony and Specificity in the Maternal and the Paternal Brain: Relations to Oxytocin and Vaso-

pressin," *Journal of the American Academy of Child and Adolescent Psychiatry* 51, no. 8 (August 2012): 798–811, https://doi.org/10.1016/j.jaac.2012.06.008; and Shir Atzil, Talma Hendler, and Ruth Feldman, "The Brain Basis of Social Synchrony," *Social Cognitive and Affective Neuroscience* 9, no. 8 (August 2014): 1193–202, https://doi.org/10.1093/scan/nst105.

9   **ability to regulate their own emotions:** Helena J. V. Rutherford, Norah S. Wallace, Heidemarie K. Laurent, and Linda C. Mayes, "Emotion Regulation in Parenthood," *Developmental Review* 36 (June 2015): 1–14, https://doi.org/10.1016/j.dr.2014.12.008.

9   **While many people experience:** Pereira and Ferreira, "Neuroanatomical and Neurochemical Basis of Parenting," https://doi.org/10.1016/j.yhbeh.2015.08.005.

9   **protect cognition:** Orchard et al., "Neuroprotective Effects of Motherhood," https://doi.org/10.1093/cercor/bhaa293.

9   **For a long time:** J. S. Rosenblatt, "Psychobiology of Maternal Behavior: Contribution to the Clinical Understanding of Maternal Behavior among Humans," supplement, *Acta Paediatrica* 83, no. s397 (June 1994): 3–8, https://doi.org/10.1111/j.1651-2227.1994.tb13259.x.

11   **He was a painter:** "Jay S. Rosenblatt—Obituary," Legacy, originally published in *New York Times*, February 19, 2014, https://www.legacy.com/amp/obituaries/nytimes/169759170.

11   **Maternal behavior was "indisputably innate":** Frank A. Beach Jr., "The Neural Basis of Innate Behavior. I. Effects of Cortical Lesions upon the Maternal Behavior Pattern in the Rat," *Journal of Comparative Psychology* 24, no. 3 (1937): 393–440, https://doi.org/10.1037/h0059606.

11   **one 1950 study:** J. P. Scott and Mary-'Vesta Marston, "Critical Periods Affecting the Development of Normal and Mal-Adjustive Social Behavior of Puppies," *Pedagogical Seminary and Journal of Genetic Psychology* 77, no. 1 (1950): 25–60, https://doi.org/10.1080/08856559.1950.10533536.

12   **Lorenz believed instinctive behavior:** Marga Vicedo, *The Nature and Nurture of Love: From Imprinting to Attachment in Cold War America*, illustrated ed. (Chicago: University of Chicago Press, 2013), 58; Konrad Z. Lorenz, "The Companion in the Bird's World," *Auk* 54, no. 3 (July 1937): 245–73, https://doi.org/10.2307/4078077; and Konrad Lorenz, *Studies in Animal and Human Behaviour*, trans. Robert Martin (Cambridge, MA: Harvard University Press, 1970), 1:244, http://archive.org/details/studiesinanimalh01lore. Lorenz was not the first to use this metaphor. By the time he wrote the article above, it had become somewhat cliché among people who studied instinct and motivation. William James used the same metaphor in his *Principles of Psychology* in 1890.

12   **He was one of three:** "3 Behavioral Science Pioneers Win Nobel Prize for Medicine," *New York Times*, October 12, 1973, https://www.nytimes.com/1973/10/12/archives/3-behavioral-science-pioneers-win-nobel-prize-for-medicine-3.html.

12   **Some of his peers:** Walter Sullivan, "Questions Raised on Lorenz's Prize," *New York Times*, December 15, 1973, https://www.nytimes.com/1973/12/15 /archives/questions-raised-on-lorenzs-prize-scientific-journal-here-cites .html.

12   **Lorenz suggested:** Vicedo, *Nature and Nurture of Love*, 58–62.

13   **There he was, bare-chested:** "An Adopted Mother Goose: Filling a Parent's Role, a Scientist Studies Goslings' Behavior," *Life*, August 22, 1955, 73.

13   **And he gained a following:** Vicedo, *Nature and Nurture of Love*, 60–64.

13   **Mothers were spending too little time:** It's worthwhile to look at the quote noted by Vicedo in a fuller context, to see how squarely Lorenz sets societal ills on parents' shoulders: "There is no doubt that through the decay of genetically anchored social behavior we are threatened by the apocalypse in a particularly horrible form. However, even this danger is easier to avert than others. . . . To prevent the genetic decline and fall of mankind, all we need do is follow the advice implied in the old Jewish story I quoted earlier. When you look for a wife or husband, do not forget the simple and obvious requirement: she must be *good*, and he no less." Konrad Lorenz, *Civilized Man's Eight Deadly Sins* (New York: Harcourt Brace Jovanovich, 1974).

13   **he told the *New York Times*:** Vicedo, *Nature and Nurture of Love*, 216–19; Paul Hofmann, "Nobel Laureate Watches Fish for Clues to Human Violence," *New York Times*, May 8, 1977, https://www.nytimes.com/1977/05/08 /archives/nobel-laureate-watches-fish-for-clues-to-human-violence.html.

14   **Schneirla believed:** T. C. Schneirla, "Behavioral Development and Comparative Psychology," *Quarterly Review of Biology* 41, no. 3 (September 1966): 283–302, https://doi.org/10.1086/405056.

14   **studied the behavior of kittens:** Jay S. Rosenblatt, Gerald Turkewitz, and T. C. Schneirla, "Development of Suckling and Related Behavior in Neonate Kittens," in *Roots of Behavior: Genetics, Instinct, and Socialization in Animal Behavior*, ed. Eugene L. Bliss (New York: Hafner, 1968), 198–210, http:// archive.org/details/rootsofbehaviorg0000blis.

15   **an incisive analysis:** Daniel S. Lehrman, "A Critique of Konrad Lorenz's Theory of Instinctive Behavior," *Quarterly Review of Biology* 28, no. 4 (December 1953): 337–63, https://doi.org/10.1086/399858.

15   **given foster pups:** Rats mother indiscriminately, meaning they will care for pups that aren't their own.

15   **in order to maintain those behaviors:** Jay S. Rosenblatt and Daniel S. Lehrman, "Maternal Behavior of the Laboratory Rat," in *Maternal Behavior in Mammals*, ed. Harriet Lange Rheingold (New York: Wiley, 1963), 8–57. In her introduction to *Maternal Behavior in Mammals*, editor Harriet L. Rheingold writes about the care taken in choosing the book's title, and why she considers the word "maternal" as applicable to mammal mothers and any other members of the species who do the work of caregiving. I also appreciate the distinction made here between maternal behavior and loving care, a subtle recognition that mothers can *and do* act in their own self-interest, and that

this is part of maternal behavior, too: "Although in mammals it is the biologic mother that is most attentive to the young, 'maternal' has been used in the title of this book in its generic sense and is not meant to exclude any other member of the species which has commerce with the young. Parental care . . . was considered as an alternative. But among mammals care is given the young not only by the mother and father but often by other members of the group, males as well as females, juveniles as well as adults. Then, under the conditions of many of the studies reported here, all but the mother and her offspring were excluded. Maternal care, a term so common that it has crept into this introduction, was rejected for the title because of its implications of solicitude for the needs of the offspring and its anthropomorphic overtones. Furthermore, it causes one to stumble over those activities of the caretaker which separate the young from her, her withdrawing from them and inflicting pain on them. Maternal behavior was chosen, then, to mean the behavior of the mother and her surrogates in the presence of the young."

16   **In 1967, Rosenblatt:** J. S. Rosenblatt, "Nonhormonal Basis of Maternal Behavior in the Rat," *Science* 156, no. 3781 (June 16, 1967): 1512–14, https://doi.org/10.1126/science.156.3781.1512.

16   **Quite by accident:** Jay S. Rosenblatt, "Views on the Onset and Maintenance of Maternal Behavior in the Rat," in *Development and Evolution of Behavior: Essays in Memory of T. C. Schneirla,* ed. Lester R. Aronson, Ethel Tobach, Daniel S. Lehrman, and Jay S. Rosenblatt (San Francisco: W. H. Freeman, 1970), 496, http://archive.org/details/developmentevolu00aron.

16   **"a basic characteristic of the rat":** Rosenblatt, "Views on the Onset and Maintenance of Maternal Behavior in the Rat," 498. I like to think that Rosenblatt and future Supreme Court Justice Ruth Bader Ginsburg were friendly acquaintances. She taught at Rutgers at the same time Rosenblatt was there, publishing his landmark work on parental behavior in rats. I imagine that they discussed their theories of how "old notions" of gender influenced science and the law. I have found no evidence for their friendship, but it seems likely they shared similar circles. Rosenblatt worked closely with Lehrman, and Lehrman's wife, Dorothy Dinnerstein, was a psychologist and feminist scholar. Dinnerstein wrote *The Mermaid and the Minotaur,* an expansive work about the social and psychological consequences of female-dominated childrearing. In 1971, the same year that Ginsburg established the ACLU Women's Rights Project, Dinnerstein and a colleague filed a federal complaint against Rutgers University alleging unequal treatment for female faculty.

16   **the same building blocks:** Lisa Feldman Barrett, *Seven and a Half Lessons about the Brain* (Boston: Houghton Mifflin Harcourt, 2020), 19–22.

17   **"father of mothering":** Alison S. Fleming, Michael Numan, and Robert S. Bridges, "Father of Mothering: Jay S. Rosenblatt," *Hormones and Behavior* 55, no. 4 (April 2009): 484–87, https://doi.org/10.1016/j.yhbeh.2009.01.001.

17   **Those papers have borne out:** Joseph S. Lonstein, Frédéric Lévy, and Alison S. Fleming, "Common and Divergent Psychobiological Mechanisms Underlying

Maternal Behaviors in Non-Human and Human Mammals," *Hormones and Behavior* 73 (July 2015): 156–85, https://doi.org/10.1016/j.yhbeh.2015.06.011.

17 **Studies of fathers:** Eyal Abraham and Ruth Feldman, "The Neurobiology of Human Allomaternal Care: Implications for Fathering, Coparenting, and Children's Social Development," in "Evolutionary Perspectives on Non-Maternal Care in Mammals: Physiology, Behavior, and Developmental Effects," ed. Stacy Rosenbaum and Lee T. Gettler, special issue, *Physiology & Behavior* 193, part A (September 1, 2018): 25–34, https://doi.org/10.1016/j.physbeh.2017.12.034.

18 **people involved in the women's liberation movement:** Kirsten Swinth, *Feminism's Forgotten Fight: The Unfinished Struggle for Work and Family* (Cambridge, MA: Harvard University Press, 2018), 42–69.

19 **In 2015, Fleming and two other:** Lonstein, Lévy, and Fleming, "Common and Divergent Psychobiological Mechanisms Underlying Maternal Behaviors," https://doi.org/10.1016/j.yhbeh.2015.06.011.

21 **published a literature review:** Pawluski, Lambert, and Kinsley, "Neuroplasticity in the Maternal Hippocampus," https://doi.org/10.1016/j.yhbeh.2015.06.004.

21 **the science of the teenage brain:** "The Teen Brain: 7 Things to Know," National Institute of Mental Health, revised 2020, https://www.nimh.nih.gov/health/publications/the-teen-brain-7-things-to-know/index.shtml.

21 **The science has become:** Frances Jensen, a neuroscientist who, with Amy Ellis Nutt, wrote *The Teenage Brain: A Neuroscientist's Survival Guide to Raising Adolescents and Young Adults* (New York: Harper, 2015), frequently speaks to high school students about their own neurobiology. "Teenagers are looking to understand themselves," she told *Time* magazine. "I think talking about this gives them more insight." Alexandra Sifferlin, "Why Teenage Brains Are So Hard to Understand," *Time*, September 8, 2017, https://time.com/4929170/inside-teen-teenage-brain/.

22 **In July 2018:** Chelsea Conaboy, "Motherhood Brings the Most Dramatic Brain Changes of a Woman's Life," *Globe Magazine, Boston Globe*, July 17, 2018, https://www.bostonglobe.com/magazine/2018/07/17/pregnant-women-care-ignores-one-most-profound-changes-new-mom-faces/CF5wyP0b5EGCcZ8fzLUWbP/story.html.

CHAPTER 2: THE MAKING OF A MOTHER'S INSTINCT

25 **Darwin was strongly influenced:** "Darwin's Women," Darwin Correspondence Project, University of Cambridge, YouTube video, 19:45, posted September 8, 2013, by Cambridge University, https://www.youtube.com/watch?v=9qZxa3WjZQg&t=595s.

25 **"What a strong feeling":** Charles Darwin, *The Descent of Man, and Selection in Relation to Sex* (repr., London: Penguin Classics, 2004), 128.

27   **There was Eve:** Carol Meyers, *Rediscovering Eve: Ancient Israelite Women in Context* (Oxford and New York: Oxford University Press, 2012), 63–65. Much of our modern understanding of the story of Eve, including that she was a temptress who deceived Adam and that her actions brought the "fall" of man, is not actually in Genesis, but came from later interpretive texts. Such misreadings have "achieved a canonicity of their own," with profound consequences, Meyers wrote.

28   **From ancient Israel to:** Laurel Thatcher Ulrich, *Good Wives: Image and Reality in the Lives of Women in Northern New England, 1650–1750,* reissue edition (New York: Vintage, 1991), 239; and Meyers, *Rediscovering Eve,* 121–25.

28   **Among the White women:** Ulrich, *Good Wives,* reissue ed., 157.

28   **Mothers counseled their husbands:** Ulrich, *Good Wives,* reissue ed., 238–40.

28   **Among the Indigenous people:** Kim Anderson, "Giving Life to the People: An Indigenous Ideology of Motherhood," in *Maternal Theory: Essential Readings,* ed. Andrea O'Reilly (Bradford, Canada: Demeter Press, 2007), 761–81.

29   **carried out largely by:** Margaret D. Jacobs, "Maternal Colonialism: White Women and Indigenous Child Removal in the American West and Australia, 1880–1940," *Western Historical Quarterly* 36, no. 4 (Winter 2005): 453–76, https://doi.org/10.2307/25443236.

29   **Many of those children:** Amanda Coletta and Michael E. Miller, "Hundreds of Graves Found at Former Residential School for Indigenous Children in Canada," *Washington Post,* June 24, 2021, https://www.washingtonpost.com /world/2021/06/23/canada-cowessess residential-school-graves/; and Brad Brooks, "Native Americans Decry Unmarked Graves, Untold History of Boarding Schools," Reuters, June 22, 2021, https://www.reuters.com/world /us/native-americans-decry-unmarked-graves-untold-history-boarding -schools-2021-06-22/.

29   **Black women enslaved:** Marie Jenkins Schwartz, *Birthing a Slave: Motherhood and Medicine in the Antebellum South* (Cambridge, MA: Harvard University Press, 2006), 13–31; and Angela Y. Davis, *Women, Race & Class* (New York: Random House, 1981), 15.

29   **It changed the nature of the home:** Meyers, *Rediscovering Eve,* 52, 121; Elinor Accampo, *Blessed Motherhood, Bitter Fruit: Nelly Roussel and the Politics of Female Pain in Third Republic France* (Baltimore: Johns Hopkins University Press, 2006), 3; and Shari L. Thurer, *The Myths of Motherhood: How Culture Reinvents the Good Mother* (Boston: Houghton Mifflin Harcourt, 1994), 183.

30   **Home became sacred:** Thurer, *Myths of Motherhood,* 184.

30   **capitalism focused work:** Stephanie Coontz, *The Way We Never Were: American Families and the Nostalgia Trap* (New York: Basic Books, 1992), 52–53.

30   **The Enlightenment:** Thurer, *Myths of Motherhood,* 195–98; and Kimberly

A. Hamlin, *From Eve to Evolution: Darwin, Science, and Women's Rights in Gilded Age America*, reprint ed. (Chicago: University of Chicago Press, 2015), 6–7.

30 **Deviation from that role:** Accampo, *Blessed Motherhood, Bitter Fruit*, 3.

30 **A close reading:** Edward Higgs and Amanda Wilkinson, "Women, Occupations and Work in the Victorian Censuses Revisited," *History Workshop Journal* 81, no. 1 (April 2016): 17–38, https://doi.org/10.1093/hwj/dbw001.

31 **Separately, economist:** Claudia Goldin, "Female Labor Force Participation: The Origin of Black and White Differences, 1870 and 1880," *Journal of Economic History* 37, no. 1 (1977): 87–108.

31 **"angel in the house":** Coventry Patmore, *The Angel in the House* (London: Cassell and Co, 1887).

31 **Middle-class families:** Coontz, *Way We Never Were*, 11–12.

31 **It empowered their bosses:** Amy Westervelt, *Forget "Having It All": How America Messed Up Motherhood—and How to Fix It* (New York: Seal Press, 2018), 66.

31 **Many men simply:** Westervelt, *Forget "Having It All,"* 66–69; and Heidi Hartmann, "The Unhappy Marriage of Marxism and Feminism: Towards a More Progressive Union," in *Marx Today: Selected Works and Recent Debates*, ed. John F. Sitton (New York: Palgrave Macmillan, 2010), 201–28, https://doi.org/10.1057/9780230117457_14.

32 **in the state's interest:** Eileen Janes Yeo, "The Creation of 'Motherhood' and Women's Responses in Britain and France, 1750–1914," *Women's History Review* 8, no. 2 (1999): 201–18, https://doi.org/10.1080/09612029900200202; and Linda Kerber, "The Republican Mother: Women and the Enlightenment—An American Perspective," in "An American Enlightenment," special issue, *American Quarterly* 28, no. 2 (Summer 1976): 187, https://doi.org/10.2307/2712349.

32 **the powerful Reverend Francis Close:** As quoted in Yeo, "The Creation of 'Motherhood,'" https://doi.org/10.1080/09612029900200202.

32 **a role for women:** Kerber, "Republican Mother," https://doi.org/10.2307/2712349.

32 **And on into the twenty-first:** Sarah Menkedick wrote in *Ordinary Insanity* that the White maternalism that was especially strong in the United States had a long-lasting effect: "This laid the groundwork for the all-or-nothing dilemma that would plague so many mothers at the end of the twentieth century and into the twenty-first: women could either accept full-time motherhood, the whole maternalist ball of fuzzy moral goodness, or reject it, establish careers, and make their way in a white man's world where motherhood had no real value." Sarah Menkedick, *Ordinary Insanity: Fear and the Silent Crisis of Motherhood in America* (New York: Pantheon, 2020), 259.

33 **That was an idea:** Hamlin, *From Eve to Evolution*, 35–42. Hamlin's book provides a fascinating history of the rift between groups of suffragists who read Darwin's work in a literal way and wanted to upend gender norms of

the day, and those who embraced social Darwinism as evidence that progress toward women's rights was inevitable as part of God's plan *and* biological destiny.

33   **Darwin believed:** Darwin, *Descent of Man*, 629.

33   **Social Darwinists seized:** Sarah Blaffer Hrdy, *Mother Nature: A History of Mothers, Infants, and Natural Selection* (New York: Pantheon, 1999), 15.

33   **Among them was Herbert Spencer:** Herbert Spencer, "Psychology of the Sexes," *Popular Science Monthly*, November 1873, 30–38, http://archive.org /details/popularsciencemo04dapprich. Spencer would eventually fall out of favor with many of the sociologists whose careers he had inspired, but his views on women persisted. It is worth noting here that Spencer himself acknowledged his own tendency to find fault over favor, especially with regard to women. He chose a life of celibacy and saw his own mother as "simple minded," someone whose intellectual development had ceased at age twenty-five, according to Spencer's autobiography. He was the oldest of nine children born to Harriet Spencer and the only one who survived beyond early childhood. Charles H. Cooley, "Reflections upon the Sociology of Herbert Spencer," *American Journal of Sociology* 26, no. 2 (1920): 129–45.

33   **opportunity in evolution:** Hamlin, *From Eve to Evolution*, 55.

34   **Antoinette Brown Blackwell:** "Antoinette Brown Blackwell," Rochester Regional Library Council, accessed March 4, 2020, https://rrlc.org/winningthevote /biographfries/antoinette-brown-blackwell/.

34   **the first feminist critique:** Hamlin, *From Eve to Evolution*, 102.

34   **Darwin, she wrote:** Antoinette Brown Blackwell, *The Sexes throughout Nature* (New York: G. P. Putnam's Sons, 1875), 234, http://archive.org/details /cu31924031174372.

34   **Blackwell looked across species:** Blackwell, *Sexes throughout Nature*, 144.

34   **According to her experience:** Blackwell, *Sexes throughout Nature*, 14.

34   **imagined a future:** Blackwell, *Sexes throughout Nature*, 14–23. Blackwell wrote, "Only a woman can approach the subject from a feminine standpoint; and there are none but beginners among us in this class of investigations. However great the disadvantages under which we are placed, these will never be lessened by waiting."

35   **Science was rapidly walled off:** Hamlin, *From Eve to Evolution*, 67–69.

35   **Darwin propelled the study:** William McDougall, *An Introduction to Social Psychology* (London: Methuen, 1926), 20, http://archive.org/details /b29815940.

35   **Included in the list:** William James, *The Principles of Psychology* (New York: Dover Publications, 1950), 2:439–40, http://archive.org/details/principles ofpsyc00will.

35   **took things one step:** McDougall, *Introduction to Social Psychology*, 56–58.

35   **In the same book:** McDougall, *Introduction to Social Psychology*, 232–33.

36   **A subtext of his writing:** McDougall, *Introduction to Social Psychology*, 58.

36   **McDougall had his dissenters:** Leta S. Hollingworth, "Social Devices for Impelling Women to Bear and Rear Children," *American Journal of Sociology* 22, no. 1 (1916): 19–29.

36   **also embraced certain eugenic ideas:** Leta S. Hollingworth, *The Psychology of Subnormal Children* (New York: Macmillan, 1920), 236–38, http://archive .org/details/psychologysubno01hollgoog.

36   **at least sixty times:** *Achievements in Public Health, 1900–1999: Healthier Mothers and Babies*, Morbidity and Mortality Weekly Report (Division of Reproductive Health, National Center for Chronic Disease Prevention and Health Promotion, Centers for Disease Control and Prevention, October 1, 1999).

37   **"the road not taken":** Hrdy, *Mother Nature*, 22.

37   **Instead, our early understanding:** Hrdy, *Mother Nature*, 535.

37   **The idea of instinct:** Mark S. Blumberg, "Development Evolving: The Origins and Meanings of Instinct," *WIREs Cognitive Science* 8, no. 1–2 (January 2017): e1371, https://doi.org/10.1002/wcs.1371.

37   **The idea survived:** Thurer, *Myths of Motherhood*, 236.

37   **a growing chorus:** Marga Vicedo, *The Nature and Nurture of Love: From Imprinting to Attachment in Cold War America*, illustrated ed. (Chicago: University of Chicago Press, 2013), 37–42.

38   **British psychoanalyst John Bowlby:** Vicedo, *Nature and Nurture of Love*, 90.

38   **effective at blocking:** Kirsten Swinth, *Feminism's Forgotten Fight: The Unfinished Struggle for Work and Family* (Cambridge, MA: Harvard University Press, 2018).

38   **Bowlby told the:** Marga Vicedo, "The Social Nature of the Mother's Tie to Her Child: John Bowlby's Theory of Attachment in Post-War America," *British Journal for the History of Science* 44, no. 3 (September 2011): 401–26, https://doi.org/10.1017/S0007087411000318; and Evelyn S. Ringold, "Bringing Up Baby in Britain," *New York Times*, June 13, 1965, http:// timesmachine.nytimes.com/timesmachine/1965/06/13/106993810.html.

38   **President Nixon vetoed it:** Jack Rosenthal, "President Vetoes Child Care Plan as Irresponsible," *New York Times*, December 10, 1971, https://www .nytimes.com/1971/12/10/archives/president-vetoes-child-care-plan-as -irresponsible-he-terms-bill.html.

39   **In March 2021:** "Klobuchar, Duckworth, Colleagues Introduce 'Marshall Plan for Moms' Resolution to Support Mothers in the American Workforce," US senator Amy Klobuchar, press release, March 3, 2021, https:// www.klobuchar.senate.gov/public/index.cfm/2021/3/klobuchar-duckworth -colleagues-introduce-marshall-plan-for-moms-resolution-to-support -mothers-in-the-american-workforce; and Betsy Z. Russell, "Governor: 'We'll Try Again' on Early Childhood Learning," *Idaho Press*, March 3, 2021, https://www.idahopress.com/news/local/governor-well-try-again-on-early -childhood-learning/article_fc643fd6-48bf-5041-bc92-58ee2ce49ab2 .html.

39 **This is the exact same:** Brigid Schulte, "The Secret to Happy, Healthy Homes? Universal Childcare," *Fast Company*, April 29, 2021, https://www.fastcompany.com/90625892/the-secret-to-happy-healthy-homes-universal-childcare.

39 **Build Back Better plan:** The White House, "President Biden Announces the Build Back Better Framework," news release, October 28, 2021, https://www.whitehouse.gov/briefing-room/statements-releases/2021/10/28/president-biden-announces-the-build-back-better-framework/.

39 **opposition to birth control and abortion:** Jill Filipovic wrote about the increased use of birth control and abortion in the nineteenth century: "With those things also came, eventually, a conservative religious backlash, led largely by men, demonizing contraception and abortion, often with the argument that it's natural for a woman to find joy in being a mother—and wholly unnatural, then, to limit the number of times in which she becomes one." Jill Filipovic, *The H-Spot: The Feminist Pursuit of Happiness* (New York: Bold Type Books, 2017), 19. Stephanie Coontz cited examples of women hospitalized as "schizophrenic" for failing to adjust to domestic life. Electric shock treatments were used on them and on women who had sought abortion, "on the assumption that failure to want a baby signified dangerous emotional disturbance." Coontz, *The Way We Never Were*, 32.

39 **It has grown the modern:** Thurer, *Myths of Motherhood*, 258–61.

40 **the reality of parenting:** Mikki Kendall, *Hood Feminism: Notes from the Women That a Movement Forgot* (New York: Viking, 2020).

40 **"Family holds a place":** Mia Birdsong, *How We Show Up: Reclaiming Family, Friendship, and Community* (New York: Hachette Go, 2020), 3.

40 **extreme attention paid:** Claire Cain Miller and Alisha Haridasani Gupta, "Why 'Supermom' Gets Star Billing on Résumés for Public Office," *New York Times*, October 14, 2020, https://www.nytimes.com/2020/10/14/upshot/barrett-harris-motherhood-politics.html?action=click&module=Top%20Stories&pgtype=Homepage.

41 **Senate Republicans "fetishized":** Lyz Lenz, "The Power—And Threat—Of Mothers Like Amy Coney Barrett," *Glamour*, October 14, 2020, https://www.glamour.com/story/threat-of-mothers-like-amy-coney-barrett.

41 **The gender pay gap:** Andrea Hsu, "Even the Most Successful Women Pay a Big Price," NPR, October 20, 2020, https://www.npr.org/2020/10/20/924566058/even-the-most-successful-women-are-sidelining-careers-for-family-in-pandemic; and Amanda Taub, "Pandemic Will 'Take Our Women 10 Years Back' in the Workplace," *New York Times*, September 26, 2020, https://www.nytimes.com/2020/09/26/world/covid-women-childcare-equality.html.

41 **even in countries:** Sarah Kliff, "A Stunning Chart Shows the True Cause of the Gender Wage Gap," Vox, February 19, 2018, https://www.vox.com/2018/2/19/17018380/gender-wage-gap-childcare-penalty.

41 **Researchers have found:** Shelley J. Correll, "Minimizing the Motherhood

Penalty: What Works, What Doesn't and Why?," *Gender & Work: Challenging Conventional Wisdom*, research symposium, Harvard Business School (Boston, 2013), https://www.hbs.edu/faculty/conferences/2013-w50 -research-symposium/Documents/correll.pdf; and Claire Cain Miller, "The Motherhood Penalty vs. the Fatherhood Bonus," *New York Times*, September 6, 2014, https://www.nytimes.com/2014/09/07/upshot/a-child-helps -your-career-if-youre-a-man.html.

42 **"That's just not true":** Hear Niles talk more about this point on the podcast *Natal*, episode 2, "Roots of the Black Birthing Crisis," https://www .natalstories.com/two.

42 **The US maternal mortality rate:** Roosa Tikkanen, Munira Z. Gunja, Molly FitzGerald, and Laurie Zephyrin, "Maternal Mortality and Maternity Care in the United States Compared to 10 Other Developed Countries," Commonwealth Fund, November 18, 2020, https://doi.org/10.26099/411v -9255; Donna Hoyert and Arialdi Miniño, *Maternal Mortality in the United States: Changes in Coding, Publication, and Data Release, 2018* (Hyattsville, MD: US Dept. of Health and Human Services, Centers for Disease Control and Prevention, National Center for Health Statistics, January 30, 2020); and Nina Martin, "The New U.S. Maternal Mortality Rate Fails to Capture Many Deaths," ProPublica, February 13, 2020, https://www.propublica.org /article/the-new-us-maternal-mortality-rate-fails-to-capture-many-deaths ?token=lZ_nPrh6oVJEnMzcTH1Jr59Ibe3K8XZC.

42 **The cause seems to be a collision:** Nina Martin and Renee Montagne, "Nothing Protects Black Women from Dying in Pregnancy and Childbirth," ProPublica, December 7, 2017, https://www.propublica.org/article/nothing -protects-black-women-from-dying-in-pregnancy-and-childbirth?token =LxlGpDTGeNkRVdBY_bX0b8KqR5dJhsIu.

43 **Evidence from around the world:** "Nursing and Midwifery," World Health Organization (WHO), January 9, 2020, https://www.who.int/news -room/fact-sheets/detail/nursing-and-midwifery; "WHO | The Case for Midwifery," WHO, accessed October 18, 2020, http://www.who.int /maternal_child_adolescent/topics/quality-of-care/midwifery/case-for -midwifery/en/; and Jane Sandall, Hora Soltani, Simon Gates, Andrew Shennan, and Declan Devane, "Midwife-Led Continuity Models of Care Versus Other Models of Care for Childbearing Women," *Cochrane Database of Systematic Reviews* 4 (2016), https://doi.org/10.1002/14651858 .CD004667.pub5.

43 **long dominated by:** Judith M. Orvos, "ACOG Releases New Study on Ob/ Gyn Workforce: Trends Similar to Those Seen in Previous Studies Expected to Continue," *Contemporary OB/GYN* 62, no. 7 (July 2017): 50–53.

43 **The shortage of maternity care providers:** Tikkanen et al., "Maternal Mortality and Maternity Care," https://doi.org/10.26099/411v-9255.

43 **patchwork system of US health insurance:** Emily Eckert, "It's Past Time to Provide Continuous Medicaid Coverage for One Year Postpartum,"

Health Affairs (blog), February 6, 2020, https://www.healthaffairs.org/do
/10.1377/hblog20200203.639479/full/. Advocates were optimistic in 2021
that, under the Biden administration and using provisions of the American
Rescue Plan, more states would choose to expand Medicaid to cover birthing parents for a year postpartum. Shefali Luthra, "How the COVID Stimulus Bill Could Help Fight Pregnancy-Related Deaths," The 19th, March
15, 2021, https://19thnews.org/2021/03/how-the-covid-stimulus-bill-could
-help-fight-pregnancy-related-deaths/.

43 **a more holistic and ongoing approach:** "ACOG Committee Opinion No.
736: Optimizing Postpartum Care," *Obstetrics & Gynecology* 131, no. 5
(2018): e140–e150.

44 **In Maine:** Matthew Stone, "Maine Has Sliced the Ranks of Nurses Who
Prevent Outbreaks, Help Drug-Affected Babies," *Bangor Daily News*, August
9, 2016, https://bangordailynews.com/2016/08/09/news/bangor/maine-has
-sliced-the-ranks-of-nurses-who-prevent-outbreaks-help-drug-affected
-babies/.

44 **captures the incredulity:** Hollie McNish, *Nobody Told Me: Poetry and Parenthood* (London: Blackfriars, 2018).

44 **Ali Wong's second Netflix special:** Ali Wong, *Hard Knock Wife* (Netflix,
2018), https://www.netflix.com/title/80186940.

45 **In February 2020:** "Frida Mom | Oscars Ad Rejected," YouTube video, 1:35,
posted February 5, 2020, by Frida Mom, https://www.youtube.com/watch?v
=3GePXGfRP04&feature=emb_title.

45 **told the *New York Times*:** Hannah Seligson, "This Is the TV Ad the Oscars
Didn't Allow on Air," *New York Times*, February 19, 2020, https://www
.nytimes.com/2020/02/19/us/postpartum-ad-oscars-frida.html.

46 **The research was publicized:** "Scientists Find Clue to 'Maternal Instinct,'"
Louisiana State University press release, EurekAlert!, July 25, 2019, https://
www.eurekalert.org/pub_releases/2019-07/lsu-sfc072519.php.

46 **In a 2017 editorial:** Tom W. J. Schulpen, "The Glass Ceiling: A Biological
Phenomenon," *Medical Hypotheses* 106 (September 2017): 41–43, https://
doi.org/10.1016/j.mehy.2017.07.002.

47 **biologists still held tight:** Hrdy, *Mother Nature*, 27.

47 **studied baboons:** Jeanne Altmann, *Baboon Mothers and Infants* (Chicago:
University of Chicago Press, 1980), 1–7.

47 **wondered about the purpose:** Barbara B. Smuts, *Sex and Friendship in
Baboons* (New York: Routledge, 2017), 7, https://doi.org/10.4324/9781315
129204.

47 **Hrdy herself began asking:** Hrdy, *Mother Nature*, xvi.

47 **A female, in Darwin's thinking:** Sarah Blaffer Hrdy, "Empathy, Polyandry,
and the Myth of the Coy Female," in *Feminist Approaches to Science*, ed.
Ruth Bleier (New York: Pergamon, 1986), 119–46.

48 **Slowly, a new picture:** Hrdy, *Mother Nature*, 29.

48 **"return to a traditional model":** Élisabeth Badinter, *The Conflict: How*

Modern Motherhood Undermines the Status of Women (New York: Metropolitan Books, 2012), 4–5.

48 **Badinter declined:** I wrote to Badinter to request an interview for this book, about whether the emerging neuroscience of motherhood has shifted her thinking at all, about whether she sees a place for it within a feminist framework. She declined the interview, saying she has not focused on neuroscience and has no expertise there. But she wrote, "Yes, I think that there may be room for neurobiology in the study of motherhood, even though I feel it comes in second, behind the societal factor. In any event, there is work to be done. Do not be afraid of feminist reactions. Scientific research must never be subjected to ideologies." (Translated from French by Paula DeFilippo.)

49 **Environmental context, social pressure:** Badinter, *Conflict*, 54–55.

49 **she told the magazine:** Élisabeth Badinter, "La femme n'est pas un chimpanzé," interview by Anne Crignon and Sophie des Déserts, *L'Obs*, February 12, 2010, https://bibliobs.nouvelobs.com/essais/20100212.BIB0270/la -femme-n-039-est-pas-un-chimpanze.html. (Translated by Paula DeFilippo.)

CHAPTER 3: ATTENTION, PLEASE

51 **The brain is like this:** Eberhard Fuchs and Gabriele Flügge, "Adult Neuroplasticity: More Than 40 Years of Research," in "Environmental Control of Adult Neurogenesis: From Hippocampal Homeostasis to Behavior," ed. Sjoukje Kuipers, Clive R. Bramham, Heather A. Cameron, Carlos P. Fitzsimons, Aniko Korosi, and Paul J. Lucassen, special issue, *Neural Plasticity* 2014 (May 4, 2014): e541870, https://doi.org/10.1155/2014/541870.

51 **eighty-six billion neurons:** Or 100 billion neurons, or 128 billion neurons, depending on whose estimate you rely on. Frederico A. C. Azevedo, Ludmila R. B. Carvalho, Lea T. Grinberg, José Marcelo Farfel, Renata E. L. Ferretti, Renata E. P. Leite, Wilson Jacob Filho, Roberto Lent, and Suzana Herculano-Houzel, "Equal Numbers of Neuronal and Nonneuronal Cells Make the Human Brain an Isometrically Scaled-Up Primate Brain," *Journal of Comparative Neurology* 513, no. 5 (2009): 532–41, https://doi.org/10.1002 /cne.21974.

51 **A neuron is made up:** Lisa Feldman Barrett, *Seven and a Half Lessons about the Brain* (Boston: Houghton Mifflin Harcourt, 2020), 31.

52 **Every part of that process:** Barrett, *Seven and a Half Lessons*, 37.

52 **whole new neurons are created:** Paul J. Lucassen, Carlos P. Fitzsimons, Evgenia Salta, and Mirjana Maletic-Savatic, "Adult Neurogenesis, Human after All (Again): Classic, Optimized, and Future Approaches," in "SI: Functions of Adult Hippocampal Neurogenesis," ed. Michael Drew and Jason Snyder, special issue, *Behavioural Brain Research* 381 (March 2, 2020): 112458, https://doi.org/10.1016/j.bbr.2019.112458.

52 **compares the complexity:** Barrett, *Seven and a Half Lessons*, 34–39.

53   **The hormonal surge:** Nicholas P. Deems and Benedetta Leuner, "Preg-
      nancy, Postpartum and Parity: Resilience and Vulnerability in Brain Health
      and Disease," *Frontiers in Neuroendocrinology* 57 (April 2020): 100820,
      https://doi.org/10.1016/j.yfrne.2020.100820; J. S. Rosenblatt, "Psychobiol-
      ogy of Maternal Behavior: Contribution to the Clinical Understanding of
      Maternal Behavior among Humans," supplement, *Acta Paediatrica* 83, no.
      S397 (June 1994): 3–8, https://doi.org/10.1111/j.1651-2227.1994.tb13259.x;
      and Johannes Kohl, Anita E. Autry, and Catherine Dulac, "The Neurobiol-
      ogy of Parenting: A Neural Circuit Perspective," *BioEssays* 39, no. 1 (January
      2017): 1–11, https://doi.org/10.1002/bies.201600159.

53   **Prenatal education typically:** "Estrogen and Progesterone," Your Guide
      to Pregnancy Hormones, What to Expect, accessed December 1, 2020,
      https://www.whattoexpect.com/pregnancy/pregnancy-health/pregnancy
      -hormones/estrogen-progesterone; and "HPL, Relaxin, and Oxytocin,"
      Your Guide to Pregnancy Hormones, What to Expect, accessed Decem-
      ber 1, 2020, https://www.whattoexpect.com/pregnancy/pregnancy-health
      /pregnancy-hormones/hpl.aspx.

54   **"a maximal state of responsiveness":** Joseph S. Lonstein, Frédéric Lévy,
      and Alison S. Fleming, "Common and Divergent Psychobiological Mech-
      anisms Underlying Maternal Behaviors in Non-Human and Human Mam-
      mals," *Hormones and Behavior* 73 (July 2015): 156–85, https://doi.org/10
      .1016/j.yhbeh.2015.06.011.

54   **Then, the babies bring the noise:** Lonstein, Lévy, and Fleming, "Common
      and Divergent Psychobiological Mechanisms Underlying Maternal Behav-
      iors," https://doi.org/10.1016/j.yhbeh.2015.06.011.

54   **But animal studies in the 1970s:** Lonstein, Lévy, and Fleming, "Common
      and Divergent Psychobiological Mechanisms Underlying Maternal Behav-
      iors," https://doi.org/10.1016/j.yhbeh.2015.06.011.

54   **the MPOA as a receiver:** Mariana Pereira and Annabel Ferreira, "Neuro-
      anatomical and Neurochemical Basis of Parenting: Dynamic Coordination
      of Motivational, Affective and Cognitive Processes," in "Parental Care," ed.
      Alison S. Fleming, Frederic Lévy, and Joe S. Lonstein, special issue, *Hor-
      mones and Behavior* 77 (January 2016): 72–85, https://doi.org/10.1016/j
      .yhbeh.2015.08.005; and Johannes Kohl and Catherine Dulac, "Neural Con-
      trol of Parental Behaviors," in "Neurobiology of Behavior," ed. Kay Tye and
      Nao Uchida, special issue, *Current Opinion in Neurobiology* 49 (April 2018):
      116–22, https://doi.org/10.1016/j.conb.2018.02.002.

55   **a critical hub:** Aya Dudin, Patrick O. McGowan, Ruiyong Wu, Alison S.
      Fleming, and Ming Li, "Psychobiology of Maternal Behavior in Nonhuman
      Mammals," in *Handbook of Parenting,* ed. Marc Bornstein, 3rd ed., vol. 2 (New
      York: Routledge, 2019), 30–77, https://doi.org/10.4324/9780429401459-2.

55   **A few years ago:** Zheng Wu, Anita E. Autry, Joseph E. Bergan, Mitsuko
      Watabe-Uchida, and Catherine G. Dulac, "Galanin Neurons in the Medial

Preoptic Area Govern Parental Behaviour," *Nature* 509, no. 7500 (May 2014): 325–30, https://doi.org/10.1038/nature13307; and Catherine Dulac, Lauren A. O'Connell, and Zheng Wu, "Neural Control of Maternal and Paternal Behaviors," *Science* 345, no. 6198 (August 15, 2014): 765–70, https://doi.org/10.1126/science.1253291.

55 **Neuropeptides are similar:** Gareth Leng and Mike Ludwig, "Neurotransmitters and Peptides: Whispered Secrets and Public Announcements," *Journal of Physiology* 586, no. 23 (December 2008): 5625–32, https://doi.org/10.1113/jphysiol.2008.159103.

55 **damage to that area:** Kohl and Dulac, "Neural Control of Parental Behaviors," https://doi.org/10.1016/j.conb.2018.02.002.

56 **follow the galanin:** Johannes Kohl, Benedicte M. Babayan, Nimrod D. Rubinstein, Anita E. Autry, Brenda Marin-Rodriguez, Vikrant Kapoor, Kazunari Miyamishi, et al., "Functional Circuit Architecture Underlying Parental Behaviour," *Nature* 556, no. 7701 (April 2018): 326–31, https://doi.org/10.1038/s41586-018-0027-0.

56 **a 2021 Breakthrough Prize in Life Sciences:** "Breakthrough Prize—Winners of the 2021 Breakthrough Prizes in Life Sciences, Fundamental Physics and Mathematics Announced," accessed October 2, 2021, https://breakthroughprize.org/News/60; and "Yuri Milner | Breakthrough Foundation," accessed October 2, 2021, https://breakthroughprize.org/Yuri_Milner.

56 **"modular architecture":** Kohl et al., "Functional Circuit Architecture Underlying Parental Behaviour," https://doi.org/10.1038/s41586-018-0027-0.

57 **Rat mothers and human mothers:** Lonstein, Lévy, and Fleming, "Common and Divergent Psychobiological Mechanisms Underlying Maternal Behaviors," https://doi.org/10.1016/j.yhbeh.2015.06.011.

58 **The mother in the fMRI:** Because this study was ongoing at the time of my visit, the lab did not allow me to interview the mother or use her name or identifying details here, citing Institutional Review Board protocol.

60 **For generation after generation:** Sarah Blaffer Hrdy, *Mother Nature: A History of Mothers, Infants, and Natural Selection* (New York: Pantheon, 1999), 303–4.

60 **Rates of infanticide:** Sandra Newman, "The Roots of Infanticide Run Deep, and Begin with Poverty," *Aeon*, November 27, 2017, https://aeon.co/essays/the-roots-of-infanticide-run-deep-and-begin-with-poverty.

60 **always been a balancing act:** Sarah B. Hrdy, "Variable Postpartum Responsiveness among Humans and Other Primates with 'Cooperative Breeding': A Comparative and Evolutionary Perspective," in "Parental Care," ed. Alison S. Fleming, Frederic Lévy, and Joe S. Lonstein, special issue, *Hormones and Behavior* 77 (January 1, 2016): 272–83, https://doi.org/10.1016/j.yhbeh.2015.10.016.

60 **"Nurturing has to be teased out":** Hrdy, *Mother Nature*, 174.

60 **One study found:** Kay Mordecai Robson and R. Kumar, "Delayed Onset of Maternal Affection after Childbirth," *British Journal of Psychiatry* 136, no. 4 (April 1980): 347–53, https://doi.org/10.1192/bjp.136.4.347.

61 **conflicting emotions:** Aurélie Athan and Lisa Miller, "Spiritual Awakening through the Motherhood Journey," *Journal of the Association for Research on Mothering* 7, no. 1 (January 1, 2005): 17–31, https://jarm.journals.yorku.ca /index.php/jarm/article/view/4951.

61 **wrote a whole book:** Rozsika Parker, *Mother Love/Mother Hate: The Power of Maternal Ambivalence* (New York: Basic Books, 1995), http://archive.org /details/motherlovemother00park.

61 **"A mother needs to know herself":** Melissa Benn, "Deep Maternal Alienation," *Guardian*, October 27, 2006, http://www.theguardian.com /lifeandstyle/2006/oct/28/familyandrelationships.family2.

61 **eighteen reasons why:** D. W. Winnicott, "Hate in the Counter-Transference," *Journal of Psychotherapy Practice and Research* 3, no. 4 (Fall 1994): 348– 56. Originally published in the *International Journal of Psycho-Analysis* 30 (1949): 69–74.

62 **Cuteness is a measurable set of characteristics:** Mayra L. Almanza-Sepúlveda, Aya Dudin, Kathleen E. Wonch, Meir Steiner, David R. Feinberg, Alison S. Fleming, and Geoffrey B. Hall, "Exploring the Morphological and Emotional Correlates of Infant Cuteness," *Infant Behavior and Development* 53 (November 2018): 90–100, https://doi.org/10.1016/j .infbeh.2018.08.001; and Morten L. Kringelbach, Eloise A. Stark, Catherine Alexander, Marc H. Bornstein, and Alan Stein, "On Cuteness: Unlocking the Parental Brain and Beyond," *Trends in Cognitive Sciences* 20, no. 7 (July 2016): 545–58, https://doi.org/10.1016/j.tics.2016.05.003.

63 **adults without children:** Christine E. Parsons, Katherine S. Young, Nina Kumari, Alan Stein, and Morten L. Kringelbach, "The Motivational Salience of Infant Faces Is Similar for Men and Women," *PLoS ONE* 6, no. 5 (May 31, 2011): e20632, https://doi.org/10.1371/journal.pone.0020632.

63 **have been found to trigger:** Morten L. Kringelbach, Annukka Lehtonen, Sarah Squire, Allison G. Harvey, Michelle G. Craske, Ian E. Holliday, Alexander L. Green, et al., "A Specific and Rapid Neural Signature for Parental Instinct," *PLoS ONE* 3, no. 2 (February 27, 2008): e1664, https://doi.org/10 .1371/journal.pone.0001664.

63 **Parents are generally really good:** Marsha Kaitz, A. Good, A. M. Rokem, and Arthur Eidelman, "Mothers' and Fathers' Recognition of Their Newborns' Photographs during the Postpartum Period," *Journal of Developmental and Behavioral Pediatrics* 9, no. 4 (August 1988): 223–26, https://doi.org/10 .1097/00004703-198808000-00008; M. Kaitz, A. Good, A. M. Rokem, and A. I. Eidelman, "Mothers' Recognition of Their Newborns by Olfactory Cues," *Developmental Psychobiology* 20, no. 6 (November 1987): 587–91, https://doi.org/10.1002/dev.420200604; and James A. Green and Gwene E.

Gustafson, "Individual Recognition of Human Infants on the Basis of Cries Alone," *Developmental Psychobiology* 16, no. 6 (November 1983): 485–93, https://doi.org/10.1002/dev.420160604.

63 **compare them to people who are not parents:** Studies comparing parents and people without children are especially tricky, because nonparents are so variable themselves. Some have extensive experience caring for siblings or other babies in their lives, or they may even be professional baby tenders. There can be very different factors shaping the brain of someone who has chosen not to have children and someone who is actively trying to have one but has not yet been pregnant. And then there are the potential hormonal and experiential factors affecting someone who has had a pregnancy that, for any number of reasons, was not carried to term. Researchers often rely on undergraduate students as a pool of potential study participants, but they don't necessarily make the best candidates for comparing with adults who have entered a phase of life that includes children. Several researchers, including Helena Rutherford, described the challenge of settling on the definition of a nonparent study group and then controlling for a wide variety of factors.

64 **These studies repeatedly found:** Erika Barba-Müller, Sinéad Craddock, Susanna Carmona, and Elseline Hoekzema, "Brain Plasticity in Pregnancy and the Postpartum Period: Links to Maternal Caregiving and Mental Health," *Archives of Women's Mental Health* 22, no. 2 (April 2019): 289–99, https://doi.org/10.1007/s00737-018-0889-z; Caitlin Post and Benedetta Leuner, "The Maternal Reward System in Postpartum Depression," *Archives of Women's Mental Health* 22, no. 3 (June 2019): 417–29, https://doi.org/10.1007/s00737-018-0926-y; and Pereira and Ferreira, "Neuroanatomical and Neurochemical Basis of Parenting," https://doi.org/10.1016/j.yhbeh.2015.08.005.

64 **It was long thought that:** Michael Numan and Thomas R. Insel, *The Neurobiology of Parental Behavior* (New York: Springer, 2003), 320–21.

65 **some indications that it's the latter:** Lonstein, Lévy, and Fleming, "Common and Divergent Psychobiological Mechanisms Underlying Maternal Behaviors," https://doi.org/10.1016/j.yhbeh.2015.06.011; and Shir Atzil, Alexandra Touroutoglou, Tali Rudy, Stephanie Salcedo, Ruth Feldman, Jacob M. Hooker, Bradford C. Dickerson, Ciprian Catana, and Lisa Feldman Barrett, "Dopamine in the Medial Amygdala Network Mediates Human Bonding," *Proceedings of the National Academy of Sciences* 114, no. 9 (February 28, 2017): 2361–66, https://doi.org/10.1073/pnas.1612233114.

65 **Scientists used to think:** John D. Salamone and Mercè Correa, "The Mysterious Motivational Functions of Mesolimbic Dopamine," *Neuron* 76, no. 3 (November 8, 2012): 470–85, https://doi.org/10.1016/j.neuron.2012.10.021.

65 **One fascinating set of studies:** Veronica M. Afonso, Waqqas M. Shams, Daniel Jin, and Alison S. Fleming, "Distal Pup Cues Evoke Dopamine Responses in Hormonally Primed Rats in the Absence of Pup Experience or Ongoing

Maternal Behavior," *Journal of Neuroscience* 33, no. 6 (February 6, 2013): 2305–12, https://doi.org/10.1523/JNEUROSCI.2081-12.2013; and Daniel E. Olazábal, Mariana Pereira, Daniella Agrati, Annabel Ferreira, Alison S. Fleming, Gabriela González-Mariscal, Frederic Lévy, et al., "New Theoretical and Experimental Approaches on Maternal Motivation in Mammals," *Neuroscience & Biobehavioral Reviews* 37, no. 8 (September 2013): 1860–74, https://doi.org/10.1016/j.neubiorev.2013.04.003.

65   **oxytocin has been shown over and over:** Ruth Feldman and Marian J. Bakermans-Kranenburg, "Oxytocin: A Parenting Hormone," in "Parenting," ed. Marinus H. van IJzendoorn and Marian J. Bakermans-Kranenburg, special issue, *Current Opinion in Psychology* 15 (June 1, 2017): 13–18, https://doi .org/10.1016/j.copsyc.2017.02.011.

65   **Rat mothers with more oxytocin projections:** Dara K. Shahrokh, Tie-Yuan Zhang, Josie Diorio, Alain Gratton, and Michael J. Meaney, "Oxytocin-Dopamine Interactions Mediate Variations in Maternal Behavior in the Rat," *Endocrinology* 151, no. 5 (May 2010): 2276–86, https://doi.org/10.1210 /en.2009-1271.

65   **In one study with a very, very small:** James E. Swain, Esra Tasgin, Linda C. Mayes, Ruth Feldman, R. Todd Constable, and James F. Leckman, "Maternal Brain Response to Own Baby-Cry Is Affected by Cesarean Section Delivery," *Journal of Child Psychology and Psychiatry* 49, no. 10 (October 2008): 1042–52, https://doi.org/10.1111/j.1469-7610.2008.01963.x; and Post and Leuner, "Maternal Reward System," https://doi.org/10.1007 /s00737-018-0926-y.

66   **Dopamine contributes to the flexibility:** Salamone and Correa, "Motivational Functions of Mesolimbic Dopamine," https://doi.org/10.1016/j .neuron.2012.10.021.

66   **The salience network:** Erika Barba-Müller et al., "Brain Plasticity in Pregnancy and the Postpartum Period," https://doi.org/10.1007/s00737-018 -0889-z; William W. Seeley, "The Salience Network: A Neural System for Perceiving and Responding to Homeostatic Demands," *Journal of Neuroscience* 39, no. 50 (December 11, 2019): 9878–82, https://doi.org/10.1523 /JNEUROSCI.1138-17.2019; and Vinod Menon and Lucina Q. Uddin, "Saliency, Switching, Attention and Control: A Network Model of Insula Function," *Brain Structure and Function* 214, no. 5–6 (June 2010): 655–67, https://doi.org/10.1007/s00429-010-0262-0.

66   **In parents, the amygdala:** Erich Seifritz, Fabrizio Esposito, John G. Neuhoff, Andreas Lüthi, Henrietta Mustovic, Gerhard Dammann, Ulrich von Bardeleben, et al., "Differential Sex-Independent Amygdala Response to Infant Crying and Laughing in Parents versus Nonparents," *Biological Psychiatry* 54, no. 12 (December 15, 2003): 1367–75, https://doi.org/10.1016/S0006 -3223(03)00697-8.

67   **One 2019 study looked at the "resting state":** Alexander J. Dufford, Andrew Erhart, and Pilyoung Kim, "Maternal Brain Resting-State Connectivity in

the Postpartum Period," in "Papers from the Parental Brain 2018 Meeting, Toronto, Canada, July 2018," special issue, *Journal of Neuroendocrinology* 31, no. 9 (September 2019): e12737, https://doi.org/10.1111/jne.12737.

67 **Recent studies in humans have found:** Seeley, "Salience Network," https://doi.org/10.1523/JNEUROSCI.1138-17.2019; and Robert A. McCutcheon, Matthew M. Nour, Tarik Dahoun, Sameer Jauhar, Fiona Pepper, Paul Expert, Mattia Veronese, et al., "Mesolimbic Dopamine Function Is Related to Salience Network Connectivity: An Integrative Positron Emission Tomography and Magnetic Resonance Study," *Biological Psychiatry* 85, no. 5 (March 1, 2019): 368–78, https://doi.org/10.1016/j.biopsych.2018.09.010.

67 **helping to tag baby cues:** Christine E. Parsons, Katherine S. Young, Alan Stein, and Morten L. Kringelbach, "Intuitive Parenting: Understanding the Neural Mechanisms of Parents' Adaptive Responses to Infants," in "Parenting," ed. Marinus H. van IJzendoorn and Marian J. Bakermans-Kranenburg, special issue, *Current Opinion in Psychology* 15 (June 1, 2017): 40–44, https://doi.org/10.1016/j.copsyc.2017.02.010.

68 **what happens when the normative changes:** Amanda J. Nguyen, Elisabeth Hoyer, Purva Rajhans, Lane Strathearn, and Sohye Kim, "A Tumultuous Transition to Motherhood: Altered Brain and Hormonal Responses in Mothers with Postpartum Depression," in "Papers from the Parental Brain 2018 Meeting, Toronto, Canada, July 2018," ed. Jodi L. Pawluski, Frances A. Champagne, and Oliver J. Bosch, special issue, *Journal of Neuroendocrinology* 31, no. 9 (September 2019): e12794, https://doi.org/10.1111/jne.12794; and Post and Leuner, "Maternal Reward System," https://doi.org/10.1007/s00737-018-0926-y.

68 **Researchers at Bar-Ilan University:** Eyal Abraham, Talma Hendler, Irit Shapira-Lichter, Yaniv Kanat-Maymon, Orna Zagoory-Sharon, and Ruth Feldman, "Father's Brain Is Sensitive to Childcare Experiences," *Proceedings of the National Academy of Sciences* 111, no. 27 (July 8, 2014): 9792–97, https://doi.org/10.1073/pnas.1402569111.

69 **written elsewhere:** Chelsea Conaboy, "A New Mother Learns to Breastfeed," *Press Herald*, May 7, 2015, https://www.pressherald.com/2015/05/06/a-new-mother-learns-to-breastfeed/.

69 **It disappeared:** Pilyoung Kim, Lane Strathearn, and James E. Swain, "The Maternal Brain and Its Plasticity in Humans," in "Parental Care," ed. Alison S. Fleming, Frederic Lévy, and Joe S. Lonstein, special issue, *Hormones and Behavior* 77 (January 2016): 113–23, https://doi.org/10.1016/j.yhbeh.2015.08.001. The finding that mothers who delivered vaginally and mothers who delivered by C-section had similar neural responses by the fourth month postpartum were published in the above review paper, but not in a separate paper subject to peer review.

69 **The same researchers:** Pilyoung Kim, Ruth Feldman, Linda C. Mayes, Virginia Eicher, Nancy Thompson, James F. Leckman, and James E. Swain,

"Breastfeeding, Brain Activation to Own Infant Cry, and Maternal Sensitivity," *Journal of Child Psychology and Psychiatry* 52, no. 8 (August 2011): 907–15, https://doi.org/10.1111/j.1469-7610.2011.02406.x.

69 **A separate study:** Elseline Hoekzema, Christian K. Tamnes, Puck Berns, Erika Barba-Müller, Cristina Pozzobon, Marisol Picado, Florencio Lucco, et al., "Becoming a Mother Entails Anatomical Changes in the Ventral Striatum of the Human Brain That Facilitate Its Responsiveness to Offspring Cues," *Psychoneuroendocrinology* 112 (February 2020): 104507, https://doi.org/10.1016/j.psyneuen.2019.104507.

70 **listening to Wendy Wood:** Shankar Vedantam, "Creatures of Habit," December 30, 2019, in *Hidden Brain*, podcast, MP3 audio, 49:40, https://podcasts.apple.com/us/podcast/creatures-of-habit/id1028908750?i=1000461145219; and Wendy Wood, *Good Habits, Bad Habits: The Science of Making Positive Changes That Stick*, illustrated ed. (New York: Farrar, Straus and Giroux, 2019), 163.

71 **ultimately came to a consensus:** Olazábal et al., "New Theoretical and Experimental Approaches on Maternal Motivation in Mammals," https://doi.org/10.1016/j.neubiorev.2013.04.003.

71 **Consider S5:** W. E. Wilsoncroft, "Babies by Bar-Press: Maternal Behavior in the Rat," *Behavior Research Methods & Instrumentation* 1, no. 6 (January 1968): 229–30, https://doi.org/10.3758/BF03208105.

72 **expanded on the results:** Anna Lee, Sharon Clancy, and Alison S. Fleming, "Mother Rats Bar-Press for Pups: Effects of Lesions of the MPOA and Limbic Sites on Maternal Behavior and Operant Responding for Pup-Reinforcement," *Behavioural Brain Research* 100, no. 1–2 (April 1999): 15–31, https://doi.org/10.1016/S0166-4328(98)00109-0.

73 **In a March 2020 interview:** Liz Tenety, "Chelsea Clinton on Motherhood, Public Health, and Advice for Families during Coronavirus," March 16, 2020, in *The Motherly Podcast*, produced by Jennifer Bassett, podcast, MP3 audio, 40:23, https://www.mother.ly/podcast/Season-3/chelsea-clinton.

75 **In Winnicott's thinking:** *The Collected Works of D. W. Winnicott*, ed. Lesley Caldwell and Helen Taylor Robinson, vol. 5, *1955–1959* (New York: Oxford University Press, 2017), 183–88.

76 **published an analysis:** J. F. Leckman, L. C. Mayes, R. Feldman, D. W. Evans, R. A. King, and D. J. Cohen, "Early Parental Preoccupations and Behaviors and Their Possible Relationship to the Symptoms of Obsessive-Compulsive Disorder," *Acta Psychiatrica Scandinavica* 100, no. S396 (February 1999): 1–26, https://doi.org/10.1111/j.1600-0447.1999.tb10951.x.

76 **find that a large majority have:** Dufford, Erhart, and Kim, "Maternal Brain Resting-State Connectivity in the Postpartum Period," https://doi.org/10.1111/jne.12737.

77 **"Parents are beset":** Leckman et al., "Early Parental Preoccupations," https://doi.org/10.1111/j.1600-0447.1999.tb10951.x.

77   **When I interviewed her:** Chelsea Conaboy, "New Mothers, Don't Fear: You Were Made for Times Like This," *Boston Sunday Globe*, May 10, 2020, https://www.bostonglobe.com/2020/05/08/opinion/new-mothers-dont -fear-you-were-made-times-like-this/.

78   **For most parents, the intense preoccupation:** Pilyoung Kim, Linda Mayes, Ruth Feldman, James F. Leckman, and James E. Swain, "Early Postpartum Parental Preoccupation and Positive Parenting Thoughts: Relationship with Parent–Infant Interaction," *Infant Mental Health Journal* 34, no. 2 (March/ April 2013): 104–16, https://doi.org/10.1002/imhj.21359; and Leckman et al., "Early Parental Preoccupations," https://doi.org/10.1111/j.1600-0447 .1999.tb10951.x.

79   **birthing parents' neural activity is shifting:** James E. Swain, P. Kim, J. Spicer, S. S. Ho, C. J. Dayton, A. Elmadih, and K. M. Abel, "Approaching the Biology of Human Parental Attachment: Brain Imaging, Oxytocin and Coordinated Assessments of Mothers and Fathers," in "Oxytocin in Human Social Behavior and Psychopathology," special issue, *Brain Research* 1580 (September 11, 2014): 78–101, https://doi.org/10.1016/j.brainres.2014 .03.007; and Katherine S. Young, Christine E. Parsons, Alan Stein, Peter Vuust, Michelle G. Craske, and Morten L. Kringelbach, "The Neural Basis of Responsive Caregiving Behaviour: Investigating Temporal Dynamics within the Parental Brain," *Behavioural Brain Research* 325, part B (May 15, 2017): 105–16, https://doi.org/10.1016/j.bbr.2016.09.012.

79   **maternal responses become "more distributed":** M. Pereira and J. I. Morrell, "Functional Mapping of the Neural Circuitry of Rat Maternal Motivation: Effects of Site-Specific Transient Neural Inactivation," in "The Parental Brain," special issue, *Journal of Neuroendocrinology* 23, no. 11 (November 2011): 1020–35, https://doi.org/10.1111/j.1365-2826.2011 .02200.x.

79   **In a pair of studies:** Madison Bunderson, David Diaz, Angela Maupin, Nicole Landi, Marc N. Potenza, Linda C. Mayes, and Helena J. V. Ruth- erford, "Prior Reproductive Experience Modulates Neural Responses to Infant Faces across the Postpartum Period," *Social Neuroscience* 15, no. 6 (November 2020): 650–54, https://doi.org/10.1080/17470919.2020 .1847729; and Angela N. Maupin, Helena J. V. Rutherford, Nicole Landi, Marc N. Potenza, and Linda C. Mayes, "Investigating the Association between Parity and the Maternal Neural Response to Infant Cues," *Social Neuroscience* 14, no. 2 (April 2019): 214–25, https://doi.org/10.1080 /17470919.2017.1422276.

80   **involved in self-regulation:** Erika Barba-Müller et al., "Brain Plasticity in Pregnancy and the Postpartum Period," https://doi.org/10.1007/s00737-018 -0889-z.

82   **bring children to the woods:** Mary Oliver, *Upstream: Selected Essays* (New York: Penguin Press, 2016), 8.

CHAPTER 4: OUR BABIES, OUR SELVES

83   **Elizabeth could tell:** Elizabeth asked that I not use her full name or Claire's to protect their privacy.

85   **surmised that the initial hypersensitivity:** *The Collected Works of D. W. Winnicott,* ed. Lesley Caldwell and Helen Taylor Robinson, vol. 5, *1955–1959* (New York: Oxford University Press, 2017), 183–88.

86   **a group of researchers in Italy:** R. Montirosso, F. Arrigoni, E. Casini, A. Nordio, P. De Carli, F. Di Salle, S. Moriconi, M. Re, G. Reni, and R. Borgatti, "Greater Brain Response to Emotional Expressions of Their Own Children in Mothers of Preterm Infants: An fMRI Study," *Journal of Perinatology* 37, no. 6 (June 2017): 716–22, https://doi.org/10.1038/jp.2017.2.

86   **previously had been implicated:** Ellen Leibenluft, M. Ida Gobbini, Tara Harrison, and James V. Haxby, "Mothers' Neural Activation in Response to Pictures of Their Children and Other Children," *Biological Psychiatry* 56, no. 4 (August 15, 2004): 225–32, https://doi.org/10.1016/j.biopsych.2004.05.017; and Paola Venuti, Andrea Caria, Gianluca Esposito, Nicola De Pisapia, Marc H. Bornstein, and Simona de Falco, "Differential Brain Responses to Cries of Infants with Autistic Disorder and Typical Development: An fMRI Study," *Research in Developmental Disabilities* 33, no. 6 (November 13, 2012): 2255–64, https://doi.org/10.1016/j.ridd.2012.06.011.

87   **In one model, called Family Integrated Care:** Karel O'Brien, Kate Robson, Marianne Bracht, Melinda Cruz, Kei Lui, Ruben Alvaro, Orlando da Silva, et al., "Effectiveness of Family Integrated Care in Neonatal Intensive Care Units on Infant and Parent Outcomes: A Multicentre, Multinational, Cluster-Randomised Controlled Trial," *Lancet: Child & Adolescent Health* 2, no. 4 (April 2018): 245–54, https://doi.org/10.1016/S2352-4642(18)30039-7.

89   **outlined their concept of allostasis:** Peter Sterling and Joseph Eyer, "Allostasis: A New Paradigm to Explain Arousal Pathology," in *Handbook of Life Stress, Cognition and Health,* ed. Shirley Fisher and James Reason (New York: John Wiley and Sons, 1988), 629–49; and Jay Schulkin and Peter Sterling, "Allostasis: A Brain-Centered, Predictive Mode of Physiological Regulation," *Trends in Neurosciences* 42, no. 10 (October 2019): 740–52, https://doi.org/10.1016/j.tins.2019.07.010.

89   **he explained in his book:** Peter Sterling, *What Is Health? Allostasis and the Evolution of Human Design* (Cambridge, MA: MIT Press, 2020), x.

90   **Allostasis suggests that:** Peter Sterling, "Allostasis: A Model of Predictive Regulation," in "Allostasis and Allostatic Load," ed. Bruce McEwen and Achim Peters, special issue, *Physiology & Behavior* 106, no. 1 (April 12, 2012): 5–15, https://doi.org/10.1016/j.physbeh.2011.06.004.

90   **Others have proposed:** Bruce S. McEwen and John C. Wingfield, "What Is in a Name? Integrating Homeostasis, Allostasis and Stress," *Hormones and*

Behavior 57, no. 2 (February 2010): 105–11, https://doi.org/10.1016/j.yhbeh
.2009.09.011.

90   **It's given researchers better insight:** Bruce S. McEwen and John C. Wingfield, "The Concept of Allostasis in Biology and Biomedicine," *Hormones
and Behavior* 43, no. 1 (January 2003): 2–15, https://doi.org/10.1016/s0018
-506x(02)00024-7.

90   **Sterling wrote that the brain keeps:** Sterling, "Allostasis: A Model of Predictive Regulation," https://doi.org/10.1016/j.physbeh.2011.06.004.

91   **Neuroscientist Lisa Feldman:** Lisa Feldman Barrett, *Seven and a Half Lessons about the Brain* (Boston: Houghton Mifflin Harcourt, 2020), 8–10.

92   **A broad network of brain regions coordinates:** Lisa Feldman Barrett and
W. Kyle Simmons, "Interoceptive Predictions in the Brain," *Nature Reviews
Neuroscience* 16, no. 7 (July 2015): 419–29, https://doi.org/10.1038/nrn3950;
and Karen S. Quigley, Scott Kanoski, Warren M. Grill, Lisa Feldman Barrett,
and Manos Tsakiris, "Functions of Interoception: From Energy Regulation
to Experience of the Self," in "The Neuroscience of Interoception," special
issue, *Trends in Neurosciences* 44, no. 1 (January 1, 2021): 29–38, https://doi
.org/10.1016/j.tins.2020.09.008.

92   **"the fundamental image of the physical self":** A. D. Craig, "How Do You
Feel? Interoception: The Sense of the Physiological Condition of the Body,"
Nature Reviews Neuroscience 3, no. 8 (August 2002): 655–66, https://doi.org
/10.1038/nrn894.

92   **Barrett and her colleagues:** Ian R. Kleckner, Jiahe Zhang, Alexandra Tou-
routoglou, Lorena Chanes, Chenjie Xia, W. Kyle Simmons, Karen S. Quigley,
Bradford C. Dickerson, and Lisa Feldman Barrett, "Evidence for a Large-Scale
Brain System Supporting Allostasis and Interoception in Humans," *Nature
Human Behaviour* 1, no. 5 (April 24, 2017): 1–14, https://doi.org/10.1038
/s41562-017-0069.

92   **In the default mode network:** Debra A. Gusnard, Erbil Akbudak, Gordon
L. Shulman, and Marcus E. Raichle, "Medial Prefrontal Cortex and Self-
Referential Mental Activity: Relation to a Default Mode of Brain Function,"
Proceedings of the National Academy of Sciences 98, no. 7 (March 27, 2001):
4259–64, https://doi.org/10.1073/pnas.071043098; and Randy L. Buckner, Jessica R. Andrews-Hanna, and Daniel L. Schacter, "The Brain's Default Network:
Anatomy, Function, and Relevance to Disease," *Annals of the New York Academy of Sciences* 1124, no. 1 (March 2008): 1–38, https://doi.org/10.1196/annals
.1440.011.

93   **with hubs generally:** The exact anatomical parameters of the default mode
network are notoriously unclear, but its role as a large-scale brain network
essential to social function is less so. For more: Felicity Callard and Daniel
S. Margulies, "What We Talk about When We Talk about the Default Mode
Network," *Frontiers in Human Neuroscience* 8 (August 25, 2014), https://doi
.org/10.3389/fnhum.2014.00619; and Chunliang Feng, Simon B. Eickhoff,
Ting Li, Li Wang, Benjamin Becker, Julia A. Camilleri, Sébastien Hétu, and

Yi Luo, "Common Brain Networks Underlying Human Social Interactions: Evidence from Large-Scale Neuroimaging Meta-Analysis," *Neuroscience & Biobehavioral Reviews* 126 (July 2021): 289–303, https://doi.org/10.1016/j .neubiorev.2021.03.025.

93   **It plays a key role:** Michael D. Greicius, Ben Krasnow, Allan L. Reiss, and Vinod Menon, "Functional Connectivity in the Resting Brain: A Network Analysis of the Default Mode Hypothesis," *Proceedings of the National Academy of Sciences* 100, no. 1 (January 7, 2003): 253–58, https://doi.org/10.1073 /pnas.0135058100; and Buckner, Andrews-Hanna, and Schacter, "Brain's Default Network," https://doi.org/10.1196/annals.1440.011.

93   **One seminal paper described:** Buckner, Andrews-Hanna, and Schacter, "Brain's Default Network," https://doi.org/10.1196/annals.1440.011.

93   **Several studies have linked motherhood:** Jin-Xia Zheng, Lili Ge, Huiyou Chen, Xindao Yin, Yu-Chen Chen, and Wei-Wei Tang, "Disruption within Brain Default Mode Network in Postpartum Women without Depression," *Medicine* 99, no. 18 (May 2020), https://doi.org/10.1097/MD .0000000000020045; Alison E. Hipwell, Chaohui Guo, Mary L. Phillips, James E. Swain, and Eydie L. Moses-Kolko, "Right Frontoinsular Cortex and Subcortical Activity to Infant Cry Is Associated with Maternal Mental State Talk," *Journal of Neuroscience* 35, no. 37 (September 16, 2015): 12725–32, https://doi.org/10.1523/JNEUROSCI.1286-15.2015; and Paola Rigo, Gianluca Esposito, Marc H. Bornstein, Nicola De Pasapia, Corinna Manzardo, and Paola Venuti, "Brain Processes in Mothers and Nulliparous Women in Response to Cry in Different Situational Contexts: A Default Mode Network Study," *Parenting* 19, no. 1–2 (February 1, 2019): 69–85, https://doi.org/10.1080/15295192.2019.1555430.

93   **Other studies have compared:** Amanda J. Nguyen, Elisabeth Hoyer, Purva Rajhans, Lane Strathearn, and Sohye Kim, "A Tumultuous Transition to Motherhood: Altered Brain and Hormonal Responses in Mothers with Postpartum Depression," in "Papers from the Parental Brain 2018 Meeting, Toronto, Canada, July 2018," ed. Jodi L. Pawluski, Frances A. Champagne, and Oliver J. Bosch, special issue, *Journal of Neuroendocrinology* 31, no. 9 (September 2019): e12794, https://doi.org/10.1111/jne.12794; and Henry W. Chase, Eydie L. Moses-Kolko, Carlos Zevallos, Katherine L. Wisner, and Mary L. Phillips, "Disrupted Posterior Cingulate–Amygdala Connectivity in Postpartum Depressed Women as Measured with Resting BOLD fMRI," *Social Cognitive and Affective Neuroscience* 9, no. 8 (August 2014): 1069–75, https://doi.org/10.1093/scan/nst083.

94   **In one remarkable study:** Elseline Hoekzema, Erika Barba-Müller, Cristina Pozzobon, Marisol Picado, Florencio Lucco, David García-García, Juan Carlos Soliva, et al., "Pregnancy Leads to Long-Lasting Changes in Human Brain Structure," *Nature Neuroscience* 20, no. 2 (2017): 287–96, https://doi .org/10.1038/nn.4458; and Magdalena Martínez-García, María Paternina-Die, Erika Barba-Müller, Daniel Martín de Blas, Laura Beumala, Romina

Cortizo, Cristina Pozzobon, et al., "Do Pregnancy-Induced Brain Changes Reverse? The Brain of a Mother Six Years after Parturition," *Brain Sciences* 11, no. 2 (January 28, 2021), https://doi.org/10.3390/brainsci11020168.

94 **The body of evidence in fathers:** Eyal Abraham and Ruth Feldman, "The Neurobiology of Human Allomaternal Care; Implications for Fathering, Coparenting, and Children's Social Development," in "Evolutionary Perspectives on Non-Maternal Care in Mammals: Physiology, Behavior, and Developmental Effects," ed. Stacy Rosenbaum and Lee T. Gettler, special issue, *Physiology & Behavior* 193, part A (September 1, 2018): 25–34, https://doi.org/10.1016/j.physbeh.2017.12.034.

94 **When researchers looked at the brains:** Jennifer S. Mascaro, Patrick D. Hackett, and James K. Rilling, "Differential Neural Responses to Child and Sexual Stimuli in Human Fathers and Non-Fathers and Their Hormonal Correlates," *Psychoneuroendocrinology* 46 (August 2014): 153–63, https://doi.org/10.1016/j.psyneuen.2014.04.014.

95 **very common experience of phantom fetal kicks:** Disha Sasan, Phillip G. D. Ward, Meredith Nash, Edwina R. Orchard, Michael J. Farrell, Jakob Hohwy, and Sharna D. Jamadar, "'Phantom Kicks': Women's Subjective Experience of Fetal Kicks after the Postpartum Period," *Journal of Women's Health* 30, no. 1 (January 2021): 36–44, https://doi.org/10.1089/jwh.2019.8191.

95 **Or in the fetal cells that cross the placenta:** Kiarash Khosrotehrani, Kirby L. Johnson, Joseph Lau, Alain Dupuy, Dong Hyun Cha, and Diana W. Bianchi, "The Influence of Fetal Loss on the Presence of Fetal Cell Microchimerism: A Systematic Review," *Arthritis & Rheumatology* 48, no. 11 (November 2003): 3237–41, https://doi.org/10.1002/art.11324; and Amy M. Boddy, Angelo Fortunato, Melissa Wilson Sayres, and Athena Aktipis, "Fetal Microchimerism and Maternal Health: A Review and Evolutionary Analysis of Cooperation and Conflict beyond the Womb," *BioEssays* 37, no. 10 (October 2015): 1106–18, https://doi.org/10.1002/bies.201500059.

95 **"as permeable as the umbilical cord":** Diane Goldenberg, Narcis Marshall, Sofia Cardenas, and Darby Saxbe, "The Development of the Social Brain within a Family Context," in *The Social Brain: A Developmental Perspective*, ed. Jean Decety (Cambridge, MA: MIT Press, 2020), 107–24.

95 **They also depend on their caregivers:** Shir Atzil, Wei Gao, Isaac Fradkin, and Lisa Feldman Barrett, "Growing a Social Brain," *Nature Human Behaviour* 2, no. 9 (September 2018): 624–36, https://doi.org/10.1038/s41562-018-0384-6.

96 **"the most primordial caregiving system":** Michael Numan and Larry J. Young, "Neural Mechanisms of Mother-Infant Bonding and Pair Bonding: Similarities, Differences, and Broader Implications," in "Parental Care," ed. Alison S. Fleming, Frederic Lévy, and Joe S. Lonstein, special issue, *Hormones and Behavior* 77 (January 2016): 98–112, https://doi.org/10.1016/j.yhbeh.2015.05.015.

96   **describes this as "biobehavioral synchrony":** Ruth Feldman, "Bio-
      Behavioral Synchrony: A Model for Integrating Biological and Microsocial
      Behavioral Processes in the Study of Parenting," *Parenting* 12, no.
      2–3 (June 14, 2012): 154–64, https://doi.org/10.1080/15295192.2012.683342.

96   **The brains of parent and infant become:** Ortal Shimon-Raz, Roy Salo-
      mon, Miki Bloch, Gabi Aisenberg Romano, Yaara Yeshurun, Adi Ulmer
      Yaniv, Orna Zagoory-Sharon, and Ruth Feldman, "Mother Brain Is Wired
      for Social Moments," *eLife* 10 (2021), e59436, https://doi.org/10.7554/eLife
      .59436.

96   **When we connect with:** Ruth Feldman, "The Neurobiology of Human
      Attachments," *Trends in Cognitive Sciences* 21, no. 2 (February 2017): 80–99,
      https://doi.org/10.1016/j.tics.2016.11.007.

97   **For the role it plays:** Ruth Feldman, "The Adaptive Human Parental Brain:
      Implications for Children's Social Development," *Trends in Neurosciences*
      38, no. 6 (June 2015): 387–99, https://doi.org/10.1016/j.tins.2015.04.004.

97   **relate this connection to allostasis:** Atzil et al., "Growing a Social Brain,"
      https://doi.org/10.1038/s41562-018-0384-6.

98   **further clarified the circuitry:** Shir Atzil, Alexandra Touroutoglou, Tali
      Rudy, Stephanie Salcedo, Ruth Feldman, Jacob M. Hooker, Bradford C. Dick-
      erson, Ciprian Catana, and Lisa Feldman Barrett, "Dopamine in the Medial
      Amygdala Network Mediates Human Bonding," *Proceedings of the National
      Academy of Sciences* 114, no. 9 (February 28, 2017): 2361–66, https://doi.org
      /10.1073/pnas.1612233114.

99   **They're still figuring out exactly where:** Daniel S. Quintana, Jaro-
      slav Rokicki, Dennis van der Meer, Dag Alnæs, Tobias Kaufmann, Aldo
      Córdova-Palomera, Ingrid Dieset, Ole A. Andreassen, and Lars T. Westlye,
      "Oxytocin Pathway Gene Networks in the Human Brain," *Nature Commu-
      nications* 10, no. 1 (February 8, 2019): 668, https://doi.org/10.1038/s41467
      -019-08503-8; Benjamin Jurek and Inga D. Neumann, "The Oxytocin
      Receptor: From Intracellular Signaling to Behavior," *Physiological Reviews*
      98, no. 3 (July 2018): 1805–908, https://doi.org/10.1152/physrev.00031
      .2017; and M. L. Boccia, P. Petrusz, K. Suzuki, L. Marson, and C. A. Peder-
      sen, "Immunohistochemical Localization of Oxytocin Receptors in Human
      Brain," *Neuroscience* 253 (December 3, 2013): 155–64, https://doi.org/10
      .1016/j.neuroscience.2013.08.048.

100   **Oxytocin is a driver of:** Atzil et al., "Dopamine Mediates Human Bonding,"
      https://doi.org/10.1073/pnas.1612233114; and Ruth Feldman and Marian J.
      Bakermans-Kranenburg, "Oxytocin: A Parenting Hormone," in "Parenting,"
      ed. Marinus H. van IJzendoorn and Marian J. Bakermans-Kranenburg, spe-
      cial issue, *Current Opinion in Psychology* 15 (June 1, 2017): 13–18, https://doi
      .org/10.1016/j.copsyc.2017.02.011.

100   **not a love hormone:** Quintana et al., "Oxytocin Pathway Gene Networks,"
      https://doi.org/10.1038/s41467-019-08503-8; and Brian Resnick, "Oxytocin,

the So-Called 'Hug Hormone,' Is Way More Sophisticated Than We Thought," Vox, February 13, 2019, https://www.vox.com/science-and-health /2019/2/13/18221876/oxytocin-morality-valentines.

100　**linked to maternal aggression:** C. F. Ferris, K. B. Foote, H. M. Meltser, M. G. Plenby, K. L. Smith, and T. R. Insel, "Oxytocin in the Amygdala Facilitates Maternal Aggression," *Annals of the New York Academy of Sciences* 652, no. 1 (June 1992): 456–57, https://doi.org/10.1111/j.1749-6632.1992.tb34382.x.

100　**oxytocin evolved to have a central role:** Daniel S. Quintana and Adam J. Guastella, "An Allostatic Theory of Oxytocin," *Trends in Cognitive Sciences* 24, no. 7 (July 1, 2020): 515–28, https://doi.org/10.1016/j.tics.2020.03.008.

101　**how groups of mothers processed infant faces:** Carla Márquez, Humberto Nicolini, Michael J. Crowley, and Rodolfo Solís-Vivanco, "Early Processing (N170) of Infant Faces in Mothers of Children with Autism Spectrum Disorder and Its Association with Maternal Sensitivity," *Autism Research* 12, no. 5 (May 2019): 744–58, https://doi.org/10.1002/aur.2102.

102　**groom the demanding pups:** This work builds on published research by Pereira and co-investigator Annabel Ferreira looking at how mother rats adjust their behavior to demanding pups. Mariana Pereira and Annabel Ferreira, "Demanding Pups Improve Maternal Behavioral Impairments in Sensitized and Haloperidol-Treated Lactating Female Rats," *Behavioural Brain Research* 175, no. 1 (November 25, 2006): 139–48, https://doi.org/10.1016/j .bbr.2006.08.013.

102　**Some have called for more studies:** Jonathan Levy, Kaisu Lankinen, Maria Hakonen, and Ruth Feldman, "The Integration of Social and Neural Synchrony: A Case for Ecologically Valid Research Using MEG Neuroimaging," *Social Cognitive and Affective Neuroscience* 16, no. 1–2 (February 2021): 143–52, https://doi.org/10.1093/scan/nsaa061; and Riitta Hari, Linda Henriksson, Sanna Malinen, and Lauri Parkkonen, "Centrality of Social Interaction in Human Brain Function," *Neuron* 88, no. 1 (October 7, 2015): 181–93, https:// doi.org/10.1016/j.neuron.2015.09.022.

103　**John Maubray cautioned:** John Maubray, *The Female Physician* (London: James Holland, 1724), 75, http://archive.org/details/femalephysicianc00maub.

104　**In his 1897 book on the topic:** Charles J. Bayer, *Maternal Impressions: A Study of Child Life before and after Birth, and Their Effect upon Individual Life and Character* (Winona, MN: Jones & Kroeger, 1897), 13, 138–39, 147, 194–95, 251, http://archive.org/details/maternalimpressi00bayeiala.

104　**Or it would be:** For more on the modern trajectory of this old idea, see Lyz Lenz, *Belabored: A Vindication of the Rights of Pregnant Women* (New York: Bold Type Books, 2020).

104　**One speaking before the:** W. T. Councilman, "Remarks on Maternal Impressions," *Boston Medical and Surgical Journal* 136, no. 2 (January 14, 1897): 32–34, https://doi.org/10.1056/NEJM189701141360203.

104　**The United States Children's Bureau would:** Sarah S. Richardson, *The*

Maternal Imprint: The Contested Science of Maternal-Fetal Effects (Chicago: University of Chicago Press, 2021), 85.

104 **A movement took hold:** Donna Bassin, Margaret Honey, and Meryle Mahrer Kaplan, eds., *Representations of Motherhood* (New Haven, CT: Yale University Press, 1994), 5.

104 **One of them, James Sully:** As quoted in Erica Burman, *Deconstructing Developmental Psychology*, 2nd ed. (London: Routledge, 2008), 16–17.

105 **Sully seems to have softened:** Marjorie Lorch and Paula Hellal, "Darwin's 'Natural Science of Babies,'" *Journal of the History of the Neurosciences* 19, no. 2 (April 2010): 140–57, https://doi.org/10.1080/09647040903504823.

105 **But as they charted the "milestones":** Sarah Menkedick, *Ordinary Insanity: Fear and the Silent Crisis of Motherhood in America* (New York: Pantheon, 2020), 199.

105 **Rima Apple documented the rise:** Rima D. Apple, *Perfect Motherhood: Science and Childrearing in America* (New Brunswick, NJ: Rutgers University Press, 2006), 6, 37–39, 53–54.

106 **like a parody of itself:** John B. Watson, *Psychological Care of Infant and Child* (London: W. W. Norton, 1928), 69–77.

106 **sold tens of thousands of copies:** B. R. Hergenhahn and Tracy Henley, *An Introduction to the History of Psychology*, 7th ed. (Belmont, CA: Wadsworth Cengage Learning, 2014), 392.

106 **shaped parenting ideals:** Robert Coughlan, "How to Survive Parenthood," *Life*, June 26, 1950.

106 **Apple wrote that he and his peers:** Apple, *Perfect Motherhood*, 134.

106 **The baby advisers reminded mothers:** Shari L. Thurer, *The Myths of Motherhood: How Culture Reinvents the Good Mother* (Boston: Houghton Mifflin Harcourt, 1994), 258–61.

107 **A lot has been written about the Searses' version:** Most notably, perhaps, this cover story: Kate Pickert, "The Man Who Remade Motherhood," *Time*, May 21, 2012, http://content.time.com/time/subscriber/article/0,33009,2114427,00.html.

107 **lay out the philosophy:** William Sears and Martha Sears, *The Attachment Parenting Book: A Commonsense Guide to Understanding and Nurturing Your Baby* (Boston: Little, Brown, 2001), 4.

109 **reading a 2011 paper:** Shir Atzil, Talma Hendler, and Ruth Feldman, "Specifying the Neurobiological Basis of Human Attachment: Brain, Hormones, and Behavior in Synchronous and Intrusive Mothers," *Neuropsychopharmacology* 36, no. 13 (December 2011): 2603–15, https://doi.org/10.1038/npp.2011.172.

111 **music training builds over time:** Ewa A. Miendlarzewska and Wiebke J. Trost, "How Musical Training Affects Cognitive Development: Rhythm, Reward and Other Modulating Variables," *Frontiers in Neuroscience* 7 (January 2014), https://doi.org/10.3389/fnins.2013.00279.

111 **In one key paper:** Christine E. Parsons, Katherine S. Young, Mikkel V.

Petersen, Else-Marie Jegindoe Elmholdt, Peter Vuust, Alan Stein, and Morten L. Kringelbach, "Duration of Motherhood Has Incremental Effects on Mothers' Neural Processing of Infant Vocal Cues: A Neuroimaging Study of Women," *Scientific Reports* 7, no. 1 (May 11, 2017): 1727, https://doi.org /10.1038/s41598-017-01776-3.

111 **among parents who were depressed:** Katherine S. Young, C. E. Parsons, A. Stein, and M. L. Kringelbach, "Interpreting Infant Vocal Distress: The Ameliorative Effect of Musical Training in Depression," *Emotion* 12, no. 6 (2012): 1200–205, https://doi.org/10.1037/a0028705.

112 **trio was at Tanglewood:** I'm With Her, "Toy Heart / Marry Me / Jerusalem," performed at *Live from Here*, June 15, 2019, YouTube video, 9:51, posted June 16, 2019, by *Live from Here*, https://www.youtube.com/watch?v=qbEfK -LsMSc.

113 **It is a favorite in our house:** Maurice Sendak, *Where the Wild Things Are*, reprint ed. (New York: HarperCollins, 1984).

CHAPTER 5: THE ANCIENT FAMILY TREE

116 **Among nonhuman primates:** Sarah Blaffer Hrdy, *Mothers and Others: The Evolutionary Origins of Mutual Understanding* (Cambridge, MA: Belknap Press, 2009), 92–93.

116 **human ancestors diverged:** Hrdy, *Mothers and Others*, 140.

116 **As a result:** Kristen Hawkes, "The Centrality of Ancestral Grandmothering in Human Evolution," *Integrative and Comparative Biology* 60, no. 3 (September 1, 2020): 765–81, https://doi.org/10.1093/icb/icaa029.

116 **To early humans:** Hrdy, *Mothers and Others*.

117 **"alloparenting":** Edward O. Wilson, *Sociobiology: The New Synthesis* (Cambridge, MA: Belknap Press, 1975), 349.

117 **global parental caregiving network:** Eyal Abraham, Talma Hendler, Irit Shapira-Lichter, Yaniv Kanat-Maymon, Orna Zagoory-Sharon, and Ruth Feldman, "Father's Brain Is Sensitive to Childcare Experiences," *Proceedings of the National Academy of Sciences* 111, no. 27 (July 8, 2014): 9792–97, https://doi.org /10.1073/pnas.1402569111; and E. R. Glasper, W. M. Kenkel, J. Bick, and J. K. Rilling, "More Than Just Mothers: The Neurobiological and Neuroendocrine Underpinnings of Allomaternal Caregiving," in "Parental Brain," ed. Susanne Brummelte and Benedetta Leuner, special issue, *Frontiers in Neuroendocrinology* 53 (April 2019): 100741, https://doi.org/10.1016/j.yfrne.2019.02.005.

118 **Prominent naturalists:** As quoted in Marion Thomas, "Are Women Naturally Devoted Mothers? Fabre, Perrier, and Giard on Maternal Instinct in France under the Third Republic," *Journal of the History of the Behavioral Sciences* 50, no. 3 (June 2014): 280–301, https://doi.org/10.1002/jhbs .21666.

118 **this characterization made it easier:** Marga Vicedo, *The Nature and Nur-*

ture of Love: From Imprinting to Attachment in Cold War America, illustrated ed. (Chicago: University of Chicago Press, 2013), 67–68.

119   **Yet Lorenz knew:** Konrad Z. Lorenz, "The Companion in the Bird's World," *Auk* 54, no. 3 (July 1937): 245–73, https://doi.org/10.2307/4078077.

119   **he chose these species:** John Bowlby, *Attachment and Loss*, vol. 1, *Attachment*, 2nd ed. (New York: Basic Books, 1982), 184.

119   **when Bowlby selected these primates:** Hrdy, *Mothers and Others*, 84.

119   **Bowlby found affirmation:** Bowlby, *Attachment and Loss*, vol. 1, *Attachment*, 199.

119   **In the wild:** Hrdy, *Mothers and Others*, 68.

119   **In many species:** Hrdy, *Mothers and Others*, 85–92.

120   **viewed as a window:** Peter Jordan, "The Ethnohistory and Anthropology of 'Modern' Hunter-Gatherers," in *The Oxford Handbook of the Archaeology and Anthropology of Hunter-Gatherers*, ed. Vicki Cummings, Peter Jordan, and Marek Zvelebil (Oxford: Oxford University Press, 2014), https://doi.org/10.1093/oxfordhb/9780199551224.013.030; and Carol R. Ember, "Hunter-Gatherers (Foragers)," in *Explaining Human Culture*, ed. C. R. Ember, Human Relations Area Files, last modified June 1, 2020, http://hraf.yale.edu/ehc/summaries/hunter-gatherers.

120   **!Kung babies were held:** Hrdy, *Mothers and Others*, 73–75.

121   **"Human mothers are just as hypervigilant":** Hrdy, *Mothers and Others*, 73.

121   **When men hunted:** Kristen Hawkes, James O'Connell, and Nicholas Blurton Jones, "Hunter-Gatherer Studies and Human Evolution: A Very Selective Review," in "Centennial Anniversary Issue of AJPA," special issue, *American Journal of Physical Anthropology* 165, no. 4 (April 2018): 777–800, https://doi.org/10.1002/ajpa.23403.

122   **A group of anthropologists:** Hawkes, O'Connell, and Blurton Jones, "Hunter-Gatherer Studies and Human Evolution," https://doi.org/10.1002/ajpa.23403.

122   **among the Hadza, older women:** Kristen Hawkes, James F. O'Connell, and Nicholas Blurton Jones, "Hardworking Hadza Grandmothers," in *Comparative Socioecology: The Behavioural Ecology of Humans and Other Mammals*, ed. V. Standen and R. A. Foley (Oxford: Blackwell Scientific Publications, 1989), 341–66; and Hawkes, O'Connell, and Blurton Jones, "Hunter-Gatherer Studies and Human Evolution," https://doi.org/10.1002/ajpa.23403.

122   **"grandmother hypothesis":** Hawkes, O'Connell, and Blurton Jones, "Hunter-Gatherer Studies and Human Evolution," https://doi.org/10.1002/ajpa.23403.

123   **Among the apes:** Hrdy, *Mothers and Others*, 101.

123   **Helpful grandmothers:** Hawkes, "Ancestral Grandmothering," https://doi.org/10.1093/icb/icaa029.

123   **Researchers in London:** Rebecca Sear and Ruth Mace, "Who Keeps Children Alive? A Review of the Effects of Kin on Child Survival," *Evolution and*

Human Behavior 29, no. 1 (January 2008): 1–18, https://doi.org/10.1016/j .evolhumbehav.2007.10.001.

124 **preindustrial Finland:** Simon N. Chapman, Jenni E. Pettay, Virpi Lummaa, and Mirkka Lahdenperä, "Limits to Fitness Benefits of Prolonged Post-Reproductive Lifespan in Women," *Current Biology* 29, no. 4 (February 18, 2019): 645–650.e3, https://doi.org/10.1016/j.cub.2018.12.052.

124 **the first French families:** Sacha C. Engelhardt, Patrick Bergeron, Alain Gagnon, Lisa Dillon, and Fanie Pelletier, "Using Geographic Distance as a Potential Proxy for Help in the Assessment of the Grandmother Hypothesis," *Current Biology* 29, no. 4 (February 18, 2019): 651–56.e3, https://doi.org /10.1016/j.cub.2019.01.027.

124 **Critics say:** Lee T. Gettler, "Direct Male Care and Hominin Evolution: Why Male–Child Interaction Is More Than a Nice Social Idea," *American Anthropologist* 112, no. 1 (March 2010): 7–21, https://doi.org/10.1111/j.1548-1433 .2009.01193.x; Kim Hill and A. Magdalena Hurtado, "Cooperative Breeding in South American Hunter–Gatherers," *Proceedings of the Royal Society B: Biological Sciences* 276, no. 1674 (November 7, 2009): 3863–70, https://doi.org/10 .1098/rspb.2009.1061; and Hillard Kaplan, Kim Hill, Jane Lancaster, and A. Magdalena Hurtado, "A Theory of Human Life History Evolution: Diet, Intelligence, and Longevity," *Evolutionary Anthropology* 9, no. 4 (2000): 156–85, https://doi.org/10.1002/1520-6505(2000)9:4<156::AID-EVAN5>3.0.CO;2-7. One long-standing obstacle to the grandmother hypothesis was the belief that ancestral human mothers would not have stayed near their own mothers in adulthood but would have moved to another group to mate. It turns out that was based—surprise, surprise—on inaccurate assumptions about the behavior of women in modern hunter-gatherer communities and an incomplete record of behavior among nonhuman apes, which do sometimes stay with their matrilineal group. See Hrdy, *Mothers and Others*, 239–47.

125 **subsidized and glorified:** Stephanie Coontz, *The Way We Never Were: American Families and the Nostalgia Trap*, reprint ed. (New York: Basic Books, 1992).

125 **ambivalence may be derived:** Hrdy, *Mothers and Others*, 119–21.

126 **the grandmother hypothesis could explain:** Hawkes, "Ancestral Grandmothering," https://doi.org/10.1093/icb/icaa029; and Kristen Hawkes and Barbara L. Finlay, "Mammalian Brain Development and Our Grandmothering Life History," in "Evolutionary Perspectives on Non-Maternal Care in Mammals: Physiology, Behavior, and Developmental Effects," ed. Stacy Rosenbaum and Lee T. Gettler, special issue, *Physiology & Behavior* 193, part A (September 1, 2018): 55–68, https://doi.org/10.1016/j.physbeh.2018 .01.013.

126 **This effort drove development:** Hrdy, *Mothers and Others*, 121.

128 **Comparing brain scans:** Elseline Hoekzema, Erika Barba-Müller, Cristina Pozzobon, Marisol Picado, Florencio Lucco, David García-García, Juan Carlos Soliva, et al., "Pregnancy Leads to Long-Lasting Changes in Human

Brain Structure," *Nature Neuroscience* 20, no. 2 (2017): 287–96, https://doi.org/10.1038/nn.4458.

129 **changes in the ventral striatum:** Elseline Hoekzema, Christian K. Tamnes, Puck Berns, Erika Barba-Müller, Cristina Pozzobon, Marisol Picado, Florencio Lucco, et al., "Becoming a Mother Entails Anatomical Changes in the Ventral Striatum of the Human Brain That Facilitate Its Responsiveness to Offspring Cues," *Psychoneuroendocrinology* 112 (February 2020): 104507, https://doi.org/10.1016/j.psyneuen.2019.104507.

129 **A later analysis:** María Paternina-Die, Magdalena Martínez-García, Clara Pretus, Elseline Hoekzema, Erika Barba-Müller, Daniel Martín de Blas, Cristina Pozzobon, et al., "The Paternal Transition Entails Neuroanatomic Adaptations That Are Associated with the Father's Brain Response to His Infant Cues," *Cerebral Cortex Communications* 1, no. 1 (2020), https://doi.org/10.1093/texcom/tgaa082.

129 **The researchers followed up at six years postpartum:** Magdalena Martínez-García, María Paternina-Die, Erika Barba-Müller, Daniel Martín de Blas, Laura Beumala, Romina Cortizo, Cristina Pozzobon, et al., "Do Pregnancy-Induced Brain Changes Reverse? The Brain of a Mother Six Years after Parturition," *Brain Sciences* 11, no. 2 (January 28, 2021), https://doi.org/10.3390/brainsci11020168.

129 *increases* **in gray matter:** Pilyoung Kim, J. F. Leckman, L. C. Mayes, R. Feldman, X. Wang, and J. E. Swain, "The Plasticity of Human Maternal Brain: Longitudinal Changes in Brain Anatomy during the Early Postpartum Period," *Behavioral Neuroscience* 124, no. 5 (October 2010): 695–700, https://doi.org/10.1037/a0020884.

130 **A 2020 study found comparable results:** Eileen Luders, Florian Kurth, Malin Gingnell, Jonas Engman, Eu-Leong Yong, Inger S. Poromaa, and Christian Gaser, "From Baby Brain to Mommy Brain: Widespread Gray Matter Gain after Giving Birth," *Cortex* 126 (May 2020): 334–42, https://doi.org/10.1016/j.cortex.2019.12.029.

130 **Both Hoekzema and Kim:** Erika Barba-Müller, Sinéad Craddock, Susanna Carmona, and Elseline Hoekzema, "Brain Plasticity in Pregnancy and the Postpartum Period: Links to Maternal Caregiving and Mental Health," *Archives of Women's Mental Health* 22, no. 2 (April 2019): 289–99, https://doi.org/10.1007/s00737-018-0889-z; and Pilyoung Kim, Alexander J. Dufford, and Rebekah C. Tribble, "Cortical Thickness Variation of the Maternal Brain in the First 6 Months Postpartum: Associations with Parental Self-Efficacy," *Brain Structure & Function* 223, no. 7 (September 2018): 3267–77, https://doi.org/10.1007/s00429-018-1688-z.

130 **The proliferation of new cells:** Benedetta Leuner and Sara Sabihi, "The Birth of New Neurons in the Maternal Brain: Hormonal Regulation and Functional Implications," *Frontiers in Neuroendocrinology* 41 (April 2016): 99–113, https://doi.org/10.1016/j.yfrne.2016.02.004; and Rand S. Eid, Jessica A. Chaiton, Stephanie E. Lieblich, Tamara S. Bodnar, Joanne Weinberg, and Liisa A. M. Galea,

"Early and Late Effects of Maternal Experience on Hippocampal Neurogenesis, Microglia, and the Circulating Cytokine Milieu," *Neurobiology of Aging* 78 (June 2019): 1–17, https://doi.org/10.1016/j.neurobiolaging.2019.01.021.

131 **with Carmona leading the analysis:** Susanna Carmona, Magdalena Martínez-García, María Paternina-Die, Erika Barba-Müller, Lara M. Wierenga, Yasser Alemán-Gómez, Clara Pretus, et al., "Pregnancy and Adolescence Entail Similar Neuroanatomical Adaptations: A Comparative Analysis of Cerebral Morphometric Changes," *Human Brain Mapping* 40, no. 7 (January 20, 2019): 2143–52, https://doi.org/10.1002/hbm.24513.

132 **developing Alzheimer's disease:** Michal Schnaider Beeri, Michael Rapp, James Schmeidler, Abraham Reichenberg, Dushyant P. Purohit, Daniel P. Perl, Hillel T. Grossman, Isak Prohovnik, Vahram Haroutunian, and Jeremy M. Silverman, "Number of Children Is Associated with Neuropathology of Alzheimer's Disease in Women," *Neurobiology of Aging* 30, no. 8 (August 2009): 1184–91, https://doi.org/10.1016/j.neurobiolaging.2007.11.011.

132 **Using new techniques:** Ann-Marie G. de Lange, Tobias Kaufmann, Dennis van der Meer, Luigi A. Maglanoc, Dag Alnæs, Torgeir Moberget, Gwenaëlle Douaud, Ole A. Andreassen, and Lars T. Westlye, "Population-Based Neuroimaging Reveals Traces of Childbirth in the Maternal Brain," *Proceedings of the National Academy of Sciences* 116, no. 44 (October 29, 2019): 22341–46, https://doi.org/10.1073/pnas.1910666116; and Ann-Marie G. de Lange, Claudia Barth, Tobias Kaufmann, Melis Anatürk, Sana Suri, Klaus P. Ebmeier, and Lars T. Westlye, "The Maternal Brain: Region-Specific Patterns of Brain Aging Are Traceable Decades after Childbirth," *Human Brain Mapping* 41, no. 16 (August 7, 2020): 4718–29, https://doi.org/10.1002/hbm.25152.

133 **In 2021, the authors published:** Irene Voldsbekk, Claudia Barth, Ivan I. Maximov, Tobias Kaufmann, Dani Beck, Genevieve Richard, Torgeir Moberget, Lars T. Westlye, and Ann-Marie de Lange, "A History of Previous Childbirths Is Linked to Women's White Matter Brain Age in Midlife and Older Age," *Human Brain Mapping* 42, no. 13 (September 2021): 4372–86, https://doi.org/10.1002/hbm.25553.

133 **used as a proxy:** Kaida Ning, Lu Zhao, Meredith Franklin, Will Matloff, Ishaan Batta, Nibal Arzouni, Fengzhu Sun, and Arthur W. Toga, "Parity Is Associated with Cognitive Function and Brain Age in Both Females and Males," *Scientific Reports* 10, no. 1 (April 8, 2020): 6100, https://doi.org/10.1038/s41598-020-63014-7.

133 **In the meantime:** De Lange et al., "Maternal Brain," https://doi.org/10.1002/hbm.25152; and Claudia Barth and Ann-Marie G. de Lange, "Towards an Understanding of Women's Brain Aging: The Immunology of Pregnancy and Menopause," in "Beyond Sex Differences: A Spotlight on Women's Brain Health," ed. Liisa Galea, Emily Jacobs, and Ann-Marie de Lange, special issue, *Frontiers in Neuroendocrinology* 58 (July 2020): 100850, https://doi.org/10.1016/j.yfrne.2020.100850.

134 **associated with a "dose" effect:** Edwina R. Orchard, Phillip G. D. Ward, Francesco Sforazzini, Elsdon Storey, Gary F. Egan, and Sharna D. Jamadar, "Relationship between Parenthood and Cortical Thickness in Late Adulthood," *PLoS ONE* 15, no. 7 (July 28, 2020): e0236031, https://doi.org/10.1371/journal.pone.0236031.

134 **Starting with the same sample:** Edwina R. Orchard, Phillip G. D. Ward, Sidhant Chopra, Elsdon Storey, Gary F. Egan, and Sharna D. Jamadar, "Neuroprotective Effects of Motherhood on Brain Function in Late Life: A Resting-State fMRI Study," *Cerebral Cortex* 31, no. 2 (February 2021): 1270–83, https://doi.org/10.1093/cercor/bhaa293.

135 **fathers among the foraging Aka:** Barry S. Hewlett, *Intimate Fathers: The Nature and Context of Aka Pygmy Paternal Infant Care* (Ann Arbor: University of Michigan Press, 1992), 126, 168; Hrdy, *Mothers and Others.*

135 **The same group of Yale researchers:** Pilyoung Kim, Paola Rigo, Linda C. Mayes, Ruth Feldman, James F. Leckman, and James E. Swain, "Neural Plasticity in Fathers of Human Infants," *Social Neuroscience* 9, no. 5 (October 2014): 522–35, https://doi.org/10.1080/17470919.2014.933713.

136 **researchers at the University of Southern California:** Ning et al., "Parity Is Associated with Cognitive Function," https://doi.org/10.1038/s41598-020-63014-7.

136 **one fascinating paper:** Marian C. Diamond, Ruth E. Johnson, and Carol Ingham, "Brain Plasticity Induced by Environment and Pregnancy," *International Journal of Neuroscience* 2, no. 4–5 (1971): 171–78, https://doi.org/10.3109/00207457109146999.

137 **But parenting comes with:** Orchard et al., "Neuroprotective Effects of Motherhood," https://doi.org/10.1093/cercor/bhaa293.

137 **Some studies—but not all:** Paula Duarte-Guterman, Benedetta Leuner, and Liisa A. M. Galea, "The Long and Short Term Effects of Motherhood on the Brain," in "Parental Brain," ed. Susanne Brummelte and Benedetta Leuner, special issue, *Frontiers in Neuroendocrinology* 53 (April 1, 2019): 100740, https://doi.org/10.1016/j.yfrne.2019.02.004; and Roksana Karim, Ha Dang, Victor W. Henderson, Howard N. Hodis, Jan St. John, Robert D. Brinton, and Wendy J. Mack, "Effect of Reproductive History and Exogenous Hormone Use on Cognitive Function in Mid- and Late Life," *Journal of the American Geriatrics Society* 64, no. 12 (December 2016): 2448–56, https://doi.org/10.1111/jgs.14658; and Michelle Heys, Chaoqiang Jiang, Kar Keung Cheng, Weisen Zhang, Shiu Lun Au Yeung, Tai Hing Lam, Gabriel M. Leung, and C. Mary Schooling, "Life Long Endogenous Estrogen Exposure and Later Adulthood Cognitive Function in a Population of Naturally Postmenopausal Women from Southern China: The Guangzhou Biobank Cohort Study," *Psychoneuroendocrinology* 36, no. 6 (July 2011): 864–73, https://doi.org/10.1016/j.psyneuen.2010.11.009.

137 **Having five or more children:** Beeri et al., "Number of Children Is Associated

with Alzheimer's Disease," https://doi.org/10.1016/j.neurobiolaging.2007.11
.011; and Hyesue Jang, Jong Bin Bae, Efthimios Dardiotis, Nikolaos Scar-
meas, Peminder S. Sachdev, Darren M. Lipnicki, Ji Won Han, et al., "Differential Effects of Completed and Incomplete Pregnancies on the Risk of
Alzheimer Disease," *Neurology* 91, no. 7 (August 14, 2018): e643–51, https://
doi.org/10.1212/WNL.0000000000006000.

137   **a small study of older British women:** Molly Fox, Carlo Berzuini, and
Leslie A. Knapp, "Cumulative Estrogen Exposure, Number of Menstrual
Cycles, and Alzheimer's Risk in a Cohort of British Women," *Psychoneuroendocrinology* 38, no. 12 (December 2013): 2973–82, https://doi.org/10
.1016/j.psyneuen.2013.08.005.

138   **Certain genotypes:** See reviews: Duarte-Guterman, Leuner, and Galea,
"Effects of Motherhood on the Brain," https://doi.org/10.1016/j.yfrne.2019
.02.004; and Nicholas P. Deems and Benedetta Leuner, "Pregnancy, Postpartum and Parity: Resilience and Vulnerability in Brain Health and Disease,"
Frontiers in Neuroendocrinology 57 (April 2020): 100820, https://doi.org/10
.1016/j.yfrne.2020.100820.

138   **rat mothers enjoy:** Liisa A. M. Galea, Wansu Qiu, and Paula Duarte-
Guterman, "Beyond Sex Differences: Short and Long-Term Implications
of Motherhood on Women's Health," in "Sex Differences," ed. Susan Howlett and Stephen Goodwin, special issue, *Current Opinion in Physiology* 6
(December 2018): 82–88, https://doi.org/10.1016/j.cophys.2018.06.003; and
Eid et al., "Early and Late Effects of Maternal Experience," https://doi.org/10
.1016/j.neurobiolaging.2019.01.021.

138   **a grandmother's brain responds:** James K. Rilling, Amber Gonzalez, and
Minwoo Lee, "The Neural Correlates of Grandmaternal Caregiving," *Proceedings of the Royal Society B* 288, no. 1963 (November 24, 2021): 20211997,
https://doi.org/10.1098/rspb.2021.1997.

140   **a group-level mechanism:** Wilson, *Sociobiology*, 349.

140   **Cooperative breeding:** Michael Griesser, Szymon M. Drobniak, Shinichi
Nakagawa, and Carlos A. Botero, "Family Living Sets the Stage for Cooperative Breeding and Ecological Resilience in Birds," *PLoS Biology* 15, no. 6 (June
2017): e2000483, https://doi.org/10.1371/journal.pbio.2000483; Judith M.
Burkart, Carel van Schaik, and Michael Griesser, "Looking for Unity in Diversity: Human Cooperative Childcare in Comparative Perspective," *Proceedings
of the Royal Society B: Biological Sciences* 284, no. 1869 (December 20, 2017):
20171184, https://doi.org/10.1098/rspb.2017.1184; and Dieter Lukas and Tim
Clutton-Brock, "Cooperative Breeding and Monogamy in Mammalian Societies," *Proceedings of the Royal Society B: Biological Sciences* 279, no. 1736 (June
7, 2012): 2151–56, https://doi.org/10.1098/rspb.2011.2468.

140   **figuring out why:** Griesser et al., "Family Living Sets the Stage," https://doi
.org/10.1371/journal.pbio.2000483.

141   **the corvid family:** Lisa Horn, Thomas Bugnyar, Michael Griesser, Marietta
Hengl, Ei-Ichi Izawa, Tim Oortwijn, Christiane Rössler, et al., "Sex-Specific

Effects of Cooperative Breeding and Colonial Nesting on Prosociality in Corvids," *eLife* 9 (October 20, 2020): e58139, https://doi.org/10.7554/eLife .58139.

141 **helpers at the nest:** "About Crows," Mass Audubon, accessed June 22, 2021, https://www.massaudubon.org/learn/nature-wildlife/birds/crows/about.

142 **economist Betsey Stevenson:** Jessica Grose, "America's Mothers Are in Crisis," *New York Times*, February 4, 2021, https://www.nytimes.com/2021/02 /04/parenting/working-moms-mental-health-coronavirus.html.

142 **the contingent of conservatives:** Mike DeBonis, "'Lefty Social Engineering': GOP Launches Cultural Attack on Biden's Plan for Day Care, Education and Employee Leave," *Washington Post*, April 30, 2021, https://www .washingtonpost.com/politics/lefty-social-engineering-gop-launches -cultural-attack-on-bidens-plan-for-day-care-education-and-employee-leave /2021/04/30/38983b6e-a9bc-11eb-8c1a-56f0cb4ff3b5_story.html; and Mical Raz, "The Secret to Passing Biden's Child Care Plan? Convincing People It Helps All Kids," *Washington Post*, May 17, 2021, https://www.washingtonpost .com/outlook/2021/05/17/secret-passing-bidens-child-care-plan-explaining -how-it-helps-all-kids/.

CHAPTER 6: INCLINED TO CARE

143 **And vice versa:** Tali Kimchi, Jennings Xu, and Catherine Dulac, "A Functional Circuit Underlying Male Sexual Behaviour in the Female Mouse Brain," *Nature* 448, no. 7157 (August 2007): 1009–14, https://doi.org/10 .1038/nature06089; and Zheng Wu, Anita E. Autry, Joseph F. Bergan, Mitsuko Watabe-Uchida, and Catherine G. Dulac, "Galanin Neurons in the Medial Preoptic Area Govern Parental Behaviour," *Nature* 509, no. 7500 (May 2014): 325–30, https://doi.org/10.1038/nature13307.

144 **presented contradictory findings:** Michael J. Baum, "Sexual Differentiation of Pheromone Processing: Links to Male-Typical Mating Behavior and Partner Preference," in "50th Anniversary of the Publication of Phoenix, Goy, Gerall & Young 1959: Organizational Effects of Hormones," ed. Kim Wallen, special issue, *Hormones and Behavior* 55, no. 5 (May 2009): 579–88, https://doi.org/10.1016/j.yhbeh.2009.02.008.

144 **a general sense had hung on:** For a good discussion about the history of the science of sexual differentiation of the brain, see Margaret M. McCarthy and Arthur P. Arnold, "Reframing Sexual Differentiation of the Brain," *Nature Neuroscience* 14, no. 6 (June 2011): 677–83, https://doi.org/10.1038 /nn.2834. It's interesting to note that a lot of the early work on the parental brain also challenged the idea of separate circuits, separate sexes.

145 **For a very long time:** Rebecca M. Shansky and Anne Z. Murphy, "Considering Sex as a Biological Variable Will Require a Global Shift in Science Culture," *Nature Neuroscience* 24, no. 4 (April 2021): 457–64, https://doi.org/10 .1038/s41593-021-00806-8; Rebecca M. Shansky, "Are Hormones a 'Female

Problem' for Animal Research?," *Science* 364, no. 6443 (May 31, 2019): 825–26, https://doi.org/10.1126/science.aaw7570; Ann-Marie G. de Lange, Emily G. Jacobs, and Liisa A. M. Galea, "The Scientific Body of Knowledge: Whose Body Does It Serve? A Spotlight on Women's Brain Health," in "Beyond Sex Differences: A Spotlight on Women's Brain Health," ed. Liisa A. M. Galea, Emily G. Jacobs, and Ann-Marie G. de Lange, special issue, *Frontiers in Neuroendocrinology* 60 (January 2021): 100898, https://doi.org/10.1016/j.yfrne.2020.100898; and Liisa A. M. Galea, "Chasing Red Herrings and Wild Geese: Sex Differences versus Sex Dimorphism," *Frontiers in Neuroendocrinology* 63 (October 2021): 100940, https://doi.org/10.1016/j.yfrne.2021.100940.

145   **controversial voice:** Larry Cahill, "Equal ≠ the Same: Sex Differences in the Human Brain," *Cerebrum* (blog), Dana Foundation, April 1, 2014, https://www.dana.org/article/equal-≠-the-same-sex-differences-in-the-human-brain/; and Cordelia Fine, Daphna Joel, Rebecca Jordan-Young, Anelis Kaiser, and Gina Rippon, "Reaction to 'Equal ≠ the Same: Sex Differences in the Human Brain,'" *Cerebrum* (blog), Dana Foundation, December 15, 2014, https://dana.org/article/reaction-to-equal-≠-the-same-sex-differences-in-the-human-brain/.

145   **stronger average sense of smell:** Piotr Sorokowski et al., "Sex Differences in Human Olfaction: A Meta-Analysis," *Frontiers in Psychology* 10 (February 13, 2019): 242, https://doi.org/10.3389/fpsyg.2019.00242.

146   **As Catherine Woolley:** Catherine S. Woolley, "His and Hers: Sex Differences in the Brain," *Cerebrum* (blog), Dana Foundation, January 15, 2021, https://dana.org/article/cerebrum-sex-differences-in-the-brain/.

146   **"bipotential male and female":** Johannes Kohl, Anita E. Autry, and Catherine Dulac, "The Neurobiology of Parenting: A Neural Circuit Perspective," *BioEssays* 39, no. 1 (January 2017): 1–11, https://doi.org/10.1002/bies.201600159.

147   **Later, in 1996:** Jay S. Rosenblatt, Senator Hazelwood, and Jekeisa Poole, "Maternal Behavior in Male Rats: Effects of Medial Preoptic Area Lesions and Presence of Maternal Aggression," *Hormones and Behavior* 30, no. 3 (September 1996): 201–15, https://doi.org/10.1006/hbeh.1996.0025.

147   **circuits might be like levers:** Catherine Dulac, Lauren A. O'Connell, and Zheng Wu, "Neural Control of Maternal and Paternal Behaviors," *Science* 345, no. 6198 (August 15, 2014): 765–70, https://doi.org/10.1126/science.1253291.

149   **"facultative rather than obligate":** James K. Rilling and Jennifer S. Mascaro, "The Neurobiology of Fatherhood," in "Parenting," ed. Marinus H. van IJzendoorn and Marian J. Bakermans-Kranenburg, special issue, *Current Opinion in Psychology* 15 (June 1, 2017): 26–32, https://doi.org/10.1016/j.copsyc.2017.02.013.

150   **Sarah Blaffer Hrdy wrote:** Sarah Blaffer Hrdy, *Mothers and Others: The Evo-*

lutionary Origins of Mutual Understanding (Cambridge, MA: Belknap Press, 2009), 161–62.

150 **looked at case studies:** Ariel Ramchandani, "She Got Pregnant. His Body Changed Too," *Atlantic*, June 3, 2021, https://www.theatlantic.com /family/archive/2021/06/when-men-get-pregnancy-symptoms-couvade -syndrome/619083/.

150 **The syndrome is well documented:** Marian J. Bakermans-Kranenburg, Anna Lotz, Kim Alyousefi-van Dijk, and Marinus van IJzendoorn, "Birth of a Father: Fathering in the First 1,000 Days," *Child Development Perspectives* 13, no. 4 (December 2019): 247–53, https://doi.org/10.1111/cdep.12347; and Hrdy, *Mothers and Others*, 98.

150 **A study published in 2000:** Anne E. Storey, Carolyn J. Walsh, Roma L. Quinton, and Katherine E. Wynne-Edwards, "Hormonal Correlates of Paternal Responsiveness in New and Expectant Fathers," *Evolution and Human Behavior* 21, no. 2 (March 2000): 79–95, https://doi.org/10.1016 /S1090-5138(99)00042-2.

151 **increased interest:** Anne E. Storey, Hayley Alloway, and Carolyn J. Walsh, "Dads: Progress in Understanding the Neuroendocrine Basis of Human Fathering Behavior," in "50th Anniversary of Hormones and Behavior: Past Accomplishments and Future Directions in Behavioral Neuroendocrinology," ed. Cheryl McCormick, special issue, *Hormones and Behavior* 119 (March 2020): 104660, https://doi.org/10.1016/j.yhbeh.2019.104660.

151 **The pattern:** Nicholas M. Grebe et al., "Pair-Bonding, Fatherhood, and the Role of Testosterone: A Meta-Analytic Review," *Neuroscience & Biobehavioral Reviews* 98 (March 2019): 221–33, https://doi.org/10.1016/j.neubiorev .2019.01.010.

151 **Some of the strongest data:** Lee T. Gettler, Thomas W. McDade, Alan B. Feranil, and Christopher W. Kuzawa, "Longitudinal Evidence That Fatherhood Decreases Testosterone in Human Males," *Proceedings of the National Academy of Sciences* 108, no. 39 (September 27, 2011): 16194–99, https://doi .org/10.1073/pnas.1105403108.

152 **followed twenty-seven heterosexual couples:** Darby E. Saxbe, Robin S. Edelstein, Hannah M. Lyden, Britney M. Wardecker, William J. Chopik, and Amy C. Moors, "Fathers' Decline in Testosterone and Synchrony with Partner Testosterone during Pregnancy Predicts Greater Postpartum Relationship Investment," *Hormones and Behavior* 90 (April 2017): 39–47, https://doi.org/10.1016/j.yhbeh.2016.07.005.

152 **cortisol levels can change together:** Darby E. Saxbe, Emma K. Adam, Christine Dunkel Schetter, Christine M. Guardino, Clarissa Simon, Chelsea O. McKinney, and Madeleine U. Shalowitz, "Cortisol Covariation within Parents of Young Children: Moderation by Relationship Aggression," *Psychoneuroendocrinology* 62 (December 2015): 121–28, https://doi.org/10 .1016/j.psyneuen.2015.08.006.

153   **the authors reviewed:** Nicholas M. Grebe, Ruth E. Sarafin, Chance R.
      Strenth, and Samuele Zilioli, "Pair-Bonding, Fatherhood, and the Role
      of Testosterone: A Meta-Analytic Review," *Neuroscience & Biobehavioral
      Reviews* 98 (March 2019): 221–33, https://doi.org/10.1016/j.neubiorev.2019
      .01.010.

153   **In a separate meta-analysis:** Willemijn M. Meijer, Marinus H. van IJzen-
      doorn, and Marian J. Bakermans-Kranenburg, "Challenging the Challenge
      Hypothesis on Testosterone in Fathers: Limited Meta-Analytic Support,"
      Psychoneuroendocrinology 110 (December 2019): 104435, https://doi.org/10
      .1016/j.psyneuen.2019.104435.

153   **That narrative:** For a fuller discussion of the cultural myths attached to testos-
      terone and a counterargument that testosterone is the driver of male-typical
      behavior, see Cordelia Fine, *Testosterone Rex: Myths of Sex, Science, and Society*
      (New York: W. W. Norton, 2017); and Carole Hooven, *T: The Story of Testos-
      terone, the Hormone That Dominates and Divides Us* (New York: Henry Holt,
      2021).

154   **study particular hormones:** Janet Shibley Hyde, R. S. Bigler, D. Joel, C. C.
      Tate, and S. M. van Anders, "The Future of Sex and Gender in Psychol-
      ogy: Five Challenges to the Gender Binary," *American Psychologist* 74, no. 2
      (March 2019): 171–93, https://doi.org/10.1037/amp0000307.

154   **There is overlap:** Hyde et al., "Future of Sex and Gender in Psychology,"
      https://doi.org/10.1037/amp0000307. See Figure 2 in Paola Sapienza, Luigi
      Zingales, and Dario Maestripieri, "Gender Differences in Financial Risk
      Aversion and Career Choices Are Affected by Testosterone," *Proceedings of
      the National Academy of Sciences* 106, no. 36 (September 8, 2009): 15268–
      73, https://doi.org/10.1073/pnas.0907352106.

154   **held out as:** Hooven, *T: The Story of Testosterone,* 112.

154   **They determined that testosterone:** David J. Handelsman, Angelica L.
      Hirschberg, and Stephane Bermon, "Circulating Testosterone as the Hor-
      monal Basis of Sex Differences in Athletic Performance," *Endocrine Reviews*
      39, no. 5 (October 2018): 803–29, https://doi.org/10.1210/er.2018-00020.

155   **in healthy elite athletes:** Anthony C. Hackney, "Hypogonadism in Exercis-
      ing Males: Dysfunction or Adaptive-Regulatory Adjustment?," *Frontiers in
      Endocrinology* 11, no. 11 (January 31, 2020), https://doi.org/10.3389/fendo
      .2020.00011.

155   **Quantifying those differences:** Grebe et al., "Pair-Bonding, Fatherhood,
      and the Role of Testosterone," https://doi.org/10.1016/j.neubiorev.2019.01
      .010.

155   **The actors, men and women:** Sari M. van Anders, Jeffrey Steiger, and Kath-
      erine L. Goldey, "Effects of Gendered Behavior on Testosterone in Women
      and Men," *Proceedings of the National Academy of Sciences* 112, no. 45
      (November 10, 2015): 13805–10, https://doi.org/10.1073/pnas.1509591112.

156   **an important, malleable component:** Hyde et al., "Future of Sex and
      Gender in Psychology," https://doi.org/10.1037/amp0000307; and Sari M.

van Anders, Katherine L. Goldey, and Patty X. Kuo, "The Steroid/Peptide Theory of Social Bonds: Integrating Testosterone and Peptide Responses for Classifying Social Behavioral Contexts," *Psychoneuroendocrinology* 36, no. 9 (October 2011): 1265–75, https://doi.org/10.1016/j.psyneuen.2011.06.001.

156 **Fathers' circulating testosterone:** Van Anders, Goldey, and Kuo, "Steroid/Peptide Theory of Social Bonds," https://doi.org/10.1016/j.psyneuen.2011.06.001; Alison S. Fleming, Carl Corter, Joy Stallings, and Meir Steiner, "Testosterone and Prolactin Are Associated with Emotional Responses to Infant Cries in New Fathers," *Hormones and Behavior* 42, no. 4 (December 2002): 399–413, https://doi.org/10.1006/hbeh.2002.1840; and Storey, Alloway, and Walsh, "Dads," https://doi.org/10.1016/j.yhbeh.2019.104660.

156 **a more nuanced model:** Van Anders, Goldey, and Kuo, "Steroid/Peptide Theory of Social Bonds," https://doi.org/10.1016/j.psyneuen.2011.06.001.

157 **see major spikes:** Robin S. Edelstein, Britney M. Wardecker, William J. Chopik, Amy C. Moors, Emily L. Shipman, and Natalie J. Lin, "Prenatal Hormones in First-Time Expectant Parents: Longitudinal Changes and Within-Couple Correlations," *American Journal of Human Biology* 27, no. 3 (May/June 2015): 317–25, https://doi.org/10.1002/ajhb.22670.

157 **to levels lower than:** Emily S. Barrett, Van Tran, Sally Thurston, Grazyna Jasienska, Anne-Sofie Furberg, Peter T. Ellison, and Inger Thune, "Marriage and Motherhood Are Associated with Lower Testosterone Concentrations in Women," *Hormones and Behavior* 63, no. 1 (January 2013): 72–79, https://doi.org/10.1016/j.yhbeh.2012.10.012; and Christopher Kuzawa, Lee T. Gettler, Yuan-yen Huang, and Thomas W. McDade, "Mothers Have Lower Testosterone Than Non-Mothers: Evidence from the Philippines," *Hormones and Behavior* 57, no. 4–5 (April 2010): 441–47, https://doi.org/10.1016/j.yhbeh.2010.01.014.

157 **fatherhood has a protective effect:** Florencia Torche and Tamkinat Rauf, "The Transition to Fatherhood and the Health of Men," *Journal of Marriage and Family* 83, no. 2 (April 2021): 446–65, https://doi.org/10.1111/jomf.12732; Craig F. Garfield, Elizabeth Clark-Kauffman, and Matthew M. Davis, "Fatherhood as a Component of Men's Health," *JAMA* 296, no. 19 (November 15, 2006): 2365–68, https://doi.org/10.1001/jama.296.19.2365; and Gettler et al., "Longitudinal Evidence That Fatherhood Decreases Testosterone," https://doi.org/10.1073/pnas.1105403108.

157 **a critical transition period:** Darby Saxbe, Maya Rossin-Slater, and Diane Goldenberg, "The Transition to Parenthood as a Critical Window for Adult Health," *American Psychologist* 73, no. 9 (December 2018): 1190–200, https://doi.org/10.1037/amp0000376.

157 **Among 149 couples:** Darby E. Saxbe, Christine Dunkel Schetter, Clarissa D. Simon, Emma K. Adam, and Madeleine U. Shalowitz, "High Paternal Testosterone May Protect against Postpartum Depressive Symptoms in Fathers, but

Confer Risk to Mothers and Children," *Hormones and Behavior* 95 (September 2017): 103–12, https://doi.org/10.1016/j.yhbeh.2017.07.014.

158 **10 percent of men:** Jonathan R. Scarff, "Postpartum Depression in Men," *Innovations in Clinical Neuroscience* 16, no. 5–6 (May 1, 2019): 11–14.

159 **He and colleagues designed a study:** Jennifer S. Mascaro, Patrick D. Hackett, and James K. Rilling, "Differential Neural Responses to Child and Sexual Stimuli in Human Fathers and Non-Fathers and Their Hormonal Correlates," *Psychoneuroendocrinology* 46 (August 2014): 153–63, https://doi.org/10.1016/j.psyneuen.2014.04.014.

159 **Yet most studies look:** Storey, Alloway, and Walsh, "Dads," https://doi.org/10.1016/j.yhbeh.2019.104660.

159 **found differences in brain activity:** Mascaro, Hackett, and Rilling, "Differential Neural Responses to Child and Sexual Stimuli," https://doi.org/10.1016/j.psyneuen.2014.04.014.

161 **fathers of daughters:** Jennifer S. Mascaro, K. E. Rentscher, P. D. Hackett, M. R. Mehl, and J. K. Rilling, "Child Gender Influences Paternal Behavior, Language, and Brain Function," *Behavioral Neuroscience* 131, no. 3 (June 2017): 262–73, https://doi.org/10.1037/bne0000199.

161 **how a first-time father's reaction:** Ting Li, Marilyn Horta, Jennifer S. Mascaro, Kelly Bijanki, Luc H. Arnal, Melissa Adams, Ronald G. Barr, and James K. Rilling, "Explaining Individual Variation in Paternal Brain Responses to Infant Cries," in "Evolutionary Perspectives on Non-Maternal Care in Mammals: Physiology, Behavior, and Developmental Effects," ed. Stacy Rosenbaum and Lee T. Gettler, special issue, *Physiology & Behavior* 193, part A (September 1, 2018): 43–54, https://doi.org/10.1016/j.physbeh.2017.12.033.

161 **small study of twenty new fathers:** James K. Rilling, Lynnet Richey, Elissar Andari, and Stephan Hamann, "The Neural Correlates of Paternal Consoling Behavior and Frustration in Response to Infant Crying," *Developmental Psychobiology* 63, no. 5 (July 2021): 1370–83, https://doi.org/10.1002/dev.22092.

161 **"along a continuum":** James K. Rilling, "The Neural and Hormonal Bases of Human Parental Care," *Neuropsychologia* 51, no. 4 (March 2013): 731–47, https://doi.org/10.1016/j.neuropsychologia.2012.12.017.

161 **A few studies have been published:** Pilyoung Kim, Paola Rigo, Linda C. Mayes, Ruth Feldman, James F. Leckman, and James E. Swain, "Neural Plasticity in Fathers of Human Infants," *Social Neuroscience* 9, no. 5 (October 2014): 522–35, https://doi.org/10.1080/17470919.2014.933713; María Paternina-Die, Magdalena Martínez-García, Clara Pretus, Elseline Hoekzema, Erika Barba-Müller, Daniel Martín de Blas, Cristina Pozzobon, et al., "The Paternal Transition Entails Neuroanatomic Adaptations That Are Associated with the Father's Brain Response to His Infant Cues," *Cerebral Cortex Communications* 1, no. 1 (November 4, 2020), https://doi.org/10.1093/texcom/tgaa082; and Françoise Diaz-Rojas, Michiko Matsunaga, Yukari Tanaka, Takefumi Kikusui, Kazutaka Mogi, Miho Nagasawa, Kohei

Asano, Nobuhito Abe, and Masako Myowa, "Development of the Paternal Brain in Expectant Fathers during Early Pregnancy," *NeuroImage* 225 (January 15, 2021): 117527, https://doi.org/10.1016/j.neuroimage.2020.117527.

162   **One early, exploratory paper:** Damion J. Grasso, Jason S. Moser, Mary Dozier, and Robert Simons, "ERP Correlates of Attention Allocation in Mothers Processing Faces of Their Children," *Biological Psychology* 81, no. 2 (May 2009): 95–102, https://doi.org/10.1016/j.biopsycho.2009.03.001.

162   **Within a larger group of foster mothers:** Johanna Bick, Mary Dozier, Kristin Bernard, Damion Grasso, and Robert Simons, "Foster Mother-Infant Bonding: Associations between Foster Mothers' Oxytocin Production, Electrophysiological Brain Activity, Feelings of Commitment, and Caregiving Quality," *Child Development* 84, no. 3 (May/June 2013): 826–40, https://doi.org/10.1111/cdev.12008.

163   **those findings came from a study:** Eyal Abraham, Talma Hendler, Irit Shapira-Lichter, Yaniv Kanat-Maymon, Orna Zagoory-Sharon, and Ruth Feldman, "Father's Brain Is Sensitive to Childcare Experiences," *Proceedings of the National Academy of Sciences* 111, no. 27 (July 8, 2014): 9792–97, https://doi.org/10.1073/pnas.1402569111.

163   **a global parental caregiving network:** Abraham et al., "Father's Brain Is Sensitive to Childcare Experiences," https://doi.org/10.1073/pnas.1402569111.

164   **Lesbians also have received:** Kristi Chin, William J. Chopik, Britney M. Wardecker, Onawa P. LaBelle, Amy C. Moors, and Robin S. Edelstein, "Longitudinal Associations between Prenatal Testosterone and Postpartum Outcomes in a Sample of First-Time Expectant Lesbian Couples," *Hormones and Behavior* 125 (September 2020): 104810, https://doi.org/10.1016/j.yhbeh.2020.104810.

168   **In a recent essay:** Thomas Page McBee, "What I Saw in My First 10 Years on Testosterone," *New York Times*, June 25, 2021, https://www.nytimes.com/2021/06/25/opinion/transgender-transition-testosterone.html.

170   **There is a backlash:** Benjamin Fearnow, "Biden Admin Replaces 'Mothers' with 'Birthing People' in Maternal Health Guidance," *Newsweek*, June 7, 2021, https://www.newsweek.com/biden-admin-replaces-mothers-birthing-people-maternal-health-guidance-1598343; John Kass, "Why Are We Calling Mothers 'Birthing Persons'?," *Baltimore Sun*, June 21, 2021, https://www.baltimoresun.com/opinion/op-ed/bs-ed-op-0621-katz-birthing-mothers-20210621-4lvc7jtpnrd37ci24oikwattc4-story.html; and Rosie Kinchen, "Antenatal Guru Milli Hill Dropped by Charity after Insisting: It's 'Women,' Not 'Birthing People,'" *Sunday Times*, July 11, 2021, https://www.thetimes.co.uk/article/antenatal-guru-milli-hill-dropped-by-charity-after-insisting-its-women-not-birthing-people-ncl88m8gx.

170   **a demeanor inspired by:** Christi Carras, "'The Mandalorian' Star Pedro Pascal Channeled Han Solo and Clint Eastwood for Disney+," *Los Angeles Times*, August 26, 2019, https://www.latimes.com/entertainment-arts/tv/story/2019-08-26/mandalorian-pedro-pascal-star-wars-disney-plus.

CHAPTER 7: START WHERE YOU ARE

174 **Between them is:** The following paper has a good representation of this spectrum in Fig. 1, though I'm unconvinced that "perinatal stress" is a separate affective state. Stress, to me, seems to be an innate part of the transition to parenthood that has variable effects across the continuum of parenting experiences. Sofia Rallis, Helen Skouteris, Marita McCabe, and Jeannette Milgrom, "The Transition to Motherhood: Towards a Broader Understanding of Perinatal Distress," *Women and Birth* 27, no. 1 (March 2014): 68–71, https://doi.org/10.1016/j.wombi.2013.12.004.

175 **thought to affect one in five:** This is a widely used statistic, but spend any time looking at prevalence and incidence data and you'll see that it varies quite a bit from study to study, with different criteria related to severity and time frame, and wide differences depending on the population studied, their access to health care, and perhaps the degree of stigma associated with reporting symptoms. Most studies look primarily at depressive symptoms. The 2014 analysis from O'Hara and Wisner, below, made perhaps the most important point: "All of these reviews and empirical studies conclude that depression is common during pregnancy and after delivery in developing and developed countries." Michael W. O'Hara and Katherine L. Wisner, "Perinatal Mental Illness: Definition, Description and Aetiology," in "Perinatal Mental Health: Guidance for the Obstetrician-Gynaecologist," ed. Michael W. O'Hara, Katherine L. Wisner, and Gerald F. Joseph Jr., special issue, *Best Practice & Research Clinical Obstetrics & Gynaecology* 28, no. 1 (January 2014): 3–12, https://doi.org/10.1016/j.bpobgyn.2013.09.002; Dara Lee Luca, Caroline Margiotta, Colleen Staatz, Eleanor Garlow, Anna Christensen, and Kara Zivin, "Financial Toll of Untreated Perinatal Mood and Anxiety Disorders among 2017 Births in the United States," *American Journal of Public Health* 110, no. 6 (June 2020): 888–96, https://doi.org/10.2105/AJPH.2020.305619; Jean Ko, Karilynn M. Rockhill, Van T. Tong, Brian Morrow, and Sherry L. Farr, "Trends in Postpartum Depressive Symptoms—27 States, 2004, 2008, and 2012," *Morbidity and Mortality Weekly Report* 66, no. 6 (February 17, 2017): 153–58, https://doi.org/10.15585/mmwr.mm6606a1; and Louise M. Howard, Emma Molyneaux, Cindy-Lee Dennis, Tamsen Rochat, Alan Stein, and Jeannette Milgrom, "Non-Psychotic Mental Disorders in the Perinatal Period," *Lancet* 384, no. 9956 (November 15, 2014): 1775–88, https://doi.org/10.1016/S0140-6736(14)61276-9.

176 **the bible of psychiatry:** Ferris Jabr, "The Newest Edition of Psychiatry's 'Bible,' the *DSM-5*, Is Complete," *Scientific American*, January 28, 2013, https://www.scientificamerican.com/article/dsm-5-update/.

176 **it's widely accepted:** Samantha Meltzer-Brody and Stephen J. Kanes, "Allopregnanolone in Postpartum Depression: Role in Pathophysiology and Treatment," in "Allopregnanolone Role in the Neurobiology of Stress and

Mood Disorders," ed. Graziano Pinna, special issue, *Neurobiology of Stress* 12 (February 3, 2020): 100212, https://doi.org/10.1016/j.ynstr.2020.100212.

176 **followed hundreds of women:** J. A. Kountanis, M. Muzik, T. Chang, E. Langen, R. Cassidy, G. A. Mashour, and M. E. Bauer, "Relationship between Postpartum Mood Disorder and Birth Experience: A Prospective Observational Study," *International Journal of Obstetric Anesthesia* 44 (November 1, 2020): 90–99, https://doi.org/10.1016/j.ijoa.2020.07.008.

176 **Scientists have begun:** Liisa A. M. Galea and Vibe G. Frokjaer, "Perinatal Depression: Embracing Variability toward Better Treatment and Outcomes," *Neuron* 102, no. 1 (April 3, 2019): 13–16, https://doi.org/10.1016/j.neuron.2019.02.023.

176 **And while postpartum generally shares:** Elizabeth O'Connor, Caitlyn A. Senger, Michelle L. Henninger, Erin Coppola, and Bradley N. Gaynes, "Interventions to Prevent Perinatal Depression: Evidence Report and Systematic Review for the US Preventive Services Task Force," *JAMA* 321, no. 6 (February 12, 2019): 588–601, https://doi.org/10.1001/jama.2018.20865.

176 **postpartum bipolar disorder:** Katherine L. Wisner, Dorothy K. Y. Sit, Mary C. McShea, David M. Rizzo, Rebecca A. Zoretich, Carolyn L. Hughes, Heather F. Eng, et al., "Onset Timing, Thoughts of Self-Harm, and Diagnoses in Postpartum Women with Screen-Positive Depression Findings," *JAMA Psychiatry* 70, no. 5 (May 2013): 490–98, https://doi.org/10.1001/jamapsychiatry.2013.87.

176 **the toll that depression can take:** Alan Stein, Rebecca M. Pearson, Sherryl H. Goodman, Elizabeth Rapa, Atif Rahman, Meaghan McCallum, Louise M. Howard, and Carmine M. Pariante, "Effects of Perinatal Mental Disorders on the Fetus and Child," *Lancet* 384, no. 9956 (November 15, 2014): 1800–819, https://doi.org/10.1016/S0140-6736(14)61277-0.

177 **Suicide is a leading cause:** Jacquelyn Campbell, Sabrina Matoff-Stepp, Martha L. Velez, Helen Hunter Cox, and Kathryn Laughon, "Pregnancy-Associated Deaths from Homicide, Suicide, and Drug Overdose: Review of Research and the Intersection with Intimate Partner Violence," in "Maternal Mortality and Morbidity," special issue, *Journal of Women's Health* 30, no. 2 (February 2021): 236–44, https://doi.org/10.1089/jwh.2020.8875; V. Lindahl, J. L. Pearson, and L. Colpe, "Prevalence of Suicidality during Pregnancy and the Postpartum," *Archives of Women's Mental Health* 8, no. 2 (May 11, 2005): 77–87, https://doi.org/10.1007/s00737-005-0080-1; Lindsay K. Admon, Vanessa K. Dalton, Giselle E. Kolenic, Susan L. Ettner, Anca Tilea, Rebecca L. Haffajee, Rebecca M. Brownlee, et al., "Trends in Suicidality 1 Year before and after Birth among Commercially Insured Childbearing Individuals in the United States, 2006–2017," *JAMA Psychiatry* 78, no. 2 (November 18, 2020): 171–76, https://doi.org/10.1001/jamapsychiatry.2020.3550; and Susan Bodnar-Deren, Kimberly Klipstein, Madeleine Fersh, Eyal Shemesh, and Elizabeth A. Howell, "Suicidal Ideation during

the Postpartum Period," *Journal of Women's Health* 25, no. 12 (December 1, 2016): 1219–24, https://doi.org/10.1089/jwh.2015.5346.

177   **a "critical window":** Darby Saxbe, Maya Rossin-Slater, and Diane Goldenberg, "The Transition to Parenthood as a Critical Window for Adult Health," *American Psychologist* 73, no. 9 (December 2018): 1190–200, https://doi.org /10.1037/amp0000376.

177   **About 40 percent of people:** Wisner et al., "Onset Timing, Thoughts of Self-Harm, and Diagnoses," https://doi.org/10.1001/jamapsychiatry.2013.87.

177   **increases a person's risk:** A. Josefsson and G. Sydsjö, "A Follow-Up Study of Postpartum Depressed Women: Recurrent Maternal Depressive Symptoms and Child Behavior after Four Years," *Archives of Women's Mental Health* 10, no. 4 (August 2007): 141–45, https://doi.org/10.1007/s00737-007-0185-9.

178   **They analyzed 291 studies:** Jennifer Hahn-Holbrook, Taylor Cornwell-Hinrichs, and Itzel Anaya, "Economic and Health Predictors of National Postpartum Depression Prevalence: A Systematic Review, Meta-Analysis, and Meta-Regression of 291 Studies from 56 Countries," *Frontiers in Psychiatry* 8 (February 2018): 248, https://doi.org/10.3389/fpsyt.2017.00248.

178   **international consortium:** Postpartum Depression: Action Towards Causes and Treatment (PACT) Consortium, "Heterogeneity of Postpartum Depression: A Latent Class Analysis," *Lancet Psychiatry* 2, no. 1 (January 2015): 59–67, https://doi.org/10.1016/S2215-0366(14)00055-8; and Karen T. Putnam, Marsha Wilcox, Emma Robertson-Blackmore, Katherine Sharkey, Veerle Bergink, Trine Munk-Olsen, Kristina M. Deligiannidis, et al., "Clinical Phenotypes of Perinatal Depression and Time of Symptom Onset: Analysis of Data from an International Consortium," *Lancet Psychiatry* 4, no. 6 (June 2017): 477–85, https://doi.org/10.1016 /S2215-0366(17)30136-0.

180   **In people with serious depressive symptoms:** Amanda J. Nguyen, Elisabeth Hoyer, Purva Rajhans, Lane Strathearn, and Sohye Kim, "A Tumultuous Transition to Motherhood: Altered Brain and Hormonal Responses in Mothers with Postpartum Depression," in "Papers from the Parental Brain 2018 Meeting, Toronto, Canada, July 2018," ed. Jodi L. Pawluski, Frances A. Champagne, and Oliver J. Bosch, special issue, *Journal of Neuroendocrinology* 31, no. 9 (September 2019): e12794, https://doi.org/10.1111/jne .12794.

180   **That's opposite from the hyperreactive effect:** E. L. Moses-Kolko, M. S. Horner, M. L. Phillips, A. E. Hipwell, and J. E. Swain, "In Search of Neural Endophenotypes of Postpartum Psychopathology and Disrupted Maternal Caregiving," in "Reviews from the 5th Parental Brain Conference, Regensburg, Germany, 11th–14th of July 2013," special issue, *Journal of Neuroendocrinology* 26, no. 10 (2014): 665–84, https://doi.org/10.1111/jne .12183.

180   **a pair of fascinating studies:** Aya Dudin, Kathleen E. Wonch, Andrew D.

Davis, Meir Steiner, Alison S. Fleming, and Geoffrey B. Hall, "Amygdala and Affective Responses to Infant Pictures: Comparing Depressed and Non-Depressed Mothers and Non-Mothers," in "Papers from the Parental Brain 2018 Meeting, Toronto, Canada, July 2018," special issue, *Journal of Neuroendocrinology* 31, no. 9 (September 2019): e12790, https://doi.org/10.1111/jne .12790; and Kathleen E. Wonch, Cynthia B. de Medeiros, Jennifer A. Barrett, Aya Dudin, William A. Cunningham, Geoffrey B. Hall, Meir Steiner, and Alison S. Fleming, "Postpartum Depression and Brain Response to Infants: Differential Amygdala Response and Connectivity," *Social Neuroscience* 11, no. 6 (December 2016): 600–17, https://doi.org/10.1080/17470919.2015 .1131193.

180 **Other studies have tried to pinpoint:** Jodi L. Pawluski, James E. Swain, and Joseph S. Lonstein, "Neurobiology of Peripartum Mental Illness," in *Handbook of Clinical Neurology,* vol. 182, *The Human Hypothalamus: Neuropsychiatric Disorders,* ed. Dick F. Swaab, Ruud M. Bujis, Felix Kreier, Paul J. Lucassen, and Ahmad Salehi (Amsterdam: Elsevier, 2021), 63–82, https:// doi.org/10.1016/B978-0-12-819973-2.00005-8; and Nguyen et al., "Tumultuous Transition to Motherhood," https://doi.org/10.1111/jne.12794.

180 **Because a person *can* be:** Chaohui Guo, Eydie Moses Kolko, Mary Phillips, James E. Swain, and Alison E. Hipwell, "Severity of Anxiety Moderates the Association between Neural Circuits and Maternal Behaviors in the Postpartum Period," *Cognitive, Affective, & Behavioral Neuroscience* 18, no. 3 (June 2018): 426–36, https://doi.org/10.3758/s13415-017-0516-x.

181 **"reciprocal inhibition":** Pawluski, Swain, and Lonstein, "Neurobiology of Peripartum Mental Illness," https://doi.org/10.1016/B978-0-12-819973 -2.00005-8; James E. Swain, S. Shaun Ho, Helen Fox, David Garry, and Susanne Brummelte, "Effects of Opioids on the Parental Brain in Health and Disease," *Frontiers in Neuroendocrinology* 54 (July 2019): 100766, https://doi.org/10.1016/j.yfrne.2019.100766; and Zheng Wu, Anita E. Autry, Joseph E. Bergan, Mitsuko Watabe-Uchida, and Catherine G. Dulac, "Galanin Neurons in the Medial Preoptic Area Govern Parental Behaviour," *Nature* 509, no. 7500 (May 2014): 325–30, https://doi.org/10 .1038/nature13307.

181 **a growing acknowledgment:** Pilyoung Kim, "How Stress Can Influence Brain Adaptations to Motherhood," *Frontiers in Neuroendocrinology* 60 (January 2021): 100875, https://doi.org/10.1016/j.yfrne.2020.100875; Mayra L. Almanza-Sepulveda, Alison S. Fleming, and Wibke Jonas, "Mothering Revisited: A Role for Cortisol?" in "50th Anniversary of Hormones and Behavior: Past Accomplishments and Future Directions in Behavioral Neuroendocrinology," ed. Cheryl McCormick, special issue, *Hormones and Behavior* 121 (May 1, 2020): 104679, https://doi.org/10.1016/j.yhbeh.2020 .104679; and Molly J. Dickens, Jodi L. Pawluski, and L. Michael Romero, "Moving Forward from COVID-19: Bridging Knowledge Gaps in Maternal

Health with a New Conceptual Model," *Frontiers in Global Women's Health* 1 (2020): 586697, https://doi.org/10.3389/fgwh.2020.586697.

182   **Cortisol is a change agent:** Bruce S. McEwen, "What Is the Confusion with Cortisol?," *Chronic Stress* 3 (February 2019): 2470547019833647, https://doi.org/10.1177/2470547019833647.

182   **In people with chronic stress:** McEwen, "What Is the Confusion with Cortisol?," https://doi.org/10.1177/2470547019833647; and Almanza-Sepulveda, Fleming, and Jonas, "Mothering Revisited," https://doi.org/10.1016/j.yhbeh.2020.104679.

182   **Psychiatric disorders related to chronic stress:** Christopher Pittenger and Ronald S. Duman, "Stress, Depression, and Neuroplasticity: A Convergence of Mechanisms," *Neuropsychopharmacology* 33 (January 2008): 88–109, https://doi.org/10.1038/sj.npp.1301574; and Bruce S. McEwen and Peter J. Gianaros, "Stress- and Allostasis-Induced Brain Plasticity," *Annual Review of Medicine* 62 (February 2011): 431–45, https://doi.org/10.1146/annurev-med-052209-100430.

182   **neuroscientist Bruce McEwen:** Randi Hutter Epstein, "Bruce McEwen, 81, Is Dead; Found Stress Can Alter the Brain," *New York Times*, February 10, 2020, https://www.nytimes.com/2020/02/10/science/bruce-s-mcewen-dead.html; and Matthew N. Hill, Ilia N. Karatsoreos, E. Ron de Kloet, Sonia Lupien, and Catherine S. Woolley, "In Memory of Bruce McEwen: A Gentle Giant of Neuroscience," *Nature Neuroscience* 23, no. 4 (April 2020): 473–74, https://doi.org/10.1038/s41593-020-0613-y.

183   **He expanded on the idea:** Bruce S. McEwen, "Protective and Damaging Effects of Stress Mediators," *New England Journal of Medicine* 338, no. 3 (January 15, 1998): 171–79, https://doi.org/10.1056/NEJM199801153380307.

183   **Central to McEwen's thinking:** McEwen, "What Is the Confusion with Cortisol?," https://doi.org/10.1177/2470547019833647; and McEwen and Gianaros, "Stress- and Allostasis-Induced Brain Plasticity," https://doi.org/10.1146/annurev-med-052209-100430.

183   **Plasma cortisol in the third trimester:** Caroline Jung, Jui T. Ho, David J. Torpy, Anne Rogers, Matt Doogue, John G. Lewis, Raymond J. Czajko, and Warrick J. Inder, "A Longitudinal Study of Plasma and Urinary Cortisol in Pregnancy and Postpartum," *Journal of Clinical Endocrinology & Metabolism* 96, no. 5 (May 1, 2011): 1533–40, https://doi.org/10.1210/jc.2010-2395.

183   **Cortisol is thought to aid:** Elizabeth C. Braithwaite, Susannah E. Murphy, and Paul G. Ramchandani, "Effects of Prenatal Depressive Symptoms on Maternal and Infant Cortisol Reactivity," *Archives of Women's Mental Health* 19, no. 4 (August 2016): 581–90, https://doi.org/10.1007/s00737-016-0611-y; Almanza-Sepulveda, Fleming, and Jonas, "Mothering Revisited," https://doi.org/10.1016/j.yhbeh.2020.104679; and Molly J. Dickens and Jodi L. Pawluski, "The HPA Axis during the Perinatal Period: Implications for Perinatal Depression," *Endocrinology* 159, no. 11 (November 2018): 3737–46, https://doi.org/10.1210/en.2018-00677.

183 **it plays a role:** Alison S. Fleming, Meir Steiner, and Carl Corter, "Cortisol, Hedonics, and Maternal Responsiveness in Human Mothers," *Hormones and Behavior* 32, no. 2 (October 1997): 85–98, https://doi.org/10.1006 /hbeh.1997.1407; Alison S. Fleming, Meir Steiner, and Veanne Anderson, "Hormonal and Attitudinal Correlates of Maternal Behaviour during the Early Postpartum Period in First-Time Mothers," *Journal of Reproductive and Infant Psychology* 5, no. 4 (1987): 193–205, https://doi.org/10.1080 /02646838708403495; Joy Stallings, Alison S. Fleming, Carl Corter, Carol Worthman, and Meir Steiner, "The Effects of Infant Cries and Odors on Sympathy, Cortisol, and Autonomic Responses in New Mothers and Non-postpartum Women," *Parenting* 1, no. 1–2 (2001): 71–100, https://doi.org /10.1080/15295192.2001.9681212; and Almanza-Sepulveda, Fleming, and Jonas, "Mothering Revisited," https://doi.org/10.1016/j.yhbeh.2020 .104679.

184 **new fathers:** Alison S. Fleming, Carl Corter, Joy Stallings, and Meir Steiner, "Testosterone and Prolactin Are Associated with Emotional Responses to Infant Cries in New Fathers," *Hormones and Behavior* 42, no. 4 (December 2002): 399–413, https://doi.org/10.1006/hbeh.2002.1840.

184 **shape early caregiving experiences:** M. Dean Graham, Stephanie L. Rees, Meir Steiner, and Alison S. Fleming, "The Effects of Adrenalectomy and Corticosterone Replacement on Maternal Memory in Postpartum Rats," *Hormones and Behavior* 49, no. 3 (March 2006): 353–61, https://doi.org/10 .1016/j.yhbeh.2005.08.014.

184 **Mothers with higher daily cortisol:** Andrea Gonzalez, Jennifer M. Jenkins, Meir Steiner, and Alison S. Fleming, "Maternal Early Life Experiences and Parenting: The Mediating Role of Cortisol and Executive Function," *Journal of the American Academy of Child & Adolescent Psychiatry* 51, no. 7 (July 1, 2012): 673–82, https://doi.org/10.1016/j.jaac.2012.04.003.

184 **the evidence on this:** Almanza-Sepulveda, Fleming, and Jonas, "Mothering Revisited," https://doi.org/10.1016/j.yhbeh.2020.104679.

184 **the HPA function of birthing parents and babies:** Almanza-Sepulveda, Fleming, and Jonas, "Mothering Revisited," https://doi.org/10.1016/j.yhbeh. 2020.104679.

184 **too much variation:** Sunaina Seth, Andrew J. Lewis, and Megan Galbally, "Perinatal Maternal Depression and Cortisol Function in Pregnancy and the Postpartum Period: A Systematic Literature Review," *BMC Pregnancy and Childbirth* 16, no. 1 (May 31, 2016): 124, https://doi.org/10.1186/s12884 -016-0915-y.

185 **Pregnancy seems to make this GABA activity:** Meltzer-Brody and Kanes, "Allopregnanolone in Postpartum Depression," https://doi.org/10.1016/j .ynstr.2020.100212; Jennifer L. Payne and Jamie Maguire, "Pathophysiological Mechanisms Implicated in Postpartum Depression," *Frontiers in Neuroendocrinology* 52 (January 2019): 165–80, https://doi.org/10.1016/j.yfrne.2018.12 .001; Jamie Maguire and Istvan Mody, "GABA$_A$R Plasticity during Pregnancy:

Relevance to Postpartum Depression," *Neuron* 59, no. 2 (July 31, 2008): 207–13, https://doi.org/10.1016/j.neuron.2008.06.019; and Pawluski, Swain, and Lonstein, "Neurobiology of Peripartum Mental Illness," https://doi.org/10.1016/B978-0-12-819973-2.00005-8.

185 **a tricky balance:** Maguire and Mody, "GABA$_A$R Plasticity during Pregnancy," https://doi.org/10.1016/j.neuron.2008.06.019; Istvan Mody and Jamie Maguire, "The Reciprocal Regulation of Stress Hormones and GABA$_A$ Receptors," *Frontiers in Cellular Neuroscience* 6 (January 30, 2012): 4, https://doi.org/10.3389/fncel.2012.00004; and Jamie Maguire and Istvan Mody, "Behavioral Deficits in Juveniles Mediated by Maternal Stress Hormones in Mice," in "The Many Faces of Stress: Implications for Neuropsychiatric Disorders," ed. Laura Musazzi and Jordan Marrocco, special issue, *Neural Plasticity* 2016 (2016): 2762518, https://doi.org/10.1155/2016/2762518.

186 **the body experiences a withdrawal state:** Miki Bloch, Peter J. Schmidt, Merry Danaceau, Jean Murphy, Lynnette Nieman, and David R. Rubinow, "Effects of Gonadal Steroids in Women with a History of Postpartum Depression," *American Journal of Psychiatry* 157, no. 6 (June 1, 2000): 924–30, https://doi.org/10.1176/appi.ajp.157.6.924; and Susanne Brummelte and Liisa A. M. Galea, "Postpartum Depression: Etiology, Treatment and Consequences for Maternal Care," in "Parental Care," ed. Alison S. Fleming, Frederic Lévy, and Joe S. Lonstein, special issue, *Hormones and Behavior* 77 (January 2016): 153–66, https://doi.org/10.1016/j.yhbeh.2015.08.008.

186 **based on animal literature:** Jodi L. Pawluski, Elseline Hoekzema, Benedetta Leuner, and Joseph S. Lonstein, "Less Can Be More: Fine Tuning the Maternal Brain," *Neuroscience & Biobehavioral Reviews* (journal pre-proof) (2021), https://doi.org/10.1016/j.neubiorev.2021.11.045.

186 **first identified:** Fleming, Steiner, and Anderson, "Hormonal and Attitudinal Correlates of Maternal Behaviour," https://doi.org/10.1080/02646838708403495.

186 **"bimodal effect":** A. M. Lomanowska, M. Boivin, C. Hertzman, and A. S. Fleming, "Parenting Begets Parenting: A Neurobiological Perspective on Early Adversity and the Transmission of Parenting Styles across Generations," in "Early Adversity and Brain Development," ed. Susanne Brummelte, special issue, *Neuroscience* 342 (February 7, 2017): 120–39, https://doi.org/10.1016/j.neuroscience.2015.09.029; and Joseph S. Lonstein, Frédéric Lévy, and Alison S. Fleming, "Common and Divergent Psychobiological Mechanisms Underlying Maternal Behaviors in Non-Human and Human Mammals," *Hormones and Behavior* 73 (July 2015): 156–85, https://doi.org/10.1016/j.yhbeh.2015.06.011.

186 **Fleming recently coauthored:** Almanza-Sepulveda, Fleming, and Jonas, "Mothering Revisited," https://doi.org/10.1016/j.yhbeh.2020.104679.

187 **since the pandemic started:** In more typical years, the mothers would share a meal at the start of each session and bring their children along, with free

childcare provided. Sometimes the setup provided opportunities for real-time practice in navigating stressful moments with kids.

188 **the animal research has acknowledged:** Alison S. Fleming and Gary W. Kraemer, "Molecular and Genetic Bases of Mammalian Maternal Behavior," *Gender and the Genome* 3 (February 2019): 1–14; and Ian C. G. Weaver, Nadia Cervoni, Frances A. Champagne, Ana C. D'Alessio, Shakti Sharma, Jonathan R. Seckl, Sergiy Dymov, Moshe Szyf, and Michael J. Meaney, "Epigenetic Programming by Maternal Behavior," *Nature Neuroscience* 7, no. 8 (August 2004): 847–54, https://doi.org/10.1038/nn1276.

188 **parenting has a physiological basis:** Gonzalez et al., "Maternal Early Life Experiences and Parenting," https://doi.org/10.1016/j.jaac.2012.04.003.

188 **A large body of evidence:** Michelle R. VanTieghem and Nim Tottenham, "Neurobiological Programming of Early Life Stress: Functional Development of Amygdala-Prefrontal Circuitry and Vulnerability for Stress-Related Psychopathology," in *Current Topics in Behavioral Neurosciences*, vol. 38, *Behavioral Neurobiology of PTSD*, ed. Eric Vermetten, Dewleen G. Baker, and Victoria B. Risbrough (Cham, Switzerland: Springer, 2018), 117–36, https://link.springer.com/chapter/10.1007/7854_2016_42.

188 **researchers have tried sorting out:** Kim, "How Stress Can Influence Brain Adaptations to Motherhood," https://doi.org/10.1016/j.yfrne.2020.100875; Pilyoung Kim, James F. Leckman, Linda C. Mayes, Michal-Ann Newman, Ruth Feldman, and James E. Swain, "Perceived Quality of Maternal Care in Childhood and Structure and Function of Mothers' Brain," *Developmental Science* 13, no. 4 (July 2010): 662–73, https://doi.org/10.1111/j.1467-7687.2009.00923.x; and Aviva K. Olsavsky, Joel Stoddard, Andrew Erhart, Rebekah Tribble, and Pilyoung Kim, "Neural Processing of Infant and Adult Face Emotion and Maternal Exposure to Childhood Maltreatment," *Social Cognitive and Affective Neuroscience* 14, no. 9 (September 2019): 997–1008, https://doi.org/10.1093/scan/nsz069.

188 **One study compared:** Emilia L. Mielke, Corinne Neukel, Katja Bertsch, Corinna Reck, Eva Möhler, and Sabine C. Herpertz, "Maternal Sensitivity and the Empathic Brain: Influences of Early Life Maltreatment," *Journal of Psychiatric Research* 77 (June 2016): 59–66, https://doi.org/10.1016/j.jpsychires.2016.02.013.

189 **Kim's lab scanned the brains of:** Pilyoung Kim, Rebekah Tribble, Aviva K. Olsavsky, Alexander J. Dufford, Andrew Erhart, Melissa Hansen, Leah Grande, and Daniel M. Gonzalez, "Associations between Stress Exposure and New Mothers' Brain Responses to Infant Cry Sounds," *NeuroImage* 223 (December 2020): 117360, https://doi.org/10.1016/j.neuroimage.2020.117360.

189 **their exposure:** VanTieghem and Tottenham, "Neurobiological Programming of Early Life Stress," https://doi.org/10.1007/7854_2016_42.

189 **Kim in particular has called for:** Kim, "How Stress Can Influence Brain Adaptations to Motherhood," https://doi.org/10.1016/j.yfrne.2020.100875.

190   **There is no certain story line:** Helena J. V. Rutherford, Sohye Kim, Sarah W.
      Yip, Marc N. Potenza, Linda C. Mayes, and Lane Strathearn, "Parenting and
      Addictions: Current Insights from Human Neuroscience," *Current Addic-
      tion Reports* 8 (September 2021): 380–88, https://doi.org/10.1007/s40429
      -021-00384-6.

190   **especially potent:** Helena J. V. Rutherford and Linda C. Mayes, "Parenting
      Stress: A Novel Mechanism of Addiction Vulnerability," in "Stress and Sub-
      stance Abuse throughout Development," ed. Roger Sorensen, Da-Yu Wu,
      Karen Sirocco, Cora lee Wetherington, and Rita Valentino, special issue,
      Neurobiology of Stress 11 (November 1, 2019): 100172, https://doi.org/10
      .1016/j.ynstr.2019.100172.

190   **recent systematic reviews:** Karen Milligan, Tamara Meixner, Monique
      Tremblay, Lesley A. Tarasoff, Amelia Usher, Ainsley Smith, Alison Niccols,
      and Karen A. Urbanoski, "Parenting Interventions for Mothers with Prob-
      lematic Substance Use: A Systematic Review of Research and Community
      Practice," *Child Maltreatment* 25, no. 3 (August 2020): 247–62, https://doi
      .org/10.1177/1077559519873047; and Allison L. West, Sarah Dauber, Laina
      Gagliardi, Leeya Correll, Alexandra Cirillo Lilli, and Jane Daniels, "Sys-
      tematic Review of Community- and Home-Based Interventions to Support
      Parenting and Reduce Risk of Child Maltreatment among Families with
      Substance-Exposed Newborns," *Child Maltreatment* 25, no. 2 (May 2020):
      137–51, https://doi.org/10.1177/1077559519866272.

191   **Mothering from the Inside Out:** Amanda F. Lowell, Elizabeth Peacock-
      Chambers, Amanda Zayde, Cindy L. DeCoste, Thomas J. McMahon, and
      Nancy E. Suchman, "Mothering from the Inside Out: Addressing the Inter-
      section of Addiction, Adversity, and Attachment with Evidence-Based Par-
      enting Intervention," *Current Addiction Reports* (July 15, 2021): 605–15,
      https://doi.org/10.1007/s40429-021-00389-1; and Nancy E. Suchman, Cindy
      L. DeCoste, Thomas J. McMahon, Rachel Dalton, Linda C. Mayes, and Jes-
      sica Borelli, "Mothering from the Inside Out: Results of a Second Random-
      ized Clinical Trial Testing a Mentalization-Based Intervention for Mothers
      in Addiction Treatment," in "Attachment in the Context of Atypical Caregiv-
      ing: Harnessing Insights from a Developmental Psychopathology Perspec-
      tive," ed. Glenn I. Roisman and Dante Cicchetti, special issue, *Development
      and Psychopathology* 29, no. 2 (May 2017): 617–36, https://doi.org/10.1017
      /S0954579417000220.

191   **About one in eight children:** Rachel N. Lipari and Struther L. Van Horn,
      "Children Living with Parents Who Have a Substance Use Disorder," *The
      CBHSQ Report* (Rockville, MD: Substance Abuse and Mental Health Ser-
      vices Administration, August 24, 2017), http://www.ncbi.nlm.nih.gov
      /books/NBK464590/.

191   **There is the separate but related fact:** Alex F. Peahl, Vanessa K. Dalton,
      John R. Montgomery, Yen-Ling Lai, Hsou Mei Hu, and Jennifer F. Waljee,

"Rates of New Persistent Opioid Use after Vaginal or Cesarean Birth among US Women," *JAMA Network Open* 2, no. 7 (July 26, 2019): e197863, https://doi.org/10.1001/jamanetworkopen.2019.7863.

191   **present an opportunity:** Marjo Susanna Flykt, Saara Salo, and Marjukka Pajulo, "'A Window of Opportunity': Parenting and Addiction in the Context of Pregnancy," *Current Addiction Reports* 8 (December 2021): 578–94, https://doi.org/10.1007/s40429-021-00394-4. Rodent studies support this idea. Mariana Pereira and Joan Morrell have conducted numerous studies that involve giving rats accustomed to cocaine a choice between the drug and pups. In the early postpartum period, rat mothers choose the pups, or pup-related environments. That effect wanes in the later postpartum period. M. Pereira and J. I. Morrell, "Functional Mapping of the Neural Circuitry of Rat Maternal Motivation: Effects of Site-Specific Transient Neural Inactivation," in "The Parental Brain," special issue, *Journal of Neuroendocrinology* 23, no. 11 (November 2011): 1020–35, https://doi.org/10.1111/j.1365-2826.2011.02200.x.

192   **Studies have found that Mom Power:** Katherine Rosenblum, Jamie Lawler, Emily Alfafara, Nicole Miller, Melisa Schuster, and Maria Muzik, "Improving Maternal Representations in High-Risk Mothers: A Randomized, Controlled Trial of the Mom Power Parenting Intervention," *Child Psychiatry & Human Development* 49, no. 3 (June 2018): 372–84, https://doi.org/10.1007/s10578-017-0757-5.

192   **Mom Power organizers worked with:** James E. Swain, S. Shaun Ho, Katherine L. Rosenblum, Diana Morelen, Carolyn J. Dayton, and Maria Muzik, "Parent–Child Intervention Decreases Stress and Increases Maternal Brain Activity and Connectivity during Own Baby-Cry: An Exploratory Study," in "Attachment in the Context of Atypical Caregiving: Harnessing Insights from a Developmental Psychopathology Perspective," ed. Glenn I. Roisman and Dante Cicchetti, special issue, *Development and Psychopathology* 29, no. 2 (May 2017): 535–53, https://doi.org/10.1017/S0954579417000165; and S. Shaun Ho, Maria Muzik, Katherine L. Rosenblum, Diana Morelen, Yoshio Nakamura, and James E. Swain, "Potential Neural Mediators of Mom Power Parenting Intervention Effects on Maternal Intersubjectivity and Stress Resilience," *Frontiers in Psychiatry* 11 (December 8, 2020): 569924, https://doi.org/10.3389/fpsyt.2020.568824.

193   **Some researchers have investigated:** Fleming and Kraemer, "Molecular and Genetic Bases of Mammalian Maternal Behavior," https://doi.org/10.1177/2470289719827306; and Viara R. Mileva-Seitz, Marian J. Bakermans-Kranenburg, and Marinus H. van IJzendoorn, "Genetic Mechanisms of Parenting," in "Parental Care," ed. Alison S. Fleming, Frederic Lévy, and Joe S. Lonstein, special issue, *Hormones and Behavior* 77 (January 2016): 211–23, https://doi.org/10.1016/j.yhbeh.2015.06.003.

193   **chance of those outcomes increases:** W. Jonas, V. Mileva-Seitz, A. W.

Girard, R. Bisceglia, J. L. Kennedy, M. Sokolowski, M. J. Meaney, A. S. Fleming, and M. Steiner, "Genetic Variation in Oxytocin rs2740210 and Early Adversity Associated with Postpartum Depression and Breastfeeding Duration," *Genes, Brain and Behavior* 12, no. 7 (October 2013): 681–94, https://doi.org/10.1111/gbb.12069.

193   **serotonin transporter gene:** Divya Mehta, Carina Quast, Peter A. Fasching, Anna Seifert, Franziska Voigt, Matthias W. Beckmann, Florian Faschingbauer, et al., "The 5-HTTLPR Polymorphism Modulates the Influence on Environmental Stressors on Peripartum Depression Symptoms," *Journal of Affective Disorders* 136, no. 3 (February 2012): 1192–97, https://doi.org/10.1016/j.jad.2011.11.042.

195   **depending on which demographic variables:** Viara Mileva-Seitz, Meir Steiner, Leslie Atkinson, Michael J. Meaney, Robert Levitan, James L. Kennedy, Marla B. Sokolowski, and Alison S. Fleming, "Interaction between Oxytocin Genotypes and Early Experience Predicts Quality of Mothering and Postpartum Mood," *PLoS ONE* 8, no. 4 (April 18, 2013): e61443, https://doi.org/10.1371/journal.pone.0061443.

195   **"There is so much noise":** Abigail Tucker, *Mom Genes: Inside the New Science of Our Ancient Maternal Instinct* (New York: Gallery Books, 2021), 145.

196   **the one that correlated a mother's "unresolved":** Sohye Kim, Peter Fonagy, Jon Allen, and Lane Strathearn, "Mothers' Unresolved Trauma Blunts Amygdala Response to Infant Distress," *Social Neuroscience* 9, no. 4 (2014): 352–63, https://doi.org/10.1080/17470919.2014.896287.

196   **"cryptic causality":** Sarah S. Richardson, *The Maternal Imprint: The Contested Science of Maternal-Fetal Effects* (Chicago: University of Chicago Press, 2021), 8.

196   **In her book *The Maternal Imprint*:** Richardson, *Maternal Imprint*, 160, 215–22.

196   **Richardson wrote that:** Richardson, *Maternal Imprint*, 24.

198   **the US Preventive Services Task Force recommended:** Albert L. Siu and the US Preventive Services Task Force, "Screening for Depression in Adults: US Preventive Services Task Force Recommendation Statement," *JAMA* 315, no. 4 (January 26, 2016): 380–87, https://doi.org/10.1001/jama.2015.18392.

198   **Most insurers in the United States:** "Preventative Services Coverage," Centers for Disease Control and Prevention, accessed October 3, 2021, https://www.cdc.gov/nchhstp/highqualitycare/preventiveservices/index.html. Note that the dozen states that have not expanded Medicaid coverage under the Affordable Care Act are not required to cover preventive services given an A or B grade by the task force, but they are offered financial incentive to do so.

199   **the same task force made another:** US Preventive Services Task Force, "Interventions to Prevent Perinatal Depression: US Preventive Services Task

Force Recommendation Statement," *JAMA* 321, no. 6 (February 12, 2019): 580–87, https://doi.org/10.1001/jama.2019.0007.

199 **screening tool:** Researchers have tested some screening tools, including a framework developed by Meltzer-Brody and colleagues at Chapel Hill that builds off the literature on Adverse Childhood Experiences to calculate a pregnant person's cumulative psychosocial risk factors. Yasmin V. Barrios, Joanna Maselko, Stephanie M. Engel, Brian W. Pence, Andrew F. Olshan, Samantha Meltzer-Brody, Nancy Dole, and John M. Thorp, "The Relationship of Cumulative Psychosocial Adversity with Antepartum Depression and Anxiety," *Depression and Anxiety* 38, no. 10 (October 2021): 1034–45, https://doi.org/10.1002/da.23206.

199 **widespread shortages of mental health providers:** Kaia Hubbard, "Many States Face Shortage of Mental Health Providers," *US News & World Report*, June 10, 2021, https://www.usnews.com/news/best-states/articles/2021-06-10/northeastern-states-have-fewest-mental-health-provider-shortages.

199 **covers more than 40 percent:** "State Health Facts: Births Financed by Medicaid," Kaiser Family Foundation, December 17, 2021, https://www.kff.org/medicaid/state-indicator/births-financed-by-medicaid/.

199 **the pandemic has been an incredible stressor:** Gus A. Mayopoulos, Tsachi Ein-Dor, Gabriella A. Dishy, Rasvitha Nandru, Sabrina J. Chan, Lauren E. Hanley, Anjali J. Kaimal, and Sharon Dekel, "COVID-19 Is Associated with Traumatic Childbirth and Subsequent Mother-Infant Bonding Problems," *Journal of Affective Disorders* 282 (March 1, 2021): 122–25, https://doi.org/10.1016/j.jad.2020.12.101; and Elizabeth L. Adams, Danyel Smith, Laura J. Caccavale, and Melanie K. Bean, "Parents Are Stressed! Patterns of Parent Stress across COVID-19," *Frontiers in Psychiatry* 12 (April 2021): 626456, https://doi.org/10.3389/fpsyt.2021.626456.

200 **"Convincing depressed postpartum women":** Lauren M. Osborne, Mary C. Kimmel, and Pamela J. Surkan, "The Crisis of Perinatal Mental Health in the Age of Covid-19," *Maternal and Child Health Journal* 25 (March 2021): 349–52, https://doi.org/10.1007/s10995-020-03114-y.

200 **In women with moderate to severe:** Stephen Kanes, Helen Colquhoun, Handan Gunduz-Bruce, Shane Raines, Ryan Arnold, Amy Schacterle, James Doherty, et al., "Brexanolone (SAGE-547 Injection) in Post-Partum Depression: A Randomised Controlled Trial," *Lancet* 390, no. 10093 (July 29, 2017): 480–89, https://doi.org/10.1016/S0140-6736(17)31264-3; and Samantha Meltzer-Brody, Helen Colquhoun, Robert Riesenberg, C. Neill Epperson, Kristina M. Deligiannidis, David R. Rubinow, Haihong Li, et al., "Brexanolone Injection in Post-Partum Depression: Two Multicentre, Double-Blind, Randomised, Placebo-Controlled, Phase 3 Trials," *Lancet* 392, no. 10152 (September 22, 2018): 1058–70, https://doi.org/10.1016/S0140-6736(18)31551-4.

201 **the company cited:** Sage Therapeutics, Inc., *Form 10-Q*, for the period ending June 30, 2021 (filed August 3, 2021), US Securities and Exchange

Commission; and Adam Feuerstein, "Biotech in the Time of Coronavirus: The Return of Biotech Mergers, Acquisitions, and Deals," STAT, April 13, 2020, https://www.statnews.com/2020/04/13/biotech-in-the-time-of-coronavirus -the-return-of-mergers-acquisitions-and-deals/.

201   **a rocky start:** Matthew Herper and Adam Feuerstein, "Sage's New Anti-depressant Faces Major Setback in New Study," STAT, December 5, 2019, https://www.statnews.com/2019/12/05/sages-new-antidepressant-faces -major-setback-in-new-study/; and Kristina M. Deligiannidis, Samantha Meltzer-Brody, Handan Gunduz-Bruce, James Doherty, Jeffrey Jonas, Sigui Li, Abdul J. Sankoh, et al., "Effect of Zuranolone vs Placebo in Postpartum Depression," *JAMA Psychiatry* 78, no. 9 (June 30, 2021): 951–59, https://doi .org/10.1001/jamapsychiatry.2021.1559.

201   **up to 10 percent:** Jodi L. Pawluski, Ming Li, and Joseph S. Lonstein, "Sero-tonin and Motherhood: From Molecules to Mood," in "Parental Brain," ed. Susanne Brummelte and Benedetta Leuner, special issue, *Frontiers in Neu-roendocrinology* 53 (April 2019): 100742, https://doi.org/10.1016/j.yfrne .2019.03.001.

201   **a big question mark:** Joseph S. Lonstein, "The Dynamic Serotonin System of the Maternal Brain," *Archives of Women's Mental Health* 22, no. 2 (April 2019): 237–43, https://doi.org/10.1007/s00737-018-0887-1.

202   **the central serotonin system:** Lonstein, "Dynamic Serotonin System of the Maternal Brain," https://doi.org/10.1007/s00737-018-0887-1.

202   **looked at how sertraline:** Jodi L. Pawluski, Rafaella Paravatou, Alan Even, Gael Cobraiville, Marianne Fillet, Nikolaos Kokras, Christina Dalla, and Thi-erry D. Charlier, "Effect of Sertraline on Central Serotonin and Hippocam-pal Plasticity in Pregnant and Non-Pregnant Rats," *Neuropharmacology* 166 (April 2020): 107950, https://doi.org/10.1016/j.neuropharm.2020.107950.

202   **serotonin interacts:** Pawluski, Li, and Lonstein, "Serotonin and Mother-hood," https://doi.org/10.1016/j.yfrne.2019.03.001.

202   **a systematic review that concluded:** Jennifer Valeska Elli Brown, Claire A. Wilson, Karyn Ayre, Lindsay Robertson, Emily South, Emma Moly-neaux, Kylee Trevillion, Louise M. Howard, and Hind Khalifeh, "Anti-depressant Treatment for Postnatal Depression," *Cochrane Database of Systematic Reviews*, no. 2 (February 2021), https://doi.org/10.1002/14651858 .CD013560.pub2.

203   **"maternity care deserts":** Martha Hostetter and Sarah Klein, "Restoring Access to Maternity Care in Rural America," *Transforming Care* (Common-wealth Fund, September 30, 2021), https://doi.org/10.26099/CYCC-FF50; and Peiyin Hung, Carrie E. Henning-Smith, Michelle M. Casey, and Katy B. Kozhimannil, "Access to Obstetric Services in Rural Counties Still Declining, with 9 Percent Losing Services, 2004–14," *Health Affairs* 36, no. 9 (September 2017): 1663–71, https://doi.org/10.1377/hlthaff.2017.0338.

203   **There is good evidence:** Kim, "How Stress Can Influence Brain Adapta-tions to Motherhood," https://doi.org/10.1016/j.yfrne.2020.100875; Nora

Ellmann, *Community-Based Doulas and Midwives: Key to Addressing the U.S. Maternal Health Crisis* (Center for American Progress, April 2020), https://www.americanprogress.org/article/community-based-doulas -midwives/; and David L. Olds, Harriet Kitzman, Elizabeth Anson, Joyce A. Smith, Michael D. Knudtson, Ted Miller, Robert Cole, Christian Hopfer, and Gabriella Conti, "Prenatal and Infancy Nurse Home Visiting Effects on Mothers: 18-Year Follow-Up of a Randomized Trial," *Pediatrics* 144, no. 6 (December 2019): e20183889, https://doi.org/10.1542/peds.2018-3889.

204   **"Postpartum depression," Menkedick argued:** Sarah Menkedick, *Ordinary Insanity: Fear and the Silent Crisis of Motherhood in America* (New York: Pantheon, 2020), 354.

204   **Something amazing happened:** Hillary Frank, "Ina May's Guide, Completely Revised and Updated," *The Longest Shortest Time* (December 10, 2019), https://longestshorttime.com/episode-218-ina-mays-guide-completely -revised-and-updated/.

205   **an updated version:** Ina May Gaskin, *Ina May's Guide to Childbirth*, revised and updated (New York: Bantam, 2003, revised 2019). Notably, this version still has a big quote on the cover from Christiane Northrup, the celebrity women's health doctor who became notorious for spreading misinformation about the pandemic and vaccines. Colin Woodard, "Instagram Blocks Account of Celebrity Maine Doctor Who Spreads Vaccine Disinformation," *Press Herald*, April 30, 2021, https://www.pressherald.com/2021/04 /30/instagram-blocks-account-of-celebrity-maine-doctor-who-spreads -vaccine-disinformation/.

205   **"the golden hour":** Gaskin, *Ina May's Guide to Childbirth*, rev. ed., 293.

206   **As much as 6 percent of mothers:** Sharon Dekel, Caren Stuebe, and Gabriella Dishy, "Childbirth Induced Posttraumatic Stress Syndrome: A Systematic Review of Prevalence and Risk Factors," *Frontiers in Psychology* 8 (April 11, 2017): 560, https://doi.org/10.3389/fpsyg.2017.00560.

206   **assess the birth and postpartum experiences:** Sharon Dekel, Tsachi Ein-Dor, Zohar Berman, Ida S. Barsoumian, Sonika Agarwal, and Roger K. Pitman, "Delivery Mode Is Associated with Maternal Mental Health Following Childbirth," *Archives of Women's Mental Health* 22, no. 6 (December 2019): 817–24, https://doi.org/10.1007/s00737-019-00968-2.

206   **Medical inductions, complicated births:** Sabrina J. Chan, Tsachi Ein-Dor, Philip A. Mayopoulos, Michelle M. Mesa, Ryan M. Sunda, Brenna F. McCarthy, Anjali J. Kaimal, and Sharon Dekel, "Risk Factors for Developing Posttraumatic Stress Disorder Following Childbirth," *Psychiatry Research* 290 (August 2020): 113090, https://doi.org/10.1016/j.psychres .2020.113090.

206   **a dissociative state:** Freya Thiel and Sharon Dekel, "Peritraumatic Dissociation in Childbirth-Evoked Posttraumatic Stress and Postpartum Mental Health," *Archives of Women's Mental Health* 23, no. 2 (April 2020): 189–97, https://doi.org/10.1007/s00737-019-00978-0.

206 **a history of sexual assault:** Zohar Berman, Freya Thiel, Anjali J. Kaimal, and Sharon Dekel, "Association of Sexual Assault History with Traumatic Childbirth and Subsequent PTSD," *Archives of Women's Mental Health* 24 (October 2021): 767–71, https://doi.org/10.1007/s00737-021-01129-0.

206 **A birthing parent's age:** Chan et al., "Risk Factors for Developing Posttraumatic Stress Disorder Following Childbirth," https://doi.org/10.1016/j.psychres.2020.113090.

206 **occurs alongside postpartum depression:** Sharon Dekel, Tsachi Ein-Dor, Gabriella A. Dishy, and Philip A. Mayopoulos, "Beyond Postpartum Depression: Posttraumatic Stress-Depressive Response Following Childbirth," *Archives of Women's Mental Health* 23, no. 4 (August 2020): 557–64, https://doi.org/10.1007/s00737-019-01006-x.

207 **Lots of brain imaging studies:** Neven Henigsberg, Petra Kalember, Zrnka Kovačić Petrović, and Ana Šećić, "Neuroimaging Research in Posttraumatic Stress Disorder—Focus on Amygdala, Hippocampus and Prefrontal Cortex," in "Theranostic Approach to PTSD," ed. Nela Pivac, special issue, *Progress in Neuro-Psychopharmacology and Biological Psychiatry* 90 (March 2, 2019): 37–42, https://doi.org/10.1016/j.pnpbp.2018.11.003; and Konstantinos Bromis, Maria Calem, Antje A. T. S. Reinders, Steven C. R. Williams, and Matthew J. Kempton, "Meta-Analysis of 89 Structural MRI Studies in Posttraumatic Stress Disorder and Comparison with Major Depressive Disorder," *American Journal of Psychiatry* 175, no. 10 (October 2018): 989–98, https://doi.org/10.1176/appi.ajp.2018.17111199.

208 **a majority of women report:** Zohar Berman, Freya Thiel, Gabriella A. Dishy, Sabrina J. Chan, and Sharon Dekel, "Maternal Psychological Growth Following Childbirth," *Archives of Women's Mental Health* 24, no. 2 (April 1, 2021): 313–20, https://doi.org/10.1007/s00737-020-01053-9.

208 **mothers who tested positive:** Gus A. Mayopoulos, Tsachi Ein-Dor, Kevin G. Li, Sabrina J. Chan, and Sharon Dekel, "COVID-19 Positivity Associated with Traumatic Stress Response to Childbirth and No Visitors and Infant Separation in the Hospital," *Scientific Reports* 11 (June 29, 2021): 13535, https://doi.org/10.1038/s41598-021-92985-4. This study paints a really stark picture of what it was like for women delivering in the first wave of the pandemic who also tested positive for the virus. They often delivered without support people. They were more likely to be separated from their infants after birth. They reported more pain during delivery and poorer outcomes for their babies, with more needing NICU care. All these factors surely contributed to their poorer psychological outcomes, too.

208 **Black and Latinx women:** Ananya S. Iyengar, Tsachi Ein-Dor, Emily X. Zhang, Sabrina J. Chan, Anjali J. Kaimal, and Sharon Dekel, "Racial and Ethnic Disparities in Maternal Mental Health during COVID-19," MedRxiv (December 2, 2021), https://doi.org/10.1101/2021.11.30.21265428.

209   **one in six women:** Saraswathi Vedam, Kathrin Stoll, Tanya Khemet Taiwo, Nicholas Rubashkin, Melissa Cheyney, Nan Strauss, Monica McLemore, et al., "The Giving Voice to Mothers Study: Inequity and Mistreatment during Pregnancy and Childbirth in the United States," *Reproductive Health* 16 (June 11, 2019): 77, https://doi.org/10.1186/s12978-019-0729-2.

209   **In May 2021, Missouri:** *Birthing While Black: Examining America's Black Maternal Health Crisis, Before the House Oversight and Reform Committee,* 117th Cong. (2021) (testimony of Cori Bush, Congresswoman from Missouri).

CHAPTER 8: THE ONE IN THE MIRROR

214   **"You watch people get pregnant":** Sian Cain, "Lucy Ellmann: 'We Need to Raise the Level of Discourse,'" *Guardian*, December 7, 2019, https://www.theguardian.com/books/2019/dec/07/lucy-ellmann-ducks-newburyport-interview.

215   **four out of five:** Matthew Brett and Sallie Baxendale, "Motherhood and Memory: A Review," *Psychoneuroendocrinology* 26, no. 4 (May 2001): 339–62, https://doi.org/10.1016/S0306-4530(01)00003-8.

215   **In 1986, researchers surveyed:** Charles M. Poser, Marilyn R. Kassirer, and Janis M. Peyser, "Benign Encephalopathy of Pregnancy: Preliminary Clinical Observations," *Acta Neurologica Scandinavica* 73, no. 1 (January 1986): 39–43, https://doi.org/10.1111/j.1600-0404.1986.tb03239.x.

215   **a handful of studies have tried:** Marla V. Anderson and Mel D. Rutherford, "Cognitive Reorganization during Pregnancy and the Postpartum Period: An Evolutionary Perspective," *Evolutionary Psychology* 10, no. 4 (October 2012): 659–87, https://doi.org/10.1177/147470491201000402.

215   **aren't always reliable reporters:** Dustin M. Logan, Kyle R. Hill, Rochelle Jones, Julianne Holt-Lunstad, and Michael J. Larson, "How Do Memory and Attention Change with Pregnancy and Childbirth? A Controlled Longitudinal Examination of Neuropsychological Functioning in Pregnant and Postpartum Women," *Journal of Clinical and Experimental Neuropsychology* 36, no. 5 (May 2014): 528–39, https://doi.org/10.1080/13803395.2014.912614.

215   **A 2012 analysis of the research:** Anderson and Rutherford, "Cognitive Reorganization during Pregnancy and the Postpartum Period," https://doi.org/10.1177/147470491201000402.

216   **A more recent analysis:** Sasha J. Davies, Jarrad A. G. Lum, Helen Skouteris, Linda K. Byrne, and Melissa J. Hayden, "Cognitive Impairment during Pregnancy: A Meta-Analysis," *Medical Journal of Australia* 208, no. 1 (January 2018): 35–40, https://doi.org/10.5694/mja17.00131.

216   **Depressive symptoms:** Elizabeth Hampson, Shauna-Dae Phillips, Sarah J. Duff-Canning, Kelly L. Evans, Mia Merrill, Julia K. Pinsonneault, Wolfgang Sadée, Claudio N. Soares, and Meir Steiner, "Working Memory in Pregnant

Women: Relation to Estrogen and Antepartum Depression," in "Estradiol and Cognition: Molecules to Mind," ed. Victoria Luine and Maya Frankfurt, special issue, *Hormones and Behavior* 74 (August 2015): 218–27, https://doi.org/10.1016/j.yhbeh.2015.07.006.

216   **fetal sex may play a role:** Claire M. Vanston and Neil V. Watson, "Selective and Persistent Effect of Foetal Sex on Cognition in Pregnant Women," *NeuroReport* 16, no. 7 (May 12, 2005): 779–82, https://doi.org/10.1097/00001756-200505120-00024.

216   **memory deficits may compound:** Laura M. Glynn, "Increasing Parity Is Associated with Cumulative Effects on Memory," *Journal of Women's Health* 21, no. 10 (October 2012): 1038–45, https://doi.org/10.1089/jwh.2011.3206.

217   **Some research has linked:** Jin-Xia Zheng, Lili Ge, Huiyou Chen, Xindao Yin, Yu-Chen Chen, and Wei-Wei Tang, "Disruption within Brain Default Mode Network in Postpartum Women without Depression," *Medicine* 99, no. 18 (May 2020): e20045, https://doi.org/10.1097/MD.0000000000020045.

217   **Remember that structural study:** Elseline Hoekzema, Erika Barba-Müller, Cristina Pozzobon, Marisol Picado, Florencio Lucco, David García-García, Juan Carlos Soliva, et al., "Pregnancy Leads to Long-Lasting Changes in Human Brain Structure," *Nature Neuroscience* 20, no. 2 (2017): 287–96, https://doi.org/10.1038/nn.4458.

218   **placed pregnant rats into a circular pool:** Liisa A. M. Galea, Brandi K. Ormerod, Sharadh Sampath, Xanthoula Kostaras, Donald M. Wilkie, and Maria T. Phelps, "Spatial Working Memory and Hippocampal Size across Pregnancy in Rats," *Hormones and Behavior* 37, no. 1 (February 2000): 86–95, https://doi.org/10.1006/hbeh.1999.1560.

218   **documented multifaceted changes:** Pawluski, Hoekzema, Leuner, and Lonstein, "Less Can Be More: Fine Tuning the Maternal Brain," https://doi.org/10.1016/j.neubiorev.2021.11.045; Jodi L. Pawluski, Kelly G. Lambert, and Craig H. Kinsley, "Neuroplasticity in the Maternal Hippocampus: Relation to Cognition and Effects of Repeated Stress," in "Parental Care," ed. Alison S. Fleming, Frederic Lévy, and Joe S. Lonstein, special issue, *Hormones and Behavior* 77 (January 2016): 86–97, https://doi.org/10.1016/j.yhbeh.2015.06.004; and J. L. Pawluski, A. Valença, A. I. M. Santos, J. P. Costa-Nunes, H. W. M. Steinbusch, and T. Strekalova, "Pregnancy or Stress Decrease Complexity of CA3 Pyramidal Neurons in the Hippocampus of Adult Female Rats," *Neuroscience* 227 (December 27, 2012): 201–10, https://doi.org/10.1016/j.neuroscience.2012.09.059.

218   **First-time rat mothers:** Paula Duarte-Guterman, Benedetta Leuner, and Liisa A. M. Galea, "The Long and Short Term Effects of Motherhood on the Brain," in "Parental Brain," ed. Susanne Brummelte and Benedetta Leuner, special issue, *Frontiers in Neuroendocrinology* 53 (April 2019): 100740, https://doi.org/10.1016/j.yfrne.2019.02.004.

218   **Studies of California mice:** Erica R. Glasper, Molly M. Hyer, Jhansi

Katakam, Robyn Harper, Cyrus Ameri, and Thomas Wolz, "Father-hood Contributes to Increased Hippocampal Spine Density and Anxiety Regulation in California Mice," *Brain and Behavior* 6, no. 1 (January 2016): e00416, https://doi.org/10.1002/brb3.416; and Erica R. Glasper, Yevgenia Kozorovitskiy, Ashley Pavlic, and Elizabeth Gould, "Paternal Experience Suppresses Adult Neurogenesis without Altering Hippocampal Function in *Peromyscus Californicus*," *Journal of Comparative Neurology* 519, no. 11 (August 1, 2011): 2271–81, https://doi.org/10.1002/cne.22628.

218 **"neuroprotective":** Pawluski, Lambert, and Kinsley, "Neuroplasticity in the Maternal Hippocampus," https://doi.org/10.1016/j.yhbeh.2015.06.004.

218 **less age-related decline:** Rand S. Eid, Jessica A. Chaiton, Stephanie E. Lieblich, Tamara S. Bodnar, Joanne Weinberg, and Liisa A. M. Galea, "Early and Late Effects of Maternal Experience on Hippocampal Neurogenesis, Microglia, and the Circulating Cytokine Milieu," *Neurobiology of Aging* 78 (June 2019): 1–17, https://doi.org/10.1016/j.neurobiolaging.2019.01.021; and Duarte-Guterman, Leuner, and Galea, "Effects of Motherhood on the Brain," https://doi.org/10.1016/j.yfrne.2019.02.004.

218 **they seem to be protected:** Lisa Y. Maeng and Tracey J. Shors, "Once a Mother, Always a Mother: Maternal Experience Protects Females from the Negative Effects of Stress on Learning," *Behavioral Neuroscience* 126, no. 1 (February 2012): 137–41, https://doi.org/10.1037/a0026707.

218 **In later life and long after:** Jessica D. Gatewood, Melissa D. Morgan, Mollie Eaton, Ilan M. McNamara, Lillian F. Stevens, Abbe H. Macbeth, Elizabeth A. A. Meyer, et al., "Motherhood Mitigates Aging-Related Decrements in Learning and Memory and Positively Affects Brain Aging in the Rat," *Brain Research Bulletin* 66, no. 2 (July 30, 2005): 91–98, https://doi.org/10.1016/j.brainresbull.2005.03.016; and Pawluski, Lambert, and Kinsley, "Neuroplasticity in the Maternal Hippocampus," https://doi.org/10.1016/j.yhbeh.2015.06.004.

219 **more efficient at foraging:** Pawluski, Lambert, and Kinsley, "Neuroplasticity in the Maternal Hippocampus," https://doi.org/10.1016/j.yhbeh.2015.06.004.

219 **One study comparing executive function:** Mayra L. Almanza-Sepulveda, Elsie Chico, Andrea Gonzalez, Geoffrey B. Hall, Meir Steiner, and Alison S. Fleming, "Executive Function in Teen and Adult Women: Association with Maternal Status and Early Adversity," *Developmental Psychobiology* 60, no. 7 (November 2018): 849–61, https://doi.org/10.1002/dev.21766.

220 **using memory tests that include:** Bridget Callaghan, Clare McCormack, Nim Tottenham, and Catherine Monk, "Evidence for Cognitive Plasticity during Pregnancy via Enhanced Learning and Memory," *Memory* (January 5, 2022): 1–18, https://doi.org/10.1080/09658211.2021.2019280.

221 **until very recently:** Todd C. Frankel, "Safety Agency Bans Range of Unregulated Baby Sleep Products Tied to at Least 90 Deaths," *Washington Post*, June 2, 2021, https://www.washingtonpost.com/business/2021/06/02/cpsc-bans-inclined-sleepers/.

221 **bad for your health:** Harvey R. Colten and Bruce M. Altevogt, eds., "Extent and Health Consequences of Chronic Sleep Loss and Sleep Disorders," in *Sleep Disorders and Sleep Deprivation: An Unmet Public Health Problem* (Washington, DC: National Academies Press, 2006), https://www.ncbi.nlm .nih.gov/books/NBK19961/.

221 **"Without sleep, our cognitive":** Adam J. Krause, Eti Ben Simon, Bryce A. Mander, Stephanie M. Greer, Jared M. Saletin, Andrea N. Goldstein-Piekarski, and Matthew P. Walker, "The Sleep-Deprived Human Brain," *Nature Reviews Neuroscience* 18, no. 7 (May 18, 2017): 404–18, https://doi .org/10.1038/nrn.2017.55.

222 **alters dopamine signaling:** Krause et al., "Sleep-Deprived Human Brain," https://doi.org/10.1038/nrn.2017.55.

222 **Both the amount of time:** David Richter, Michael D. Krämer, Nicole K. Y. Tang, Hawley E. Montgomery-Downs, and Sakari Lemola, "Long-Term Effects of Pregnancy and Childbirth on Sleep Satisfaction and Duration of First-Time and Experienced Mothers and Fathers," *Sleep* 42, no. 4 (April 2019), https://doi.org/10.1093/sleep/zsz015.

223 **Robert Sapolsky told journalist:** Katherine Ellison, *The Mommy Brain: How Motherhood Makes Us Smarter* (New York: Basic Books, 2005), 22.

223 **Lots of studies:** Sue Bhati and Kathy Richards, "A Systematic Review of the Relationship between Postpartum Sleep Disturbance and Postpartum Depression," *Journal of Obstetric, Gynecologic & Neonatal Nursing* 44, no. 3 (May–June 2015): 350–57, https://doi.org/10.1111/1552-6909.12562.

223 **measured depressive symptoms and sleep:** Eliza M. Park, Samantha Meltzer-Brody, and Robert Stickgold, "Poor Sleep Maintenance and Subjective Sleep Quality Are Associated with Postpartum Maternal Depression Symptom Severity," *Archives of Women's Mental Health* 16, no. 6 (December 2013): 539–47, https://doi.org/10.1007/s00737-013-0356-9.

224 **total hours of sleep:** Hawley E. Montgomery-Downs, Salvatore P. Insana, Megan M. Clegg-Kraynok, and Laura M. Mancini, "Normative Longitudinal Maternal Sleep: The First 4 Postpartum Months," *American Journal of Obstetrics and Gynecology* 203, no. 5 (November 2010): 465.e1–465.e7, https://doi.org/10.1016/j.ajog.2010.06.057.

224 **Others have suggested:** Lily K. Gordon, Katherine A. Mason, Emily Mepham, and Katherine M. Sharkey, "A Mixed Methods Study of Perinatal Sleep and Breastfeeding Outcomes in Women at Risk for Postpartum Depression," *Sleep Health* 7, no. 3 (June 2021): 353–61, https://doi.org/10.1016/j.sleh.2021.01.004; and Jessica L. Obeysekare, Zachary L. Cohen, Meredith E. Coles, Teri B. Pearlstein, Carmen Monzon, E. Ellen Flynn, and Katherine M. Sharkey, "Delayed Sleep Timing and Circadian Rhythms in Pregnancy and Transdiagnostic Symptoms Associated with Postpartum Depression," *Translational Psychiatry* 10, 14 (January 21, 2020), https://doi.org/10.1038/s41398-020-0683-3.

225 **fifteen mothers and fifteen fathers:** Shir Atzil, Talma Hendler, Orna Zagoory-Sharon, Yonatan Winetraub, and Ruth Feldman, "Synchrony and Specificity

in the Maternal and the Paternal Brain: Relations to Oxytocin and Vasopressin," *Journal of the American Academy of Child & Adolescent Psychiatry* 51, no. 8 (August 1, 2012): 798–811, https://doi.org/10.1016/j.jaac.2012.06.008.

225 **The findings were nuanced, but among them:** Eyal Abraham, Gadi Gilam, Yaniv Kanat-Maymon, Yael Jacob, Orna Zagoory-Sharon, Talma Hendler, and Ruth Feldman, "The Human Coparental Bond Implicates Distinct Corticostriatal Pathways: Longitudinal Impact on Family Formation and Child Well-Being," *Neuropsychopharmacology* 42, no. 12 (November 2017): 2301–13, https://doi.org/10.1038/npp.2017.71.

226 **Human relationships don't exist as:** Elizabeth Redcay and Leonhard Schilbach, "Using Second-Person Neuroscience to Elucidate the Mechanisms of Social Interaction," *Nature Reviews Neuroscience* 20, no. 8 (August 2019): 495–505, https://doi.org/10.1038/s41583-019-0179-4; and Mattia Gallotti and Chris D. Frith, "Social Cognition in the We-Mode," *Trends in Cognitive Sciences* 17, no. 4 (April 2013): 160–65, https://doi.org/10.1016/j.tics.2013 .02.002.

226 **Two-person neuroscience:** Redcay and Schilbach, "Using Second-Person Neuroscience to Elucidate the Mechanisms of Social Interaction," https:// doi.org/10.1038/s41583-019-0179-4.

226 **In one recent study:** Atiqah Azhari, Mengyu Lim, Andrea Bizzego, Giulio Gabrieli, Marc H. Bornstein, and Gianluca Esposito, "Physical Presence of Spouse Enhances Brain-to-Brain Synchrony in Co-Parenting Couples," *Scientific Reports* 10, no. 1 (May 5, 2020): 7569, https://doi.org/10.1038/s41598 -020-63596-2.

227 **how mothers relate to:** Shir Atzil, Talma Hendler, and Ruth Feldman, "The Brain Basis of Social Synchrony," *Social Cognitive and Affective Neuroscience* 9, no. 8 (August 2014): 1193–202, https://doi.org/10.1093/scan/nst105.

228 **wrote a group of researchers:** Morten L. Kringelbach, Eloise A. Stark, Catherine Alexander, Marc H. Bornstein, and Alan Stein, "On Cuteness: Unlocking the Parental Brain and Beyond," *Trends in Cognitive Sciences* 20, no. 7 (July 2016): 545–58, https://doi.org/10.1016/j.tics.2016.05.003.

228 **Kringelbach and colleagues propose:** Kringelbach et al., "On Cuteness," https://doi.org/10.1016/j.tics.2016.05.003.

229 **One series of studies:** Michael Gilead and Nira Liberman, "We Take Care of Our Own: Caregiving Salience Increases Out-Group Bias in Response to Out-Group Threat," *Psychological Science* 25, no. 7 (July 2014): 1380–87, https://doi.org/10.1177/0956797614531439.

230 **Feldman wrote that Darwin's:** Ruth Feldman, "The Neurobiology of Mammalian Parenting and the Biosocial Context of Human Caregiving," in "Parental Care," ed. Alison S. Fleming, Frederic Lévy, and Joe S. Lonstein, special issue, *Hormones and Behavior* 77 (January 2016): 3–17, https://doi .org/10.1016/j.yhbeh.2015.10.001.

231 **enriched environment:** Marian C. Diamond, Ruth E. Johnson, and Carol Ingham, "Brain Plasticity Induced by Environment and Pregnancy," *International*

Journal of Neuroscience 2, no. 4–5 (1971): 171–78, https://doi.org/10.3109 /00207457109146999.

231 **"evolutionary division of labor"**: Alison Gopnik, *The Philosophical Baby: What Children's Minds Tell Us about Truth, Love, and the Meaning of Life* (New York: Picador USA, 2010).

231 **to elicit awe:** Marianna Graziosi and David Yaden, "Interpersonal Awe: Exploring the Social Domain of Awe Elicitors," *Journal of Positive Psychology* 16, no. 2 (2021): 263–71, https://doi.org/10.1080/17439760.2019.1689422.

232 **And awe is thought to be:** Alice Chirico, Vlad Petre Glaveanu, Pietro Cipresso, Giuseppe Riva, and Andrea Gaggioli, "Awe Enhances Creative Thinking: An Experimental Study," *Creativity Research Journal* 30, no. 2 (April 2018): 123–31, https://doi.org/10.1080/10400419.2018.1446491.

232 **"The part that enraged me"**: Molly Dickens, "Baby's First Race: An Interview with Olympian Alysia Montaño," Preg U, June 26, 2017, https://preg-u .bloomlife.com/interview-with-alysia-montano-ce0dcbc6f286.

232 **this time for the *New York Times*:** Alysia Montaño (video by Max Cantor, Taige Jensen, and Lindsay Crouse), "Nike Told Me to Dream Crazy, Until I Wanted a Baby," *New York Times*, May 12, 2019, https://www.nytimes.com /2019/05/12/opinion/nike-maternity-leave.html.

232 **Less than two weeks later:** Allyson Felix (video by Lindsay Crouse, Taige Jensen, and Max Cantor), "Allyson Felix: My Own Nike Pregnancy Story," *New York Times*, May 22, 2019, https://www.nytimes.com/2019/05/22 /opinion/allyson-felix-pregnancy-nike.html.

234 **The barriers to balancing:** Katherine Goldstein, "Where Are the Mothers?," *Nieman Reports*, July 26, 2017, https://niemanreports.org/articles/where- are-the-mothers/.

234 **Mothers in competition:** Dave Sheinin, Bonnie Berkowitz, and Rick Maese, "They Are Olympians. They Are Mothers. And They No Longer Have to Choose," *Washington Post*, July 20, 2021, https://www.washingtonpost.com /sports/olympics/interactive/2021/olympics-mothers/.

CHAPTER 9: BETWEEN US

235 **T. Berry Brazelton:** I first told this story for the Sunday magazine of the *Boston Globe*. See Chelsea Conaboy, "Motherhood Brings the Most Dramatic Brain Changes of a Woman's Life," *Globe Magazine, Boston Globe*, July 17, 2018, https://www.bostonglobe.com/magazine/2018/07/17/pregnant -women-care-ignores-one-most-profound-changes-new-mom-faces /CF5wyP0b5EGCcZ8fzLUWbP/story.html.

235 **"I am angry"**: Louisa May Alcott, *Little Women; or Meg, Jo, Beth, and Amy* (Boston: Little, Brown, 1916), 92.

236 **according to the obituary:** Sandra Blakeslee, "Dr. T. Berry Brazelton, Who Explored Babies' Mental Growth, Dies at 99," *New York Times*,

March 14, 2018, https://www.nytimes.com/2018/03/14/obituaries/dr-t-berry -brazelton-dies.html.

238 **one such app:** Amy O'Connor, "'Pregnancy Brain' or Forgetfulness During Pregnancy," What to Expect, October 2, 2020, https://www.whattoexpect .com/pregnancy/symptoms-and-solutions/forgetfulness.aspx.

239 **skips over labor and delivery:** Orli Dahan, "The Birthing Brain: A Lacuna in Neuroscience," *Brain and Cognition* 150 (June 2021): 105722, https://doi .org/10.1016/j.bandc.2021.105722.

239 **an increasing understanding:** Timothy G. Dinan and John F. Cryan, "Microbes, Immunity, and Behavior: Psychoneuroimmunology Meets the Microbiome," *Neuropsychopharmacology* 42, no. 1 (January 2017): 178–92, https://doi.org/10.1038/npp.2016.103.

239 **But what happens in a person's gut:** Nusiebeh Redpath, Hannah S. Rackers, and Mary C. Kimmel, "The Relationship between Perinatal Mental Health and Stress: A Review of the Microbiome," *Current Psychiatry Reports* 21, no. 3 (March 2, 2019): 18, https://doi.org/10.1007/s11920-019-0998-z.

239 **the microbiome changes:** Omry Koren, Julia K. Goodrich, Tyler C. Cullender, Aymé Spor, Kirsi Laitinen, Helene Kling Bäckhed, Antonio Gonzalez, et al., "Host Remodeling of the Gut Microbiome and Metabolic Changes during Pregnancy," *Cell* 150, no. 3 (August 3, 2012): 470–80, https://doi.org/10.1016 /j.cell.2012.07.008; and Hannah S. Rackers, Stephanie Thomas, Kelsey Williamson, Rachael Posey, and Mary C. Kimmel, "Emerging Literature in the Microbiota-Brain Axis and Perinatal Mood and Anxiety Disorders," *Psychoneuroendocrinology* 95 (September 2018): 86–96, https://doi.org/10.1016/j .psyneuen.2018.05.020.

240 **in the Greek tradition:** *Encyclopedia Britannica Online*, s.v. "Chimera," accessed October 31, 2021, https://www.britannica.com/topic/Chimera -Greek-mythology.

240 **"cell trafficking":** Diana W. Bianchi, Kiarash Khosrotehrani, Sing Sing Way, Tippi C. MacKenzie, Ingeborg Bajema, and Keelin O'Donoghue, "Forever Connected: The Lifelong Biological Consequences of Fetomaternal and Maternofetal Microchimerism," *Clinical Chemistry* 67, no. 2 (February 2021): 351–62, https://doi.org/10.1093/clinchem/hvaa304.

240 **Babies carry cells from the parents:** Jeremy M. Kinder, Ina A. Stelzer, Petra C. Arck, and Sing Sing Way, "Immunological Implications of Pregnancy-Induced Microchimerism," *Nature Reviews Immunology* 17, no. 8 (August 2017): 483–94, https://doi.org/10.1038/nri.2017.38.

240 **intact fetal cells:** Kinder et al., "Immunological Implications of Pregnancy-Induced Microchimerism," https://doi.org/10.1038/nri.2017.38.

240 **100 percent:** Bianchi et al., "Forever Connected," https://doi.org/10.1093 /clinchem/hvaa304.

240 **might be a kind of biological envoy:** Amy M. Boddy, Angelo Fortunato, Melissa Wilson Sayres, and Athena Aktipis, "Fetal Microchimerism and

Maternal Health: A Review and Evolutionary Analysis of Cooperation and Conflict beyond the Womb," *BioEssays* 37, no. 10 (October 2015): 1106–18, https://doi.org/10.1002/bies.201500059.

241   **the brains of fifty-nine:** William F. N. Chan, Cécile Gurnot, Thomas J. Montine, Joshua A. Sonnen, Katherine A. Guthrie, and J. Lee Nelson, "Male Microchimerism in the Human Female Brain," *PLoS ONE* 7, no. 9 (September 26, 2012): e45592, https://doi.org/10.1371/journal.pone.0045592.

241   **"grossly overlooked":** Liisa A. M. Galea, Wansu Qiu, and Paula Duarte-Guterman, "Beyond Sex Differences: Short and Long-Term Implications of Motherhood on Women's Health," in "Sex Differences," ed. Susan Howlett and Stephen Goodwin, special issue, *Current Opinion in Physiology* 6 (December 2018): 82–88, https://www.sciencedirect.com/science/article/pii/S2468867318300865.

241   **In 1997, the US Food and Drug Administration:** "Gender Studies in Product Development: Historical Overview," US Food and Drug Administration, February 16, 2018, https://www.fda.gov/science-research/womens-health-research/gender-studies-product-development-historical-overview;   and Londa Schiebinger, "Women's Health and Clinical Trials," *Journal of Clinical Investigation* 112, no. 7 (October 2003): 973–77, https://doi.org/10.1172/JCI19993.

242   **In 1993, Congress mandated:** Anna C. Mastroianni, Ruth Faden, and Daniel Federman, eds., *Women and Health Research*, vol. 1, *Ethical and Legal Issues of Including Women in Clinical Studies* (Washington, DC: National Academies Press, 1994).

242   **In the two decades after:** Rowena J. Dolor, Chiara Melloni, Ranee Chatterjee, Nancy M. Allen LaPointe, Judson B. Williams Jr., Remy R. Coeytaux, Amanda J. McBroom, et al., *Treatment Strategies for Women with Coronary Artery Disease*, in *Comparative Effectiveness Review* (Agency for Healthcare Research and Quality, August 2012), https://www.ncbi.nlm.nih.gov/books/NBK100775/.

242   **In 2016, the NIH:** Matthew E. Arnegard, Lori A. Whitten, Chyren Hunter, and Janine Austin Clayton, "Sex as a Biological Variable: A 5-Year Progress Report and Call to Action," in "Incorporating Sex and Gender throughout Scientific Endeavors: Update and Call to Action," special issue, *Journal of Women's Health* 29, no. 6 (June 2020): 858–64, https://doi.org/10.1089/jwh.2019.8247.

242   **Other major funding agencies:** "Sex and Gender Analysis Policies of Major Granting Agencies," Gendered Innovations, accessed November 2, 2021, https://www.genderedinnovations.se/page/en-US/72/Major_Granting_Agencies.

242   **There are indications:** Nicole C. Woitowich, Annaliese Beery, and Teresa Woodruff, "A 10-Year Follow-Up Study of Sex Inclusion in the Biological Sciences," *eLife* 9 (June 9, 2020): e56344, https://doi.org/10.7554/eLife

.56344; and Jenna Haverfield and Cara Tannenbaum, "A 10-Year Longitudinal Evaluation of Science Policy Interventions to Promote Sex and Gender in Health Research," *Health Research Policy and Systems* 19 (June 15, 2021): 94, https://doi.org/10.1186/s12961-021-00741-x.

242   **a recent analysis:** Rebecca K. Rechlin, Tallinn F. L. Splinter, Travis E. Hodges, Arianne Y. Albert, and Liisa A. M. Galea, "Harnessing the Power of Sex Differences: What a Difference Ten Years Did Not Make," *BioRxiv* (November 4, 2021), https://doi.org/10.1101/2021.06.30.450396.

242   **When the Society for Women's Health Research:** Ansley Waters, Society for Women's Health Research Alzheimer's Disease Network, and Melissa H. Laitner, "Biological Sex Differences in Alzheimer's Preclinical Research: A Call to Action," *Alzheimer's & Dementia: Translational Research & Clinical Interventions* 7, no. 1 (February 14, 2021): e12111, https://doi.org/10.1002/trc2.12111.

243   **Until January 2019:** "Basic HHS Policy for Protection of Human Research Subjects," *Code of Federal Regulations*, title 45, part 46, effective July 14, 2009 (Rockville, MD: Office for Human Research Protections), https://www.hhs.gov/ohrp/regulations-and-policy/regulations/regulatory-text/index.html; and Carolyn Y. Johnson, "Long Overlooked by Science, Pregnancy Is Finally Getting Attention It Deserves," *Washington Post*, March 6, 2019, https://www.washingtonpost.com/national/health-science/long-overlooked-by-science-pregnancy-is-finally-getting-attention-it-deserves/2019/03/06/a29ae9bc-3556-11e9-af5b-b51b7ff322e9_story.html.

243   **The FDA has issued:** Center for Drug Evaluation and Research, "Pregnant Women: Scientific and Ethical Considerations for Inclusion in Clinical Trials," Draft Guidance Document, docket FDA-2018-D-1201 (US Food and Drug Administration, April 2018), https://www.fda.gov/regulatory-information/search-fda-guidance-documents/pregnant-women-scientific-and-ethical-considerations-inclusion-clinical-trials.

243   **little information to guide them:** Task Force on Research Specific to Pregnant Women and Lactating Women, *Report to Secretary, Health and Human Services, Congress*, September 2018, https://www.nichd.nih.gov/sites/default/files/2018-09/PRGLAC_Report.pdf.

243   **journalist Carolyn Y. Johnson:** Johnson, "Pregnancy Is Finally Getting Attention," https://www.washingtonpost.com/national/health-science/long-overlooked-by-science-pregnancy-is-finally-getting-attention-it-deserves/2019/03/06/a29ae9bc-3556-11e9-af5b-b51b7ff322e9_story.html?utm_term=.362cb58e9639.

243   **Around 83 percent:** Gladys M. Martinez, Kimberly Daniels, and Isaedmarie Febo-Vazquez, "Fertility of Men and Women Aged 15–44 in the United States: National Survey of Family Growth, 2011–2015," in *National Health Statistics Reports*, no. 113 (Hyattsville, MD: National Center for Health Statistics, 2018), 1–17.

243   **Fetal microchimerism has been implicated:** Bianchi et al., "Forever Connected," https://doi.org/10.1093/clinchem/hvaa304.

244   **a 2021 review led by Diana Bianchi:** Bianchi et al., "Forever Connected," https://doi.org/10.1093/clinchem/hvaa304.

244   **with estrogen and prolactin levels:** Victoria C. Musey, Delwood C. Collins, Paul I. Musey, D. Martino-Saltzman, and John R. K. Preedy, "Long-Term Effect of a First Pregnancy on the Secretion of Prolactin," *New England Journal of Medicine* 316, no. 5 (January 29, 1987): 229–34, https://doi.org /10.1056/NEJM198701293160501; and Caitlin M. Taylor et al., "Applying a Women's Health Lens to the Study of the Aging Brain," *Frontiers in Human Neuroscience* 13 (2019): 224, https://doi.org/10.3389/fnhum.2019.00224.

244   **Those hormonal changes, along with:** Paula Duarte-Guterman, Benedetta Leuner, and Liisa A. M. Galea, "The Long and Short Term Effects of Motherhood on the Brain," in "Parental Brain," ed. Susanne Brummelte and Benedetta Leuner, special issue, *Frontiers in Neuroendocrinology* 53 (April 2019): 100740, https://doi.org/10.1016/j.yfrne.2019.02.004; and Nicholas P. Deems and Benedetta Leuner, "Pregnancy, Postpartum and Parity: Resilience and Vulnerability in Brain Health and Disease," *Frontiers in Neuroendocrinology* 57 (April 2020): 100820, https://doi.org/10.1016/j.yfrne.2020 .100820.

244   **Studies of rats and humans:** Samantha Tang and Bronwyn M. Graham, "Hormonal, Reproductive, and Behavioural Predictors of Fear Extinction Recall in Female Rats," *Hormones and Behavior* 121 (May 2020): 104693, https://doi.org/10.1016/j.yhbeh.2020.104693.

245   **What they found:** Tang and Graham, "Predictors of Fear Extinction Recall in Female Rats," https://doi.org/10.1016/j.yhbeh.2020.104693; and J. S. Milligan-Saville and B. M. Graham, "Mothers Do It Differently: Reproductive Experience Alters Fear Extinction in Female Rats and Women," *Translational Psychiatry* 6, no. 10 (October 2016): e928, https://doi.org/10 .1038/tp.2016.193.

246   **Only five other countries:** Claire Cain Miller, "The World 'Has Found a Way to Do This': The U.S. Lags on Paid Leave," *New York Times*, October 25, 2021, https://www.nytimes.com/2021/10/25/upshot/paid-leave-democrats .html.

247   **more than a century after:** Mona L. Siegel, "The Forgotten Origins of Paid Family Leave," *New York Times*, November 29, 2019, https://www.nytimes .com/2019/11/29/opinion/mothers-paid-family-leave.html.

247   **paid leave checks each of those boxes:** Isabel V. Sawhill, Richard V. Reeves, and Sarah Nzau, "Paid Leave as Fuel for Economic Growth," Middle Class Memos, Brookings Institution, June 27, 2019, https://www.brookings.edu /blog/up-front/2019/06/27/paid-leave-as-fuel-for-economic-growth/; Alexandra Boyle Stanczyk, "Does Paid Family Leave Improve Household Economic Security Following a Birth? Evidence from California," *Social Service Review* 93, no. 2 (June 2019): 262–304, https://doi.org/10.1086/703138; *Paid*

Family and Medical Leave: Good for Business, fact sheet (Washington, DC: National Partnership for Women & Families, September 2018), https://www .nationalpartnership.org/our-work/resources/economic-justice/paid-leave /paid-leave-good-for-business.pdf; and "Evaluation of the California Paid Family Leave Program," executive summary (San Francisco: Bay Area Council Economic Institute, June 19, 2020), http://www.bayareaeconomy.org /report/evaluation-of-the-california-paid-family-leave-program/.

247   **paid leave has been linked to:** Jenna Stearns, "The Effects of Paid Maternity Leave: Evidence from Temporary Disability Insurance," *Journal of Health Economics* 43 (September 2015): 85–102, https://doi.org/10.1016/j.jhealeco .2015.04.005.

247   **Birthing parents who have:** Shirlee Lichtman-Sadot and Neryvia Pillay Bell, "Child Health in Elementary School Following California's Paid Family Leave Program," *Journal of Policy Analysis and Management* 36, no. 4 (2017): 790–827, https://doi.org/10.1002/pam.22012.

247   **several studies have found:** Maureen Sayres Van Niel, Richa Bhatia, Nicholas S. Riano, Ludmila de Faria, Lisa Catapano-Friedman, Simha Ravven, Barbara Weissman, et al., "The Impact of Paid Maternity Leave on the Mental and Physical Health of Mothers and Children: A Review of the Literature and Policy Implications," *Harvard Review of Psychiatry* 28, no. 2 (April 2020): 113–26, https://doi.org/10.1097/HRP.0000000000000246.

247   **For mothers, the health benefits:** Van Niel et al., "Impact of Paid Maternity Leave," https://doi.org/10.1097/HRP.0000000000000246.

248   **The higher breastfeeding rates:** "Infant and Toddler Nutrition: Recommendations and Benefits," Centers for Disease Control and Prevention, July 9, 2021, https://www.cdc.gov/nutrition/infantandtoddlernutrition /breastfeeding/recommendations-benefits.html.

248   **found, over and over:** Van Niel et al., "Impact of Paid Maternity Leave," https://doi.org/10.1097/HRP.0000000000000246.

248   **protecting against depression:** Mauricio Avendano, Lisa F. Berkman, Agar Brugiavini, and Giacomo Pasini, "The Long-Run Effect of Maternity Leave Benefits on Mental Health: Evidence from European Countries," *Social Science & Medicine* 132 (May 2015): 45–53, https://doi.org/10.1016/j .socscimed.2015.02.037.

248   **wrote in a 2021 commentary:** Joia Crear-Perry, "Paid Maternity Leave Saves Lives," *Bloomberg Opinion*, June 24, 2021, https://www.bloomberg .com/opinion/articles/2021-06-24/paid-maternity-leave-would-help -relieve-america-s-maternal-mortality-crisis.

249   **wrote in 2015:** Danielle Kurtzleben, "Lots of Other Countries Mandate Paid Leave. Why Not the U.S.?," NPR, July 15, 2015, https://www.npr.org /sections/itsallpolitics/2015/07/15/422957640/lots-of-other-countries -mandate-paid-leave-why-not-the-us.

249   **"In terms of bonding":** Matt Walsh (@MattWalshBlog), "In terms of bonding with dad, the most important time is a little later in the child's life. Dads will do

much more bonding in toddler years than in early infancy. Infants are focused almost entirely on mommy. It's biological. Not sure why this point is upsetting to people," Twitter, October 15, 2021, https://twitter.com/MattWalshBlog/status/1449068469627105281; and Matt Walsh (@MattWalshBlog), "You can also still bond with your child while working. I'm very well bonded with all four of my kids and I had no paternity leave for any of them," Twitter, October 15, 2021, https://twitter.com/MattWalshBlog/status/1449029551359725586.

249   **fathers can support their partners:** Sofia I. Cardenas, Michaele Francesco Corbisiero, Alyssa R. Morris, and Darby E. Saxbe, "Associations between Paid Paternity Leave and Parental Mental Health across the Transition to Parenthood: Evidence from a Repeated-Measure Study of First-Time Parents in California," *Journal of Child and Family Studies* 30 (December 2021): 3080–94, https://doi.org/10.1007/s10826-021-02139-3.

249   **fathers help to shape:** Eva Diniz, Tânia Brandão, Lígia Monteiro, and Manuela Veríssimo, "Father Involvement during Early Childhood: A Systematic Review of the Literature," *Journal of Family Theory & Review* 13, no. 1 (March 2021): 77–99, https://doi.org/10.1111/jftr.12410; and Jeffrey Rosenberg and W. Bradford Wilcox, "The Importance of Fathers in the Healthy Development of Children" (Washington, DC: U.S. Department of Health and Human Services, Children's Bureau, 2006), https://www.childwelfare.gov/pubs/usermanuals/fatherhood/.

250   **In her 2021 book:** Nancy Folbre, *The Rise and Decline of Patriarchal Systems: An Intersectional Political Economy* (New York: Verso, 2021), 34–37.

251   **dramatically more engaged:** Gretchen Livingston and Kim Parker, "8 Facts about American Dads," *Pew Research Center* (blog), June 12, 2019, https://www.pewresearch.org/fact-tank/2019/06/12/fathers-day-facts/.

251   **"The safest dose":** John Bowlby, *Attachment and Loss*, vol. 2, *Separation: Anxiety and Anger* (New York: Basic Books, 1973), 73.

253   **Weisner's early research:** Thomas S. Weisner, "Sibling Interdependence and Child Caretaking: A Cross-Cultural View," in *Sibling Relationships: Their Nature and Significance across the Lifespan*, ed. Michael E. Lamb and Brian Sutton-Smith (Hillsdale, NJ: Psychology Press, 1982), 305–25.

253   **observed the behavior:** Marc H. Bornstein, Diane L. Putnick, Paola Rigo, Gianluca Esposito, James E. Swain, Joan T. D. Suwalsky, Xueyun Su, et al., "Neurobiology of Culturally Common Maternal Responses to Infant Cry," *Proceedings of the National Academy of Sciences* 114, no. 45 (November 7, 2017): E9465–73, https://doi.org/10.1073/pnas.1712022114.

255   **her theory of "maternal thinking":** Sara Ruddick, *Maternal Thinking: Toward a Politics of Peace* (Boston: Beacon Press, 1995), 9–11, 18, 69–72, 119–23.

255   **"Attention is akin":** Ruddick, *Maternal Thinking*, 121.

255   **not only women:** Ruddick, *Maternal Thinking*, xii, 70.

256   **"work of conscience":** Ruddick, *Maternal Thinking*, 123.

258   **the idea of *matrescence*:** Dana Raphael, "Matrescence, Becoming a Mother, a 'New/Old' *Rite de Passage*," in *Being Female: Reproduction, Power, and*

Change, ed. Dana Raphael (Chicago: Aldine, 1975), 65–71, http://archive .org/details/beingfemalerepro0000inte.

258 **parenthood is one:** Aurelie Athan and Lisa Miller, "Motherhood as Opportunity to Learn Spiritual Values: Experiences and Insights of New Mothers," *Journal of Prenatal and Perinatal Psychology and Health* 27, no. 4 (2013): 220–53.

258 **acceleration of development:** Aurélie Athan and Lisa Miller, "Spiritual Awakening through the Motherhood Journey," *Journal of the Association for Research on Mothering* 7, no. 1 (January 2005): 17–31, https://jarm.journals .yorku.ca/index.php/jarm/article/view/4951.

259 **reproductive identity development:** Aurélie M. Athan, "Reproductive Identity: An Emerging Concept," *American Psychologist* 75, no. 4 (2020): 445–56, https://doi.org/10.1037/amp0000623.

260 **celebrated in Simmons's time:** "Jochebed," *Art-Journal* 35, no. 12 (January 1873): 304.

260 **as one early-twentieth-century art writer:** Lilian Whiting, *Italy: The Magic Land* (Boston: Little, Brown, 1910), 121.

ACKNOWLEDGMENTS

It seems a book like this one must be imagined into being before it can be written. Thank you to the many people who helped me do just that, including Celia Johnson, who told me, "I'd read that book," and made it real. To Melissa Danaczko at the Stuart Krichevsky Literary Agency for seeing it, too, and for holding my hand along the way. I'm so grateful for your guidance and for your friendship. Thank you to Serena Jones, Anita Sheih, and everyone at Holt who helped take the ideas that lived in my head and on my computer screen out into the world, including Molly Bloom, Flora Esterly, Jane Haxby, Julianna Lee, Devon Mazzone, Catryn Silbersack, and Kelly Too.

This book was made possible with generous support from the Alfred P. Sloan Foundation's program on the Public Understanding of Science, Technology & Economics; with precious time and space created by Pamela Moulton and the people who make the Hewnoaks artist colony a reality; and with the extraordinary effort by the South Portland Public Library to keep us all in books throughout the pandemic. Thank you to Adriana Galván for serving as science advisor on this project and to Laura Thompson for careful fact-checking—you made this book better on every page. Thanks to Mary Robbins for transcription and neighborliness, to Paula DeFilippo for fast and helpful translation, and to Dan Kany for sharing his art history knowledge. Thanks to Paula Rizzo for helping me to find my confidence.

Thank you to all the parents interviewed for this book who gener-
ously shared their stories and made the science come alive, and to the
many researchers who made the science make sense. Special thanks to
Alison Fleming and Jodi Pawluski, whose insights and time shaped this
book, and to Sarah Blaffer Hrdy for breaking the trail and for providing
encouragement and advice early on in this project. Rely on the allo-
mothers, she told me. Thank you to Martha Baldwin and Ethan Somer-
man, who set the standard, and to Cora Boothby-Akilo, who helped us
through crunch time. Thanks to Susanna Dubois and Jess Townsend for
clear-eyed perspective when I've needed it most.

This book was written at a desk that sits on the ancestral land of the
Wabanaki Confederacy, in a state where the people of the confederacy,
including the Penobscot and the Passamaquoddy, continue to grapple
with the legacy of child removal and residential schools. Acknowledging that in the context of this book is important, because the emerging
science of the parental brain further reveals that many of the ideals that
White settlers held up as godly and used to eradicate or assimilate Indigenous people, including the moral certainty of the nuclear family, were
false and damaging. Indigenous people here and across North America
deserve acknowledgment for the harm that was done to them and their
ancestors, as well as a bigger voice in policy making that affects young
families and communities.

Because this is my first book, I want to thank the editors and men-
tors who helped me get here and who continue to support me, either
directly or because their voices still live in my head, most especially
Meredith Hall, Jane Harrigan, Hans Schulz, and Larry Tye. I'm grateful
to Veronica Chao for giving me the encouragement and space to first
write about this topic.

To the friends without whom I couldn't have found my way in parenthood or this project, including Marie and David Boneparth, Alli Grap-
pone, Liz Szeliga, Annie Moskov, Lori Duff, Anna Stoessinger, Cecilia De
Giorgi, Holly Tavano, Ashley Keiser, Liz Yarrington, Anna Berke, Lauren
Tarantino, Mira Ptacin, Erin Masterson, and Jodi Ferry—I'm grateful
beyond measure. Thank you to my parents-in-law for their encouragement. To my parents and siblings, and their families, for their support,
now and always—thank you. I love you. Thanks especially to Marie and

to my sister, Kristin Edwards, who offered meals, babysitting, and much-needed cheerleading, and who read every word.

To my Yoon: I couldn't have asked for a better partner in raising our boys. I'm so proud of the father you've grown to be and so grateful we get to keep growing together. In every way, this book wouldn't have been possible without your patience and your love.

One Friday night, late in the process of writing this book, when I was leaving our house to go to my office and missing out on family movie night, Hartley asked me to think of him and his brother, Ashley, every time I hit the H key or the A key. So, here they are. All the Hs and all the As for the two boys who changed my brain—and my heart—forever. All the other letters, too.

INDEX

ABOUT THE AUTHOR

CHELSEA CONABOY is a journalist specializing in personal and public health. She was part of the *Boston Globe*'s Pulitzer Prize-winning team for coverage of the Boston Marathon bombing and more recently has worked as a magazine writer with bylines at *Mother Jones, Politico, The Week, Globe Magazine* and others. She lives in Maine with her husband and their two children.